Turner and McIlwraith's Techniques in Large Animal Surgery

4th Edition

Turner and McIlwraith's Techniques in Large Animal Surgery

4th Edition

Dean A. Hendrickson
DVM, MS, DACVS
Colorado State University
College of Veterinary Medicine
and Biomedical Sciences
Fort Collins, Colorado

A. N. (Nickie) Baird
DVM, MS, DACVS
Purdue University
College of Veterinary Medicine
West Lafayette, Indiana

WILEY Blackwell

This edition first published 2013 © 2013 by John Wiley & Sons, Inc.

First and Second editions, © Lea & Febiger
Third edition, © Blackwell Publishing Ltd.

Editorial offices: 2121 State Avenue, Ames, Iowa 50014-8300, USA
The Atrium, Southern Gate, Chichester, West Sussex, PO19 8SQ, UK
9600 Garsington Road, Oxford, OX4 2DQ, UK

For details of our global editorial offices, for customer services and for information about how to apply for permission to reuse the copyright material in this book please see our website at www.wiley.com/wiley-blackwell.

Library of Congress Cataloging-in-Publication Data
Hendrickson, Dean A.
  Turner and McIlwraith's techniques in large animal surgery. – 4th ed. / Dean A. Hendrickson, A.N. (Nickie) Baird.
     p. ; cm.
  Techniques in large animal surgery
  Rev. ed. of: Techniques in large animal surgery / Dean A. Hendrickson. 3rd ed. c2007.
  Includes bibliographical references and index.
  ISBN 978-1-118-27323-4 (hardback : alk. paper) – ISBN 978-1-118-68399-6 (PDF) –
ISBN 978-1-118-68404-7 – ISBN 978-1-118-68405-4 (Mobi) – ISBN 978-1-118-68429-0 –
ISBN 978-1-118-68439-9
  I. Baird, A.N. (Aubrey Nickie)   II. Hendrickson, Dean A. Techniques in large animal
surgery.   III. Turner, A. Simon (Anthony Simon) Techniques in large animal
surgery.   IV. Title.   V. Title: Techniques in large animal surgery.
  [DNLM: 1. Surgery, Veterinary–methods.   2. Goats–surgery.   3. Horses–surgery.   4. Surgical Procedures, Operative–veterinary.   5. Swine–surgery. SF 911]
  636.089'7–dc23

                                                    2013007056

A catalogue record for this book is available from the British Library.

Wiley also publishes its books in a variety of electronic formats. Some content that appears in print may not be available in electronic books.

Cover design by Modern Alchemy LLC

Set in 10.5/12 pt Minion-Regular by Toppan Best-set Premedia Limited

1 2013

CONTENTS

About the Companion Website   viii

Contributors   ix

Preface to the First Edition   xi

Preface to the Second Edition   xiii

Preface to the Third Edition   xv

Preface to the Fourth Edition   xvii

1. Presurgical Considerations   3
Dean A. Hendrickson, DVM, MS, DACVS
Preoperative Evaluation of the Patient   3
Surgical Judgment   4
Principles of Asepsis and Antisepsis   4
Surgical Classifications   4
Role of Antibiotics   5
Preoperative Planning   5
Preparation of the Surgical Site   5
Postoperative Infection   6
References   6

2. Anesthesia and Fluid Therapy   7
Khursheed Mama, DVM, DACVA
Anesthesia   7
Fluid Therapy   23
References   29

3. Surgical Instruments   33
Dean A. Hendrickson, DVM, MS, DACVS
Use of Surgical Instruments   33
Preparation of Instruments   38
General Surgical Instruments   39
Instruments Used Specifically in Large Animal Surgery   52

4. Suture Materials and Needles   61
Dean A. Hendrickson, DVM, MS, DACVS
Suture Materials   61
Needles   67
References   69

5. Knots and Ligatures   71
Dean A. Hendrickson, DVM, MS, DACVS
Principles of Knot Tying   71
Ligatures   73
References   76

6. Suture Patterns   77
Dean A. Hendrickson, DVM, MS, DACVS
Basic Suture Patterns   77
Suture Patterns Used for Closure of Hollow Organs   83

Stent Bandages (Tie-Over Dressings)   88
Suture Patterns for Severed Tendons   88
References   91

7. **Principles of Wound Management and the Use of Drains**   93
   Dean A. Hendrickson, DVM, MS, DACVS
   Wound Management   93
   Methods of Closure and Healing   96
   Use of Drains   97
   References   101

8. **Reconstructive Surgery of Wounds**   103
   Dean A. Hendrickson, DVM, MS, DACVS
   References   111

9. **Equine Orthopedic Surgery**   113
   Dean A. Hendrickson, DVM, MS, DACVS
   Medial Patellar Desmotomy   113
   Lateral Digital Extensor Tenotomy   114
   Inferior (Distal) Check Ligament Desmotomy   119
   Superior Check Ligament Desmotomy (After Bramlage)   122
   Superficial Digital Flexor Tenotomy   124
   Deep Digital Flexor Tenotomy   126
   Sectioning of the Palmar (or Plantar) Annular Ligament of the Fetlock   127
   Palmar Digital Neurectomy   129
   Amputation of the Splint (II and IV Metacarpal and Metatarsal) Bones   131
   Arthrotomy of the Fetlock Joint and Removal of an Apical Sesamoid Chip Fracture   134
   References   136

10. **Equine Urogenital Surgery**   139
    Dean A. Hendrickson, DVM, MS, DACVS
    Castration   139
    Cryptorchidectomy by the Inguinal, Parainguinal, and Flank Approach   152
    Laparoscopic Cryptorchidectomy   155
    Caslick's Operation for Pneumovagina in the Mare   156
    Urethroplasty by Caudal Relocation of the Transverse Fold   159
    Cesarean Section in the Mare   160
    Circumcision of the Penis (Reefing)   164
    Amputation of the Penis   166
    Aanes' Method of Repair of Third-Degree Perineal Laceration   169
    References   174

11. **Surgery of the Equine Upper Respiratory Tract**   177
    Dean A. Hendrickson, DVM, MS, DACVS
    Tracheostomy   177
    Laryngotomy, Laryngeal Ventriculectomy, and Ventriculocordectomy   179
    Partial Resection of the Soft Palate   183
    Surgical Entry and Drainage of the Guttural Pouches   186
    References   189

12. **Equine Dental and Gastrointestinal Surgery**   191
    Dean A. Hendrickson, DVM, MS, DACVS
    Repulsion of Cheek Teeth   191
    Ventral Midline Laparotomy and Abdominal Exploration   196
    Standing Flank Laparotomy   202
    Umbilical Herniorrhaphy in the Foal   207
    References   210

13. **Bovine Gastrointestinal Surgery**   211
    A. N. Baird, DVM, MS, DACVS
    Principles of Laparotomy   211
    Flank Laparotomy and Abdominal Exploration   212
    Rumenotomy   215
    Rumenostomy (Rumenal Fistulation)   219

Surgical Corrections of Abomasal Displacements and Torsion   221
Surgical Correction of Cecal Dilatation/Volvulus   231
Small Intestinal Resection and Anastomosis   231
References   232

14. **Bovine Urogenital Surgery**   235
    A. N. Baird, DVM, MS, DACVS
    Calf Castration   235
    Urethrostomy   236
    Hematoma Evacuation of the Bovine Penis   241
    Preputial Resection and Anastomosis in the Bull   245
    Surgical Techniques for Teaser Bull Preparation   248
    Inguinal Herniorrhaphy in the Mature Bull   252
    Unilateral Castration   257
    Cesarean Section in the Cow   258
    Retention Suturing of the Bovine Vulva (Buhner's Method)   265
    Cervicopexy for Vaginal Prolapse (after Winkler)   266
    References   270

15. **Bovine General Surgery**   273
    A. N. Baird, DVM, MS, DACVS
    Digit Amputation   273
    Digit Amputation via Disarticulation   274
    Eye Enucleation   276
    Cosmetic Dehorning   277
    Rib Resection and Pericardiotomy   280
    Repair of Teat Lacerations   283
    Third Eyelid Resection   288
    Tracheotomy   288
    Umbilical Surgery   289
    References   290

16. **Small Ruminant Surgery**   293
    A. N. Baird, DVM, MS, DACVS
    Dehorning the Mature Goat   293
    Disbudding the Young Goat   295
    Obstructive Urolithiasis   296
    Mastectomy   297
    Vasectomy   298
    Cesarean Section   299
    Rectal Prolapse Resection in Small Ruminants   300
    References   301

17. **Camelid Surgery**   303
    A. N. Baird, DVM, MS, DACVS
    Castration of the Llama   303
    Cesarean Section in the Camelid   304
    Tooth Removal in the Llama   305
    References   309

18. **Swine Surgery**   311
    A. N. Baird, DVM, MS, DACVS
    Castration of the Piglet   311
    Inguinal Herniorrhaphy in the Piglet   312
    Cryptorchid Castration of Piglets   314
    Preputial Diverticulum Ablation   316
    Cesarean Section in the Sow   317
    Ovariohysterectomy in the Pot-Bellied Pig   319
    Rectal Prolapse Ring Placement   319
    References   320

Index   323

ABOUT THE COMPANION WEBSITE

This book is accompanied by a companion website:

www.wiley.com/go/hendrickson/techniques

The website includes:

- Multiple Choice Questions
- Powerpoints of all figures from the book for downloading

CONTRIBUTORS

Dean A. Hendrickson, DVM, MS, DACVS
Editor-in Chief
Colorado State University
College of Veterinary Medicine and Biomedical Sciences
Fort Collins, Colorado

A. N. (Nickie) Baird, DVM, MS, DACVS
Associate Editor
Purdue University
College of Veterinary Medicine
West Lafayette, Indiana

Khursheed Mama, DVM, DACVA
Colorado State University
College of Veterinary Medicine and Biomedical Sciences
Fort Collins, Colorado

PREFACE TO THE FIRST EDITION

The purpose of this book is to present some fundamental techniques in large animal surgery to both veterinary students and large animal practitioners. It is designed to be brief, discussing only the major steps in a particular operation, and each discussion is accompanied by appropriate illustrations. Most of the techniques presented in this book can be performed without the advantages of a fully equipped large animal hospital or teaching institution.

The book assumes a basic understanding of anatomy and physiology. Those who wish to know more about a particular technique are encouraged to consult the bibliography.

We and our colleagues at the Colorado State University Veterinary Teaching Hospital consider the procedures discussed in this book to be time honored. Some practitioners may perform certain techniques in slightly different ways. We would be happy to receive input about modifications of these techniques for future editions of this book.

All of the drawings in the book are original and based on rough sketches and photographs taken at various points during actual surgery. Occasionally, dissections were performed on cadavers.

The surgical procedures described in this text represent not only our thoughts, but suggestions from many of our colleagues as well. Their help was an important contribution to the production of this book. We are indebted to Dr. Wilbur Aanes, Professor of Surgery, Colorado State University, who unselfishly shared 30 years of his personal experience in large animal surgery with us. We are proud to be able to present in Chapter 10 of this book "Aanes' Method of Repair of Third-Degree Perineal Laceration" in the mare, a technique that he pioneered over 15 years ago. We also wish to give credit to the following faculty members at Colorado State University Veterinary Teaching Hospital who willingly gave us advice on the diagrams and manuscript of various techniques discussed in this book: Dr. Leslie Ball, Dr. Bill Bennett, Dr. Bruce Heath, Dr. Tony Knight, Dr. LaRue Johnson, Dr. Gary Rupp, Dr. Ted Stashak, Dr. Gayle Trotter, Dr. James Voss, and Dr. Mollie Wright. We also wish to express appreciation to Dr. John Baker, Purdue University, and Dr. Charles Wallace, University of Georgia, for their comments on some questions we had. Dr. McIlwraith is also grateful to Dr. John Fessler, Professor of Surgery, Purdue University, for his inspiration and training.

We are particularly grateful to Dr. Robert Kainer, Professor of Anatomy, Colorado State University, for checking the manuscript and the illustrations and advising us on nomenclature. His input impressed upon us the importance of the relationship between the dissection room and the surgery room.

The terrific amount of time and effort involved with the illustrations will be clear to the reader who cares only to leaf through the book. For these illustrations, we are indebted to Mr. Tom McCracken, Director, Office of Biomedical Media, Colorado State University. We are thankful for his expertise, as well as his cooperation and understanding. The diagrams for "Aanes' Method of Repair of Third-Degree Perineal Laceration" were done by Mr. John Daughtery, Medical Illustrator, Colorado State University. We must also thank Kathleen Jee, who assisted with various aspects of the artwork. We would also like to thank Messrs. Al Kilminster and Charles Kerlee for taking photographs during the various surgical procedures that were used to assist with the artwork of this text.

The manuscript was typed by Mrs. Helen Mawhiney, Ms. Teresa Repphun, and Mrs. Jan Schmidt. We thank them for their patience and understanding during the many changes we made during the generation of the final manuscript.

We are grateful to the following instrument companies for allowing us to use some of the diagrams from their sales catalogs for inclusion in Chapter 3, "Surgical Instruments": Schroer Manufacturing Co., Kansas City, MO; Intermountain Veterinary Supply, Denver, CO; Miltex Instrument Co., Lake Success, NY; J. Skyler Manufacturing Co., Inc., Long Island, NY.

The idea for this book was conceived in 1978 when one of us (AST) was approached by Mr. George Mundroff,

Executive Editor, Lea & Febiger. We would like to thank him for his encouragement and guidance. We are also grateful to Mr. Kit Spahr, Jr., Veterinary Editor; Diane Ramanauskas, Copy Editor; Tom Colaiezzi, Production Manager; and Samuel A. Rondinelli, Assistant Production Manager, Lea & Febiger, for their assistance, as well as to others at the Publisher who assisted in the production of this book.

A. Simon Turner
C. Wayne McIlwraith
Fort Collins, Colorado

PREFACE TO THE SECOND EDITION

The second edition of *Techniques in Large Animal Surgery* is in response to the acceptance of the first edition and the continued need for such a book for both veterinary students and large animal practitioners. In many instances, the techniques are time honored and require no change from 5 years ago. In other instances, however, refinements in technique as well as improved perception of indications, limitations, and complications have made changes appropriate.

A significant change is the addition of Dr. R. Bruce Hull, Professor of Veterinary Clinical Sciences, The Ohio State University, as a contributor. He has carefully analyzed the entire bovine section, and his suggested changes and additions have been incorporated into the text. In addition, two procedures, "teaser bull preparations by penile fixation" and "treatment of vaginal prolapse by fixation to the prepubic tendon," have been added. We are most grateful in having Dr. Hull's help and expertise. Among the introductory chapters, the section on anesthesia required the most updating, and we are grateful to our colleague Dr. David Hodgson at Colorado State University for his review and advice. Two new procedures, "superior check ligament desmotomy" and "deep digital flexor tenotomy," were considered appropriate additions to this edition. We are grateful to Dr. Larry Bramlage, Ohio State University, for his comments and help with the first of these procedures. Many of the other changes in this edition are in response to the book reviews and comments on the first edition returned to Lea & Febiger. To these people, we appreciate your feedback.

A chapter on llama tooth removal was added because of the increased popularity of this species, especially in our own part of the country. Although we only discuss this one technique, it should not be inferred that other operations are unheard of in llamas. We have corrected angular limb deformities, repaired fractures, and performed gastrointestinal surgery, among other procedures, but tooth removal is the most common. Descriptions of these other procedures in llamas are beyond the scope of this book at this stage.

The need for more sophisticated equine techniques prompted us to produce the textbook *Equine Surgery: Advanced Techniques* in 1987. It is envisioned that the book will be used as a companion to this second edition, to provide a full spectrum of equine procedures, with the well-accepted format of concise text and clear illustrations.

Again, we are thankful to Mr. Tom McCracken, Assistant Professor, Department of Anatomy and Neurobiology, Colorado State University, for his talent in capturing the techniques described in his line drawings. We are also indebted to Helen Acvedo for typing our additions and to Holly Lukens for copyediting. Finally, our thanks again to the excellent staff at Lea & Febiger for the production of this edition.

A. Simon Turner
C. Wayne McIlwraith
Fort Collins, Colorado

PREFACE TO THE THIRD EDITION

The first two editions of *Techniques in Large Animal Surgery* have been well accepted, much to the credit of Drs. Turner and McIlwraith. They have been excellent texts for the veterinary student and the large animal practitioner. I was fortunate to be able to take on the task when it came time to update the information for a third edition. I am deeply appreciative of the opportunity to take such an excellent text and update it with new information and techniques.

The third edition of *Techniques in Large Animal Surgery* has been updated in response to the continued need for such a book for both veterinary students and large animal practitioners. There are some techniques that are time tested and continue to be included. There are other techniques that have been refined or replaced, and these are included in the new text.

New information has been included in essentially every chapter. We have made extensive use of tables to simplify the information. The anesthesia section includes new and updated information on sedation and anesthetic agents. The instrument section has been evaluated, adding new instruments where applicable and removing outdated or unavailable instruments. The section on suture materials has been updated to include new materials. There are new illustrations in the suture pattern section to better aid the practitioner with surgical techniques. The sections on wound management and reconstructive surgery have been increased to provide up-to-date information on wound care. Tables of required instrumentation have been added to all sections of the remaining surgical chapters to aid in surgical planning and preparation.

I am very grateful for our new illustrator Anne Rains; she has done an excellent job and has made my life very easy. I am indebted to Joanna Virgin who has done the lion's share of the research to make sure this text was as up-to-date and accurate as possible. I could not have done this work without her. Thanks to the folks at Blackwell for their help and assistance in the production of this edition.

Dean A. Hendrickson
Fort Collins, Colorado

PREFACE TO THE FOURTH EDITION

The first two editions of *Techniques in Large Animal Surgery* have been well accepted much to the credit of Drs. Turner and McIlwraith. They have been excellent texts for the veterinary student and the large animal practitioner. I was fortunate in that when it came time to update the information for a third edition, I was able to take on the task; and now we have added a fourth edition.

The fourth edition of *Techniques in Large Animal Surgery* has been updated in response to the continued need for such a book for both veterinary students and large animal practitioners. As with the third edition, we have gone through the entire text to make sure the information was reliable. The "tried-and-true" procedures have been retained, the outdated procedures have been removed, and new procedures have been added. As we thoroughly researched each of the chapters in the text, we did a major overhaul of the references.

Probably the most important changes in this text are the addition of two authors. Nickie Baird joined me in co-authoring the fourth edition. His expertise in livestock animal surgery was a perfect fit for this textbook. He brings a great deal of new information to the text and has been a great partner. Dr. Khursheed Mama joined us as the author of Chapter 2, *Anesthesia and Fluid Therapy*. She did an excellent job updating all of the information.

We added a considerable amount of new information in the text and retained the table format to simplify information. New figures have been added, where needed, to support the updated information.

I am very grateful for Grahm Hendrickson for illustrating the new procedures, as well as Katie Hunsucker and Joy Fuhrman for providing a lot of the background research. Thanks as well to the folks at Wiley for their help and assistance in the production of this edition.

Dean A. Hendrickson
Fort Collins, Colorado

A. N. (Nickie) Baird
West Lafayette, Indiana

Turner and McIlwraith's Techniques in Large Animal Surgery

4th Edition

Chapter 1

PRESURGICAL CONSIDERATIONS

Dean A. Hendrickson, DVM, MS, DACVS

Objectives

1. Discuss some of the presurgical considerations that can affect the success of a procedure, including the physiological state and condition of the patient; the predisposing factors for infection; and the limitations of the surgeon, facilities, and equipment.
2. Describe the methods of asepsis and antisepsis.
3. Describe the classification of different procedures with regard to risk of infection and degree of contamination.
4. Discuss the judicious use of antibiotics and their applications prophylaxis and postoperative infection.
5. Describe proper techniques for surgical site preparation.

Preoperative Evaluation of the Patient

Before a surgical procedure, a physical examination is generally indicated. This applies to both emergency and elective surgery. The following are laboratory tests that are generally indicated for horses based upon animal age and systemic status at our clinic:

- For horses younger than 4 years old and healthy:
  - Packed cell volume (PCV)
  - Total protein
- Appropriate for horses greater than 4 years old or those that are systemically ill:
  - Complete blood count (CBC)
  - Chemistry

Exactly where to draw the line on laboratory tests is largely a matter of judgment on the part of the surgeon. Obviously, if the surgery consists of castration of several litters of piglets, then for purely economic reasons laboratory tests prior to surgery may not be performed. In many cases, however, additional tests will be necessary. The following are examples of other optional tests and their indications:

- Electrolyte measurement for right-sided abomasal diseases of the dairy cow
- Urinalysis in the dairy cow to evaluate the presence of ketosis
- Measurement of blood urea nitrogen (BUN) and creatinine if urinary problems are suspected
- Analysis of peritoneal fluid prior to laparotomy for horses with colic
- Full chemistry panels when there are age or systemic considerations

If any laboratory parameters are abnormal, the underlying causes should be investigated and efforts made to correct them. In "elective" surgery this is possible, but it may not be possible in an emergency. The owner should be made aware of any problems prior to subjecting the animal to surgery. Risks are always present in normal elective surgery, and these should be explained to the owner. It is always better to have an early, frank discussion with the owner about the possible risks associated with the surgery than to have the discussion after the risk has been realized.

Fluid replacement should be performed if necessary. In the elective case, the surgical procedure should be postponed if the animal's physical condition or laboratory parameters are abnormal. In some animals, internal and external parasitism may have to be rectified to achieve this goal.

Medical records should be kept at all times. Obviously this can be difficult in such cases as castration of several litters of piglets. However, record keeping should become

Turner and McIlwraith's Techniques in Large Animal Surgery, 4th Edition. Dean A. Hendrickson and A. N. (Nickie) Baird.
© 2013 John Wiley & Sons, Inc. Published 2013 by John Wiley & Sons, Inc.

an essential part of the procedure for horses and cattle in a hospital, and herd records should be kept in all other situations. Finally, if the animal is insured, the insurance company must be notified of any surgical procedure; otherwise, the policy may be void.

Surgical Judgment

Surgical judgment cannot be learned overnight by reading a surgery textbook, nor is it necessarily attained by years of experience. The surgeon who continually makes the same mistake will probably never possess good surgical judgment. Not only should the surgeon learn from his own mistakes; he also should learn from the mistakes of others, including those documented in the surgical literature. As part of surgical judgment, the surgeon must ask the following questions:

* Is the surgery necessary?
* What would happen if the surgery were not performed?
* Is the procedure within the capabilities of the surgeon, the facilities, and the technical help?

If the surgeon finds that the procedure is too advanced for his or her capabilities and/or facilities, the surgery should be referred. Some veterinarians have a fear that this will mean loss of the client's business in the future, but this is rarely the case. If the surgeon explains why the case should be referred elsewhere, most clients will be grateful for such frankness and honesty. It is inexcusable to operate on a patient and then have complications arise due to inadequate training and facilities, when the surgery could easily have been referred to a well-equipped, well-staffed hospital with specially qualified personnel. Clearly, this rule has exceptions—mainly the emergency patient, which may fare better by undergoing immediate surgery than being subjected to a long trailer ride to another facility.

Many of the procedures described in this book can be done "on the farm." Some, such as arthrotomy for removal of chip fractures of the carpal and sesamoid bones in horses, should be done in a dust-free operating theater. If clients want these latter procedures to be done "in the field," they should understand the disastrous consequences of postsurgical infection. The surgeon must be the final judge of whether his facilities or experience are suitable.

Principles of Asepsis and Antisepsis

There are four main determinants for a surgical site infection (SSI): host defense, physiologic derangement, bacterial contamination risk at surgery, and prolonged surgical time.[1] Other factors that impact infection of deep structures and organs include hypoalbuminemia and a prior

Table 1.1.   Surgical classifications.

Classification	Description	Examples
Clean	Gastrointestinal, urinary, or respiratory tract is not entered.	Arthrotomy for removal of a chip fracture of a carpal bone of a horse
Clean-contaminated	Gastrointestinal, respiratory, or urinary tract is entered. There is no spillage of contaminated contents.	Abomasopexy for displaced abomasum in the dairy cow
Contaminated-dirty	Gross spillage of contaminated body contents or acute inflammation occurs.	Wounds Abscesses Devitalized bowel

operation.[2] Perioperative blood loss also contributes to SSI.[3] Control methods include aseptic surgical practices as well as identification of the high-risk patient, correction of systemic imbalances prior to surgery, and the proper use of prophylactic antibiotics.

We are sometimes reminded by fellow veterinarians in the field that we must teach undergraduates how to do surgery in the real world. By this they mean that we must ignore aseptic draping and gloving and lower the standard to a "practical" level. This is fallacious in our opinion. Although we recognize that while the ideal may be unattainable in private practice, one should always strive for the highest possible standard; otherwise, the final standard of practice may be so low that the well-being of the patient is at risk, not to mention the reputation of the veterinarian as a surgeon. For this reason, we believe that it behooves us as instructors of undergraduates to teach the *best possible methods with regard to asepsis as well as technique.*

The extent to which the practice of asepsis or even antisepsis is carried out depends on the classification of the operation, as shown in Table 1.1. This classification may also help the veterinarian decide whether antibiotics are indicated or whether postoperative infection can be anticipated.

Surgical Classifications

Once the surgeon has categorized the surgical procedure, appropriate precautions to avoid postoperative infection can be determined. In all cases, however, the surgical site is prepared properly, including clipping and aseptic scrubbing.

Whatever category of surgery is performed, clean clothing should be worn. The wearing of surgical gloves is good policy even if only to protect the operator from infectious organisms that may be present at the surgical site. Surgical gowns, gloves, and caps are recommended for clean surgical procedures, although such attire has obvious practical limitations for the large animal surgeon operating in the field. The purpose of this book is to present guidelines rather than to lay down hard-and-fast rules. For example, the decision between wearing caps, gowns, and gloves and wearing just gloves can be made only by the surgeon. Good surgical judgment is required. In general, it is better to be more careful than what may appear necessary in order to be better prepared when problems arise.

Role of Antibiotics

Antibiotics should never be used to cover flaws in surgical technique. The young surgeon is often tempted, sometimes under pressure from the client, to use antibiotics prophylactically. However, the disadvantages of antimicrobial therapy often outweigh its benefits. Extended periods of antimicrobial therapy can select for resistant organisms and adversely affect the gastrointestinal tract by eliminating many of the normal enteric organisms and allowing outgrowths of pathogenic bacteria, such as *Clostridia* spp., which can result in colitis and diarrhea.[4] When selecting an antibiotic regimen, the surgeon should consider the following aspects:

- Does the diagnosis warrant antibiotics?
- Which organisms are most likely to be involved, and what is their in-vitro antimicrobial susceptibility?
- What is the location or likely location of the infection?
- How accessible is the location of the infection to the drug?
- What possible adverse reactions and toxicities to the drug could occur?
- What dosage and duration of treatment are necessary to obtain sufficient concentrations of the drug?

Again, some judgment is required, but suffice it to say, antibiotics should never be substitutes for "surgical conscience." *Surgical conscience* consists of the following: dissection along tissue planes, gentleness in handling tissues, adequate hemostasis, selection of the best surgical approach, correct choice of suture material (both size and type), closure of dead space, and short operating time.

If the surgeon decides that antibiotics are indicated, special attention should be given to selecting the type of antimicrobial drug, the dosage, and the duration of use. Ample scientific literature indicates that for maximum benefit, antimicrobials should be administered prophylactically prior to surgery and, at the latest, during surgery. Beyond 4 hours postsurgically, the administration of prophylactic antibiotics has little to no effect on the incidence of postoperative infection.[1] The duration of treatment should not exceed 24 hours because most research indicates that antimicrobial use after this period of time does not confer further benefits. If longer duration of antimicrobial coverage is necessary, the full duration of the specific antimicrobial drug selected should be given. This varies depending on the drug; however, in most cases the duration is at least 3 and up to 5 days. If the surgeon is operating on a food animal, there are regulations for withdrawal times from different antimicrobial drugs prior to slaughter that must be taken into account.

If topical antibiotics are used during surgery, they should be nonirritating to the tissues; otherwise, tissue necrosis from cellular damage will outweigh any advantageous effects of the antibiotics. It is also beneficial when using topical antibiotics to use antibiotics that are not generally used systemically.

All equine surgical patients should have tetanus prophylaxis. If the immunization program is doubtful, the horse can receive 1500–3000 units of tetanus antitoxin. Horses on a permanent immunization program that have not had tetanus toxoid within the previous 6 months should receive a booster injection.

Tetanus prophylaxis is generally not provided for food animals, but an immunization program may be considered, especially if a specific predisposition is thought to exist.

Preoperative Planning

The surgeon should be thoroughly familiar with the regional anatomy. In this book we illustrate what we consider to be the important structures in each technique. If more detail is required, a suitable anatomy text should be consulted. Not only should the procedure be planned prior to the surgery, but the surgeon also should visit the dissection room and review local anatomy on cadavers prior to attempting surgery on a client's animal. We are fortunate in veterinary surgery to have greater access to cadavers than our counterparts in human surgery.

Preparation of the Surgical Site

For the large animal surgeon, preparation of the surgical site can present major problems, especially in the winter and spring when farms can be muddy. Preparation for surgery may have to begin with removal of dirt and manure. Some animals that have been recumbent in mud and filth for various reasons may have to be hosed off. Hair should then be removed, not just from the surgical site, but from an adequate area surrounding the surgical site.

The clipping should be done in a neat square or rectangular shape with straight edges. Surprisingly, this, along with the neatness of the final suture pattern in the skin, is how the client judges the skill of the surgeon. Clipping may be done initially with a no. 10 clipper blade, and then the finer no. 40 blade may be used. The incision site can be shaved with a straight razor in horses and cattle, but debate exists regarding the benefit or problems associated with this procedure. In sheep and goats, in which the skin is supple and pliable, it is difficult to shave the edges.

Preparation of the surgical site, such as the ventral midline of a horse about to undergo an exploratory laparotomy, may have to be performed when the animal is anesthetized. If surgery is to be done with the animal standing, an initial surgical scrub, followed by the appropriate local anesthetic technique and a final scrub, is standard procedure.

For cattle or pigs, the skin of the surgical site can be prepared for surgery with the aid of a stiff brush. For horses, gauze sponges are recommended. Sheep may require defatting of the skin with alcohol prior to the actual skin scrub. The antiseptic scrub solution used is generally a matter of personal preference. Either povidone-iodine scrub (Betadine Scrub) alternated with a 70% alcohol rinse, or Chlorhexidine alternated with water, can be used. Finally, the skin can be sprayed with povidone-iodine solution (Betadine Solution) and allowed to dry.

Scrubbing of the proposed surgical site is done immediately prior to the operation. Scrubbing should commence at the proposed site of the incision and progress toward the periphery; one must be sure not to come back onto a previously scrubbed area. Some equine surgeons clip and shave the surgical site the night before the surgery, perform an aseptic preparation as previously described, and wrap the limb in a sterile bandage until the next day. A shaving nick made the day before surgery may be a pustule on the day of surgery, however, so this is generally not recommended for anything proximal to the pastern region.

When aseptic surgery is to be performed, an efficient draping system is mandatory. Generally, time taken to drape the animal properly is well spent. The draping of cattle in the standing position can be difficult, especially if the animal decides to move or becomes restless. It can be difficult to secure drapes with towel clamps in the conscious animal because only the operative site is anesthetized. However, if the surgeon applies slow pressure when closing the towel clamps, most animals will tolerate their application, even if the local site is not desensitized. If draping is not done, the surgeon must minimize contact with parts of the animal that have not been scrubbed. The tail must be tied to prevent it from flicking into the surgical field.

Several operations described in this book require the strictest of aseptic technique; sterile, antimicrobial, adhe-sive, incise drapes are indicated. Characteristics of sterile plastic adhesive drapes include their ability to adhere, their antimicrobial activity, and their clarity when applied to the skin. Probably the most desirable feature is the one first mentioned. With excessive traction or manipulation, some brands of drapes quickly separate from the skin surfaces, and this separation instantly defeats their purpose.

Rubberized drapes are helpful when large amounts of fluids (such as peritoneal and amniotic fluid) are encountered during the procedure. Rubberized drapes are also useful to isolate the bowel or any other organ that is potentially contaminated, to prevent contamination of drapes. Newer fluid-impermeable paper drapes that are disposable make the surgeon's job even easier.

Postoperative Infection

Prevention of postoperative infection should be the goal of the surgeon, but infection may occur despite all measures taken to prevent it. If infection occurs, the surgeon must decide whether antibiotic treatment is indicated, or whether the animal is strong enough to fight it using its own defense mechanisms. Some surgical wounds require drainage at their most ventral part, whereas others require more aggressive treatment. If, in the judgment of the surgeon, the infection appears to be serious, a Gram stain, culture, and sensitivity testing of the offending microorganism(s) will be indicated. A Gram stain may give the surgeon a better idea of what type of organism is involved and may in turn narrow the selection of antibiotics. Sometimes in-vitro sensitivities have to be ignored because the antibiotic of choice would be prohibitively expensive. This is especially true for adult cattle and horses. A broad-spectrum antibiotic should be given, if possible, as soon as practical.

References

1. Barie, P.S. Modern surgical antibiotic prophylaxis and therapy—less is more. *Surgical Infections*, 1:23–29, 2000.
2. Haridas, M., and Malangoni, M.A. Predictive factors for surgical site infection in general surgery. *Surgery*, 144:496–503, 2008.
3. Sorensen, L.T., Hemmingsen, U., Kallehave, F., Wille-Jorgensen, P., Kjoergaard, J., Moller, L.N., and Jorgensen, T. Risk factors for tissue and wound complications in gastrointetstinal surgery. *Annals of Surgery*, 241:654–658, 2005.
4. Papich, M.G. Antimicrobial therapy for gastrointestinal disease. *The Veterinary Clinics of North America. Equine Practice*, 19: 645–663, 2003.

Chapter 2

ANESTHESIA AND FLUID THERAPY

Khursheed Mama, DVM, DACVA

Objectives

1. Describe routine regional anesthetic techniques in large animals.
2. Discuss selected species differences in reference to anesthetic techniques.
3. Describe the indications for, advantages of, and disadvantages of general anesthesia in large animal species.
4. Provide a basic discussion of the fundamentals of fluid therapy including methods for ascertaining fluid deficits, acid-base imbalances, and electrolyte abnormalities.
5. Discuss specific fluid therapies in patients undergoing elective surgery and in compromised patients, either with or without preliminary data.

Anesthesia

The purpose of this section is not to present an in-depth discussion of all aspects of anesthesia. Details on the principles of anesthesia, recognition of stages of anesthesia, monitoring during anesthesia, and the pharmacology and physiology associated with anesthesia are well documented in other texts.[1-3] Rather, information pertaining to routinely used anesthetic techniques for large animals is provided. The interested reader is referred to additional sources for more in depth information.[4,5]

Local and Regional Anesthesia (Analgesia)

Regional anesthesia results from desensitization of sensory nerves to a given area. This may be performed by infiltration into the desired location or by "blocking" sensory nerve(s) innervating a region. Both techniques may be used to desensitize the surgical site. Depending on the required duration of anesthesia, local anesthetic agents including lidocaine hydrochloride (shortest onset and duration), mepivacaine hydrochloride and bupivacaine hydrochloride (longest onset and duration) may be used. Due to cardiovascular toxicity with vascular absorption, bupivacaine use is usually limited to epidural and perineural administration; lidocaine and mepivacaine may be used by any route. Mepivacaine is often selected because of its rapid onset, intermediate duration, and reduced tissue reactivity.[6]

Regional anesthesia techniques are still commonly used as primary means to facilitate noxious intervention in many ruminant species. Sedation may be used as an adjunct. In horses, while these techniques may be used in sedated patients, they are also commonly used as adjuncts to general anesthesia. A description of selected regional anesthesia techniques follows.

Infiltration Analgesia

The principles of infiltration anesthesia are simple and similar for all species. Following definition of the area to be desensitized, local anesthetic is injected at an initial site with a small gauge needle and then a longer needle is inserted through the initial region of desensitization. Repeat injections are usually made through a region that has already been desensitized. When possible, the skin and subcutis should be infiltrated first and then the deeper layers, such as muscle and peritoneum. The injection of significant amounts of local anesthetic into the peritoneal

Turner and McIlwraith's Techniques in Large Animal Surgery, 4th Edition. Dean A. Hendrickson and A. N. (Nickie) Baird.
© 2013 John Wiley & Sons, Inc. Published 2013 by John Wiley & Sons, Inc.

cavity should be avoided as rapid vascular absorption can result in toxicity. Infiltrating injections should be made in straight lines; "fanning" should be avoided as much as possible because of the potential for tissue trauma.

Infiltration analgesia is commonly used for suturing wounds and for removing cutaneous lesions in all large animal species. It may also be used in the form of a "line block" for laparotomy, in which case the analgesic agent is infiltrated along the line of incision. Although convenient, the infiltration of the analgesic agent into the incision line causes edema in the tissues and may affect wound healing. In this respect, regional anesthetic techniques that are removed from the surgical site are generally preferred.

Techniques of Regional Analgesia

Inverted L Block

This is the simplest technique of regional anesthesia for laparotomy and laparoscopy in large animal species. It may be used to facilitate flank or paramedian interventions. The principles of the technique are illustrated for cattle in Figure 2.1. Local anesthetic agent is administered nonspecifically in the form of an inverted L with a goal of blocking nerves entering the surgical field. The procedure is facilitated by the use of an 8- to 10-cm, 16- to 18-gauge needle. It is generally recommended that a dose of local anesthetic is limited to 2 mg/kg. However, up to 100 ml of 2% lidocaine has been used for adult horses and cows (4 mg/kg for 500-kg patient). The vertical portion of the inverted L is caudal to the last rib, and the horizontal portion is just ventral to the transverse processes of the lumbar vertebrae. Ten to fifteen minutes should be allowed for the drug to take effect.

Systemic toxicity following inadvertent intravenous administration or absorption from regional sites is reported. Experiments in sheep have shown that convulsions occur in adult sheep at a dose of lidocaine hydrochloride of 5.8 ± 1.8 mg/kg intravenously.[7] Sub-convulsive doses of lidocaine hydrochloride produce drowsiness. Above convulsive doses, hypotension, respiratory arrest, and circulatory collapse occur progressively. If convulsions do occur, they can be controlled with an intravenous dose of 0.5 mg/kg of diazepam (Valium). To minimize the occurrence, it is recommended that diluted local anesthetic is used for smaller sized animals such as sheep and goats.[1,8] Toxicity following inadvertent intravenous bupivacaine administration manifests in cardiovascular collapse.

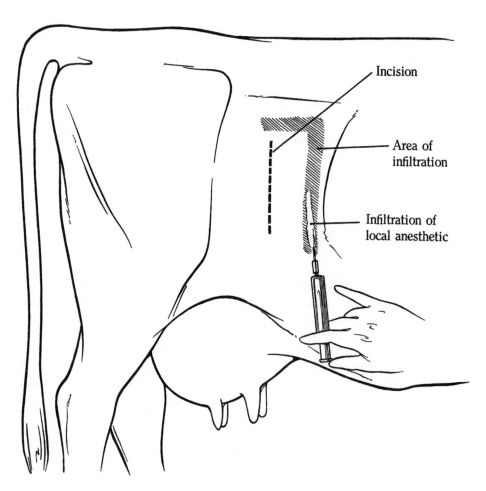

Fig. 2.1. Inverted L block.

Paravertebral Block

While not common, the paravertebral block has been described and utilized to desensitize the flank area for standing procedures in horses.[9] It is however more commonly performed in cattle, sheep, and goats.[8,10] In ruminants, the thirteenth thoracic nerve (T13), the first and second lumbar nerves (L1 and L2), and the dorsolateral branch of the third lumbar nerve (L3) supply sensory and motor innervation to the skin, fascia, muscles, and peritoneum of the flank. Regional analgesia of these nerves is the basis of the paravertebral block. For practical purposes with flank laparotomy, blocking of the dorsolateral branch of L3 is not generally considered necessary and may be contraindicated because, if one has miscounted the vertebrae, one may actually block L4, where sensory and motor nerve fibers to the hind limbs originate.

Two approaches to performing the paravertebral block have been described for cattle. The first consists of walking the needle off the transverse process, as illustrated in Figure 2.2. As the nerve is most distinct at its intervertebral foramen, walking the needle off the transverse process closer to this site allows one to block the nerve before or close to the split into individual dorsal and ventral branches. As the transverse processes slope forward, the transverse process of L1 is used as a landmark to block T13, and the transverse processes of L2 and L3 are similarly used to locate nerves L1 and L2, respectively. When the transverse process has been located, a line is drawn from its cranial edge to the dorsal midline. The site for injection is 3 to 5 cm from the midline (Figure 2.2) caudal to transverse processes of L1, L2 and L3. The transverse process of L1 is difficult to locate in fat animals, in which case the site is estimated relative to the distance between the processes of L2 and L3. Following subcutaneous infiltration of local anesthetic, a 1-inch, 16-gauge needle is inserted to act as a guide in placing a 10-cm, 20-gauge needle perpendicular to the transverse process is encountered. The needle is then walked off the cranial border of the transverse process and advanced 0.75 cm (will generally feel penetration of the intertransverse ligament); and

Farquharson method

T13   L1   L2   L3   L4

Dorsal branch of first lumbar nerve

Ventral branch of first lumbar nerve

Ventral branch of second lumbar nerve

Magda's method

Site of deposition of anesthetic (N.T13)

Site of deposition of anesthetic (N.L1)

Site of deposition of anesthetic (N.L2)

Transverse process of third lumbar vertebra

Fig. 2.2. Paravertebral block.

approximately 10 ml of local anesthetic solution (typically 2% lidocaine or mepivacaine) is administered below the ligament. An additional 5 ml is placed dorsal to the ligament. If the drug has been administered correctly, desensitization will be effective within a few minutes. In testing the block, one must remember that the distribution of the nerves is such that T13 innervates the ventral flank area, whereas L2 innervates the more dorsal region closer to the transverse processes. A temporary lateral deviation of the spine due to muscle paralysis is observed in association with paravertebral analgesia. Vasodilation of surface vessels may also be observed.

An alternate technique favored by some was developed by Magda and modified by Cakala.[11] It uses a lateral approach to the nerves and is sometimes referred to as the distal paravertebral or paralumbar approach. The branches of T13, L1, and L2 are blocked close to the ends of the first, second, and fourth transverse processes, respectively, as illustrated in Figure 2.2. The skin is clipped and prepared at the ends of the first, second, and fourth lumbar transverse processes. An 18-gauge needle is inserted under each transverse process towards the midline, and 10 ml of solution is injected. The needle is then withdrawn a short distance and is redirected both cranially and caudally and additional local anesthetic solution is injected. In this fashion, a diffuse region ventral to the transverse process is infiltrated, to block the ventral branch of the nerve. The needle is then redirected slightly dorsal and caudal to the transverse process to block the dorsolateral branch of each nerve. In adult cattle, up to 25 ml of local anesthetic solution has been administered at each site without adverse effect. Because the paralumbar technique does not paralyze the lumbar muscles, lateral deviation of the spine does not occur.

The technique for paravertebral nerve block is the same in sheep and goats as it is in cattle. Up to 5 ml of 1% or 2% lidocaine is recommended for each of the injection sites.[1] While the total dose should not exceed 6 mg/kg, a lower dose (2 mg/kg) is usually recommended.

Epidural Analgesia

Epidural analgesia is used frequently to facilitate standing surgical interventions in cattle and horses, for cesarean sections in swine, for urogenital surgery in goats, and for postoperative analgesia. Drug selection varies depending on the goal (e.g., local anesthetics for anesthesia of the area, opioids or alpha-2's for analgesia without motor blockade) Species differences also influence the choice of epidural drug and need for systemic administration of sedatives or tranquilizers. Sheep can be easily handled and may only require administration of a local anesthetic and physical restraint for some procedures. Goats and pigs tend to be more curious and less amenable to physical restraint so may require concurrent sedation. Site of administration of the epidural drug(s) also varies with species and procedure to be performed and commonly includes either the lumbosacral or caudal epidural space.

The lumbosacral space is commonly used in sheep, goats, and pigs, whereas in cattle and horses the caudal epidural site is more typical and facilitates "standing" procedures as motor control of the hind legs is generally not affected (as it often is with lumbosacral administration of local anesthetic); but the anal sphincter relaxes, and tenesmus and obstetric straining is prevented.

Caudal epidural administration describes the injection of analgesic and anesthetic agents between either the first and second coccygeal vertebrae or in the sacrococcygeal space. The former site is 1–2 inches cranial to the long tail hairs in the horse. To locate the space, the tail is grasped and is moved up and down; the first obvious articulation caudal to the sacrum is the first intercoccygeal space. After clipping and skin preparation, a skin bleb is made with 2% lidocaine using a 2.5-cm, 25-gauge needle, to facilitate needle placement. An 18- or 19-gauge, 3- to 5-cm needle (or a spinal needle) is introduced through the center of the space on the midline at a 45° angle in cattle until its point hits the floor of the spinal canal (Figure 2.3). The needle is then retracted slightly to ensure that the end is not embedded in the intervertebral disc. In the horse, this needle may be inserted at an angle of 30° from a perpendicular line through the vertebrae or at an angle of 60° as illustrated in Figure 2.4. If a regular needle (versus a spinal needle with a stilette) is utilized, aspiration of sterile fluid placed in the needle hub is a practical indicator of entry into the epidural space especially with first-time injections. Additionally, if the needle is correctly placed in the epidural space, there should be no resistance to injection. The bevel of the needle is usually directed cranially. In cattle and small ruminants, 2% lidocaine may be used for epidural anesthesia. Doses are shown in Table 2.1. Injections of 2% lidocaine can also be used in the sacrococcygeal space of sheep and goats to provide caudal epidural analgesia for obstetric procedures. The total volume of drug administered via the caudal epidural space should not exceed 3 ml in sheep and goats and 10 ml in cattle if the goal is to avoid hind limb incoordination or recumbency.[12] Alpha-2 agents can be used with 2% lidocaine in cattle to achieve a longer duration of analgesia.[1,12,13]

In horses, caudal epidural administration of lidocaine has been similarly used for certain procedures (e.g., Caslicks). This provides surgical anesthesia for a duration of 87.2 ± 7.5 minutes, which is considered fairly short for many procedures performed in horses. Volumes greater than 5–7 ml may extend duration of the block but are not typically recommended as they increase the likelihood of recumbency.[1,14] As in cattle, alpha-2 agonists such as detomidine, xylazine, and medetomidine are therefore often administered in combination to increase the duration of analgesia and potentially decrease ataxia.[6,15] Systemic effects may, however, be observed. Alternative anesthetic/analgesic combinations are shown in Table 2.2.

To achieve anesthesia for more rostral perineal and hind limb surgical procedures in small ruminants and

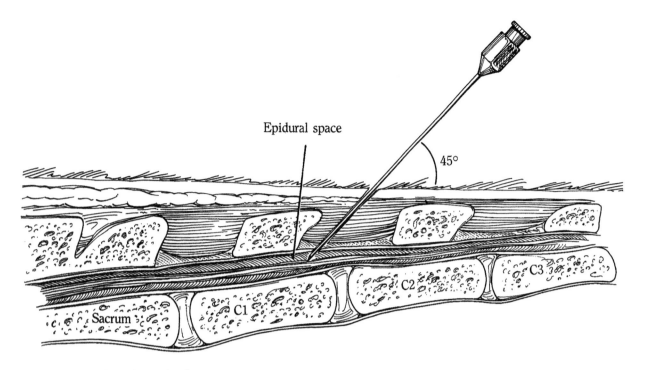

Epidural space

45°

C3

C2

C1

Sacrum

Fig. 2.3. Bovine epidural anesthesia.

pigs, the drug is administered at the lumbosacral space. In sheep and goats, a volume of 1 ml/5–7 kg lean body weight has been suggested depending on the desired cranial extent of the block; recumbency should be expected. While generally contraindicated and challenging to perform in horses, this technique has been used to provide 2–4 hours of analgesia in cattle for laparotomy, pelvic limb surgery, or udder amputation. Recognize that the animal will become recumbent if high volumes of local anesthetic are injected into the lumbosacral space. Accidental spinal injection in any species will extend the block further cranially which could result in respiratory compromise and worsening hypotension from vasodilation.[16] Ruminal atony and bloat may also be observed in cattle.

Continuous caudal epidural anesthesia using a commercial epidural catheter kit (continuous epidural tray) is also used in horses and, in some instances, ruminants for repeated delivery of epidural delivery of analgesics and postoperative pain relief.[15,17,18] The kit contains a Huber-point directional needle with stilette (Tuohy spinal needle) inserted through a pilot hole at 45° to the horizontal until one encounters an abrupt reduction in resistance. The catheter is then inserted through the needle, it is advanced a distance beyond the end of the needle, and the needle is withdrawn. Combinations of either a local anesthetic or an alpha-2 adrenergic agonist and morphine administered in the caudal epidural space have been shown to have useful clinical applications for postoperative and long-term pain relief in both humans and animals. Preoperative epidural administration of detomidine (30 µg/kg) and morphine (0.2 mg/kg) provides effective,

long-lasting pain relief and decreases postoperative lameness in horses that undergo bilateral stifle arthroscopy.[19]

Lumbosacral epidural analgesia has been used in both young and adult pigs and in particular for cesarean section in the sow. This technique is reported to result in maternal immobilization and analgesia, with minimal fetal depression. The lumbosacral space is located at the intersection of the spine with a line drawn through the cranial borders of the ilium. An 18-gauge needle is inserted 1–2 cm caudal to this line in small pigs and 2.5–5 cm caudal to the line in larger animals. The needle is then directed ventrally until it is felt to pass through the dorsal ligament of the vertebrae and into the epidural space. The needle size varies with the size of the pig: 8 cm is used for the pig weighing up to 75 kg; and 15 cm is used for pigs heavier than 75 kg. The dose is about 1 ml/5–10 kg of 2% lidocaine for pelvic limb block; the higher dose rate is used in small pigs; and the smaller dose rate is used in large pigs. Other drug combinations used for epidural anesthesia in swine are listed in Table 2.3.

Although epidural analgesia may have advantages based on a requirement for minimal depression of the central nervous system and decreased expense, its use in swine practice has been limited by the time required to perform the technique and the temperament of the animal.

As a cautionary note, Food and Drug Administration regulations must also be considered in any milk-producing animals and those destined for market. Few analgesics are approved for use in ruminant species and swine, and withdrawal and food residue values are not consistently available.

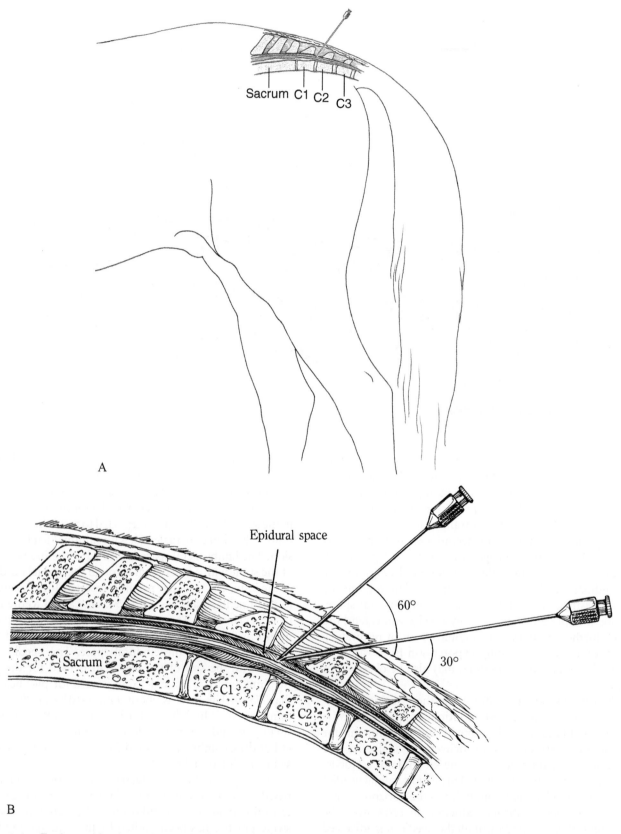

A

B

Fig. 2.4. Equine epidural anesthesia. **A.** Overall view of hindquarters. **B.** Close-up of caudal vertebra.

Table 2.1. Epidural anesthesia and analgesia in cattle and small ruminants.

Drug	Indications	Dosage	Comments
2% Lidocaine	Cranial and caudal epidural anesthesia. Caudal epidural anesthesia in sheep and goats	Cattle: 1 ml/10 lb or 0.5–1 ml/100 lb. Sheep/goats: 2–3 ml	Short onset and duration (20–180 minutes). Commonly used in cattle. Doses greater than 10 ml in cattle and 3 ml in sheep and goats can cause hind limb incoordination and recumbency.[3,12]
2% Lidocaine/xylazine	Caudal epidural anesthesia in cattle	0.22 mg/kg lidocaine, 0.05 mg/kg xylazine. Total volume: 5–7 ml[13,72]	The addition of xylazine lengthens the duration of analgesia (303 ± 11 minutes) compared to either drug alone.[29] The onset is also quicker than for lidocaine alone. Xylazine should be avoided in pregnant cows.
Medetomidine	Caudal epidural anesthesia in cattle. Lumbosacral epidural anesthesia in goats	Cattle: 15 μg/kg diluted to 5 ml with 0.9% saline[73]. Sheep/goats: 20 μg/kg diluted to 5 ml in sterile water[74]	Greatest duration of analgesia (412 ± 156 minutes) and comparable onset time to lidocaine/xylazine in cattle.[73] Systemic effects may be seen.
Medetomidine/ Mepivacaine	Caudal epidural anesthesia in cattle	Medetomidine: 15 υg/kg. Mepivacaine: 0.5–1 ml/100 lb	
Morphine	Epidural analgesia/ postoperative pain relief in goats and sheep	15 mg/ml morphine diluted to 0.15–0.20 ml/kg in 0.9% saline[75]	Provides perioperative analgesia without paralysis.[75] Pruritis reported with spinal injection of morphine in sheep.

Table 2.2. Caudal epidural analgesic agents in the horse.

Drug	Indications	Dosage	Comments
Detomidine	Sedation/analgesia	20–60 μg/kg. Dilute with 0.9% saline to total volume of 10–15 ml.	Detomidine is more potent in horses than xylazine. Associated with moderate ataxia, mild cardiopulmonary depression, and renal diuresis. Detomidine may be combined with morphine to provide longer-lasting analgesia and to provide postoperative pain relief.[19]
Detomidine/morphine	Sedation/analgesia	Detomidine: 20–40 μg/kg with Morphine: 0.1–0.2 mg/kg. Dilute with 0.9% saline to total volume of 10–15 ml.	Systemic effects likely with epidural detomidine. Ileus possible with higher doses of morphine.
Xylazine/2% lidocaine	Sedation/analgesia	0.22 mg/kg lidocaine, 0.17 mg/kg xylazine	Local anesthetics alone are not ideal for caudal epidural analgesia due to their undesirable level of hind limb ataxia and weakness in horses. They are commonly combined with an alpha-2 agonist.[1,14] Ataxia may, however, be observed with xylazine.
2% Mepivacaine	Anesthesia	4–4.5 ml of 2% solution (80–90 mg)[6]	Rapid onset (5–10 minutes) and medium duration (70–210 minutes). Reported to cause less tissue irritation than lidocaine.[6]

Table 2.3.   Epidural analgesic agents in swine.

Drug	Indication	Dosage	Comments
Detomidine	Lumbosacral epidural anesthesia in swine	0.05–0.1 mg/kg in 5 ml 0.9% saline	Onset of 10 minutes, duration of 30 minutes. Minimal analgesia caudal to umbilicus.[3,12]
2% Lidocaine	Lumbosacral epidural anesthesia in swine	0.5–1 ml/5 kg, depending on the size of the pig	2% lidocaine has been used successfully for castration of boars and cesarean section in sows.[3,12]
Xylazine	Lumbosacral epidural anesthesia in swine	1–2 mg/kg diluted in 5 ml of 0.9% saline	Xylazine produces bilateral analgesia from the anus to the umbilicus within 5–10 minutes and lasting for at least 120 minutes.[76] Addition of lidocaine may increase duration to 5–8 hours. Typically used for cesarean sections.
10% Xylazine and 2% lidocaine		Xylazine (10%): 1 mg/kg Lidocaine (2%): 10 ml	

Regional Analgesia of the Eye

The main indication for analgesia of the eye in cattle is for orbital exenteration. For this purpose, the technique of local infiltration using the retrobulbar (four-point) block is convenient and satisfactory. The technique is described and illustrated under eye enucleation in Chapter 15.

An alternate technique for regional analgesia to the eye is the Peterson block. For this technique, an 11-cm, 18-gauge needle bent to a curvature of a 10-inch circle is required. A skin bleb is made at the point where the supraorbital process meets the zygomatic arch, and a puncture wound is made in this bleb with a short 14-gauge needle. The 11-cm needle is then directed medially, with the concavity of the needle directed caudally. In this fashion, the point of the needle will pass around the cranial border of the coronoid process of the mandible, and the needle is then directed further medially until it hits the pterygoid crest. The needle is then moved slightly rostral and down to the pterygopalatine fossa at the foramen orbitorotundum, and 15–20 ml of local analgesic solution are injected. The needle is withdrawn and is directed caudally just beneath the skin, to infiltrate the subcutaneous tissues along the zygomatic arch. A small region just dorsal to the medial canthus should also be infiltrated.

Although the Peterson block is preferred by some practitioners for eye analgesia, it is unpredictable, and the injection of 15 ml of local anesthetic inadvertently into the internal maxillary artery can have fatal results. The latter problem can be avoided by injecting 5 ml in one place, repositioning the needle slightly, aspirating and injecting another 5 ml, and then repeating this procedure. Placing a subcutaneous line block across (perpendicular) to the medial canthus of the eye (resulting in likely block of a branch of the infratrochlear nerve) may be a useful adjunct when this block is used to achieve complete desensitization of the eye and adnexa.

Regional Analgesia of the Horn

The cornual block is a simple technique that provides analgesia for dehorning cattle and goats. An imaginary line is drawn from the lateral canthus of the eye to the base of the horn along the crest dorsal to the temporal fossa. On this line, an 18-gauge, 2.5-cm needle is inserted halfway from the lateral canthus to the horn, and an injection is made under the skin and through the frontalis muscle at the lateral border of the crest. Generally, 5 ml of 2% lidocaine is sufficient, but up to 10 ml may be used in a larger animal.

Unlike cattle, goats have two cornual branches, one arising from the lacrimal nerve and one from the infratrochlear nerve. The locations of these branches and the technique for blocking are described in Chapter 16. Some exotic breeds of cattle, especially the Simmental, also require additional blockade of the infratrochlear nerve, which innervates the medial aspect of the horn.[20] This can be achieved by using a line block subcutaneously from the midline of the head to the facial crest across the forehead dorsal to the eye.

Intravenous Limb Anesthesia of Ruminants

For anesthesia of the distal limb, the technique of intravenous administration of local anesthetic drugs is considered superior to specific nerve blocks or ring blocks. The technique involves intravenous injection of local anesthetic solution distal to a tourniquet.[21] The animal is restrained, and the tourniquet (e.g., rubber tubing/penrose drain) is applied distal to the carpus or hock (Figure 2.5). A protective pad may be placed under the tourniquet. Following tourniquet placement, a superficial vein is identified, typically either the dorsal common digital vein III in the metacarpus or the cranial branch of the lateral saphenous vein in the metatarsus. An intravenous injection of 10–20 ml of 2% lidocaine or mepivacaine is administered to adult cattle after the area has been clipped and prepared. For sheep and particularly goats, a

Fig. 2.5. Intravenous limb anesthesia. **A.** Forelimb, dorsal aspect. **B.** Hind limb, dorsal aspect.

lower dose of 2–3 ml (preferably not to exceed 2 mg/kg) should be used initially. It is important to avoid the use of lidocaine with epinephrine because the combination may cause regional vasoconstriction and systemic release of epinephrine upon release of the tourniquet may result in adverse effects. Following injection, the needle is with-

drawn, and the injection site is wrapped to prevent hematoma formation. Alternatively a small gauge catheter may be secured and left in place until the procedure is completed. Anesthesia of the distal limb is complete in 5 minutes and persists 1–2 hours if the tourniquet remains in place. At the end of the operation, the tourniquet is

Table 2.4. Tranquilizers and sedatives used in cattle.

Drug	Indications	Dosage	Comments
Detomidine	Standing sedation in cattle	0.01–0.03 mg/kg IV	No associations with drug residues in milk after dosing in dairy cows or increased risk of abortion.[23,77]
Medetomidine	Deep sedation and recumbency at high doses in cattle	0.002–0.01 mg/kg IV	The lower dose results in deep sedation while the higher dose produces recumbency.
Xylazine	Casting agent or standing sedation in cattle	0.11–0.22 mg/kg IM 0.055–0.11 mg/kg IV	Profound effects in cattle, causes recumbency at the higher intramuscular dose and standing sedation with the lower intravenous dose. Gastrointestinal side effects in large bulls have been noted with xylazine.[78] Increased risk of spontaneous abortion during the third trimester in pregnant cows.[25] This combination is used to provide chemical restraint in standing cattle.
Xylazine/butorphanol	Standing sedation/analgesia Standing sedation.	Xylazine: 0.02 mg/kg IV Butorphanol: 0.05–0.07 mg/kg IV[24]	
Xylazine/butorphanol ketamine	Ket-Stun	Xylazine 0.02–0.05 mg/kg Butorphanol 0.01–0.025 mg/kg Ketamine 0.04–0.1 mg/kg	

released slowly over a period of 10 seconds, and the limb will regain normal sensation and motor function in about 5 minutes. Toxicity related to the entrance of the local anesthetic into the circulation at these doses has not been observed.[21]

Other Nerve Blocks

Nerve blocks and ring blocks are usually performed in the limb for lameness diagnosis and wound repair. Specific nerve blocks for different areas of the limbs and intra-articular analgesic techniques also have an important place in the diagnosis of lameness and are well described elsewhere.[22] These techniques are not repeated in this text.

Tranquilization and Sedation

There are three general purposes for the tranquilization or sedation of large animals: (1) sedation of intractable animals for routine diagnostic and therapeutic procedures; (2) sedation for minor surgical procedures in conjunction with local anesthesia; and (3) preanesthetic medication. The terms tranquilization and sedation in the horse imply that the animal is standing, whereas in the bovine patient, it commonly implies that the animal will be placed in recumbency and secured with ropes or restrained on a tilt table. Selected drugs with referenced dosages are found in Table 2.4. The phenothiazine tranquilizer most commonly used in the horse is acetylpromazine maleate (Acepromazine Maleate Injectable). Hypotension, tachycardia, and rarely persistent penile paralysis are potential side effects.[23] Additionally, acepromazine has no analgesic properties. Use of alpha-2 adrenoceptor agonists, such as xylazine hydrochloride, detomidine, medetomidine, dexmedetomidine, and romifidine in place of acepromazine is common as these

drugs provide both sedation and analgesia. They do, however, have side effects including a drug-, dose-, and route-dependent period of hypertension (followed by hypotension), decreased heart rate and decreased cardiac output. Effects on respiratory rate and character are more variable. Ruminal atony or ileus is also reported. To minimize the sudden responsiveness (e.g., phantom kick) by some animals, alpha-2 agonist drugs are frequently combined with opioids. The potential for respiratory depression and ileus is, however increased when these drugs are used in combination. Table 2.4 and Table 2.5 depict a few of the commonly used drugs for sedation in cattle and horses.

Sedation in swine can be achieved with azaperone (a safe, inexpensive drug used by herdsman to control fighting and aggression). Droperidol also produces a similar quality of sedation in pigs. Opioids are often used with alpha-2 agents in pigs to provide preanesthetic sedation and analgesia.

The benzodiazepines diazepam or midazolam provide short-acting sedation in goats and sheep. While alpha-2 agents may be used in these species, they have significant negative cardiopulmonary effects. Opioids such as morphine and fentanyl have been used in sheep and goats to provide analgesia. Dosages for selected drugs are listed in Table 2.6 and Table 2.7.

General Anesthesia

General anesthesia should be used whenever it is considered the optimal technique. Many surgical procedures have either been cancelled or performed under compromised circumstances because of reluctance to anesthetize the patient. General anesthesia offers the ultimate in restraint and, therefore, the ideal situation for aseptic

Table 2.5. Tranquilizers and sedatives used in horses.

Drug	Indications	Dosage	Comments
Acepromazine/ May be used with any opioid or alone.	Sedation	Ace: 0.03–0.06 mg/kg Butorphanol: 0.01–0.04 mg/kg, IV or IM Morphine (0.03–0.09 mg/kg IV or IM)	Acepromazine at a dose of 0.05 mg/kg IV or IM can be used for mild sedation that lasts approximately 90 minutes and begins within 15–20 minutes.[2] Acepromazine should not be used after recent treatment with organophosphate anthelmintics. Due to its alpha-adrenergic blocking effect, this drug should not be used in cases of hypovolemic shock, except when volume replacement has been adequate and when peripheral vasodilation to increase perfusion is desired.
Detomidine Detomidine/opioid	Sedation	4–20 µg/kg IV Detomidine: 5–20 µg/kg Butorphanol: 0.01–0.04 mg/kg, IV or IM Morphine: 0.03–0.09 mg/kg, IV or IM	Cardiovascular effects are longer lasting than with xylazine or dex/medetomidine. Duration of 60–120 minutes.[6] Detomidine can be administered with a loading dose of 7.5 µg/kg IV followed by constant rate infusion to effect.
Medetomidine	Sedation	5 µg/kg IV	Similar/slightly longer duration than xylazine.[6] As with other alpha-2 agents it may be infused intravenously to effect to achieve the desired length of sedation.
Romifidine	Sedation	40–120 µg/kg IV	Produces sedation of a similar duration to detomidine and longer than xylazine.[6]
Xylazine	Premedication and standing sedation	1.1 mg/kg IV[79] 0.3–0.6 mg/kg IV for preanesthetic	Bradycardia and transient cardiac arrhythmias (usually atrioventricular block) occur when xylazine is given intravenously. At high doses, significant ataxia may complicate standing procedures. Animal behavior under heavy sedation may be unpredictable. Good for short procedures.
Xylazine/ Acepromazine	Sedation	Xylazine: 0.5 mg/kg Ace: 0.05 mg/kg IV	Addition of acepromazine, similar to opioids, results in more reliable sedation. However, this is considered "off-label" use.
Xylazine/ Butorphanol tartate		Xylazine: 0.3–1 mg/kg Butorphanol: 0.01–0.05 mg/kg IV	Xylazine in combination with opioids facilitates restraint and minimizes sudden arousal seen with xylazine alone.
Xylazine/ morphine		Xylazine: 0.3–1 mg/kg Morphine: 0.03–0.9 mg/kg IV[80,81]	

Table 2.6. Tranquilizers and sedatives used in swine.

Drug	Indications	Dosage	Comments
Azaperone	Tranquilization	1–8 mg/kg	Not recommended for use in boars at doses greater than 1 mg/kg due to the risk of penile protrusion and subsequent injury.[1] Onset is approximately 20 minutes.
Droperidol	Tranquilization.	0.1–0.4 mg/kg	Produces sedation similar to azaperone.
Ketamine/diazepam	Sedation in swine.	10–15 mg/kg ketamine, 0.5–2.0 mg/kg diazepam IM	Heavy sedation with longer duration than previous drugs (1–2 hours).
Ketamine/Midazolam		10–20 mg/kg ketamine, 0.1–0.5 mg/kg midazolam IM 1–2 mg/kg IM	Ketamine dose may be reduced to facilitate mild sedation.
Xylazine	Sedation and analgesia in swine	May be used with opioids for additional analgesia and sedation	

Table 2.7. Tranquilizers and sedatives used in small ruminants.

Drug	Indications	Dosage	Comments
Acepromazine	Mild sedation	0.05–0.1 mg/kg IM	May be used for restraint prior to induction.
Ketamine/diazepam	Sedation	2–5 mg/kg ketamine, 0.1–0.2 mg/kg diazepam IV	Mild sedation with ketamine and benzodiazepine combinations at these doses. Higher dosages are used for anesthesia. Diazepam is generally given by IV whereas midazolam may be given by either the IV or IM route. Midazolam may also be used in combination with opioids such as butorphanol or morphine to provide sedation and analgesia.
Ketamine/midazolam		2–5 mg/kg ketamine, 0.1–0.2 mg/kg midazolam IM	
Xylazine	Sedation	0.1–0.4 mg/kg in sheep 0.05–0.1 mg/kg IV	Significant negative cardiopulmonary effects are noted with xylazine in ruminants. Similar considerations exist for other alpha-2 agents such as medetomidine.

surgery, proper handling of tissues, and hemostasis. It also affords the opportunity to provide analgesia for the patient. General anesthesia should never be done casually, however, and the operator should be experienced in performing general anesthesia before electing to use the technique.

Many procedures in horses are performed under general anesthesia. Most surgical procedures in cattle can be performed with the animal standing or with physical and chemical restraint and regional anesthesia in lateral or dorsal recumbency. This is done in part because general anesthesia in ruminants presents many challenges due to their physiological characteristics. Prolonged recumbency in cattle may cause the abdominal contents to interfere with normal diaphragm movement and result in hypoventilation, hypoxia, hypercarbia, and respiratory acidosis.[24,25] Regurgitation and postoperative bloat are also concerns in ruminants under general anesthesia. Fasting patients prior to anesthesia and surgery and placement of a cuffed endotracheal tube will minimize the risk of regurgitation and subsequent aspiration during recumbency. Additionally an oro-ruminal tube may be placed to facilitate displacement of gas and liquid contents to reduce bloat.

In many practice situations due to the absence of appropriate support and monitoring tools, sedation with regional anesthesia is still used in small ruminants in place of general anesthesia.[1] However, these patients may be safely and effectively anesthetized in a hospital circumstance. A common protocol would include premedication with an opioid or opioid and benzodiazepine, intravenous induction with ketamine, and a benzodiazepine and maintenance with an inhaled anesthetic. Cardiovascular and respiratory function is monitored and supported.

Prior to general anesthesia in any patient, a thorough preanesthetic evaluation should be completed, followed by appropriate preoperative preparation. The preanesthetic patient evaluation should include a history, clinical examination, and a complete blood count (CBC) or at least a packed cell volume (PCV)/total protein determina-

tion. Complete serum chemistry profiles are indicated in older and debilitated patients. All anesthetized patients should be carefully monitored during the procedure and throughout postoperative recovery.

Feed should be withheld from all patients before general anesthesia unless the urgency of the problem precludes it. This is especially crucial in ruminants, where bloat, regurgitation, and aspiration of ingesta are concerns. Adult cattle should be kept off feed for 48 hours prior to surgery, especially grain and concentrates. Water may be removed for 12 hours if environmental temperature permits. Regurgitation is less of a problem in younger cattle, and feed need only be withheld for 12–24 hours and water withheld overnight prior to surgery.[26] Feed should be withheld from sheep and goats 12–24 hours prior to surgery and from pigs 8–12 hours prior to surgery. Water should be withheld 6–12 hours prior to surgery in sheep and goats and 2 hours prior to surgery for pigs. Feed should be withheld from horses for 12 hours prior to surgery, while water can be available free choice.

Premedication

Sedation or tranquilization of the equine patient is almost always indicated prior to inducing general anesthesia, but is not consistently required for cattle or small ruminants. Most tranquilizers and sedatives are not approved for use in ruminants by the Food and Drug Administration, and the veterinarian must assume responsibility when using theses drugs. Compromised horses, such as a patient with an acute abdominal disorder, may preclude the need for sedation prior to induction. However, analgesic drugs are still warranted. Preanesthetic tranquilizers may be omitted from the anesthetic plan for neonatal foals because of inadequate development of the microsomal enzyme system in the liver and the consequent slow metabolism of these drugs. The alpha-2 agonists are commonly used as preinduction agents in horses and occasionally in unruly cattle (refer to Table 2.5).

Table 2.8. Anesthetic induction regimens in the equine patient.

Drug	Dosage	Comments
Guaifenesin/ketamine	5–10% solution of guaifenesin IV (50–100 mg/kg) followed by bolus of ketamine (1.8–2.2 mg/kg)	Excellent for debilitated patients. Provides relatively smooth induction of anesthesia with little cardiopulmonary depression.[29] In healthy patients, a low to moderate dose of an alpha-2 agent may be administered prior to induction with guaifenesin and ketamine.
Tiletamine/zolazepam (Telazol®)	0.7–1.0 mg/kg IV	Given following sedation with alpha-2 agonist drugs or guaifenesin. Considered to have superior induction quality and produce greater muscle relaxation than some other agents, but is also associated with a prolonged ataxia during recovery.[82]
Xylazine/ketamine	1.1 mg/kg xylazine IV followed 2–3 minutes later by 2.2 mg/kg ketamine IV	This regimen provides anesthesia for a short duration (12–15 minutes) and eliminates the need for large-volume administration through a catheter or needle. Induction is smooth when xylazine takes effect before ketamine is administered. Disadvantages include the short duration, maintenance of reflex activity, and inability to judge anesthetic depth. Active palpebral, corneal, and swallowing reflexes are maintained; passing an endotracheal tube can be difficult. Diazepam (0.02–0.1 mg/kg) concurrently with ketamine will reduce reflex activity and facilitate intubation.[83] Other alpha-2 agents (romifidine 80–100 μg/kg), detomidine 20–30 μg/kg) may be similarly used with benzodiazepines (diazepam or midazolam) and ketamine.

Anticholinergic drugs, such as atropine, are not used frequently as preanesthetic agents in horses or large ruminants as the advantages do not typically outweigh the disadvantages, which include postoperative ileus, increased myocardial oxygen consumption, tachycardia, and ocular effects in sheep and goats.[1,23,27] Anticholinergics are thought to reduce salivation in the small ruminant but also to render it more viscous. While this may facilitate visual intubation, in smaller patients endotracheal tube occlusion is also possible. Atropine or glycopyrrolate is useful in pigs to control excessive salivation during general anesthesia especially when ketamine or tiletamine are used.[1]

Induction of Anesthesia

There are many possible regimens for the intravenous induction of anesthesia in ruminants and horses. The methods discussed here currently receive the most use. Common induction agents and doses are included in Table 2.8 and Table 2.9.

Traditionally, thiobarbiturates were used to induce recumbency in sedated horses, but as a result of their lack of availability (at least in the United States) and other concerns with their use in nonhospital circumstances, they have been largely replaced by dissociative drugs such as ketamine and tiletamine. Guaifenesin has been used alone as a casting agent[28] or in combination with ketamine for induction of anesthesia in sedated or tranquilized horses.[87,23] This drug is a muscle relaxant that acts at the level of the internuncial neurons in the spinal cord and brainstem and provides a calm state similar to sleep, but it is not an anesthetic. At appropriate doses it has minimal depressant effects on the respiratory and cardiac systems, and the transition to recumbency is generally smooth, without involuntary movements of the forelimbs (dog paddling). The drug is administered as a 5% solution in dextrose or as a 10% solution in sterile distilled water.[29,30]

While foals may be induced to anesthesia with inhaled anesthetics, it has been shown that cardiovascular function is better maintained when ketamine and diazepam are used.[31] If using an inhaled agent, both nasotracheal and mask applications are possible. Premedication may be required to facilitate an inhaled anesthetic induction. For both nasotracheal and mask applications, it is suggested that following placement the foal is allowed to adjust to the mask or tube with oxygen alone (5–6 L/min) and that the vaporizer is then gradually turned up in 0.5–1% increments first to introduce the foal to the inhalant, and then until anesthesia is induced. Excitement may be observed during inhaled anesthetic induction and caution is advised as depth changes occur rapidly. Following recumbency, the foal may be orotracheally intubated with a tube (or larger tube following nasotracheal intubation) and maintained with the inhalant.

Similar to the horse, combinations of guaifenesin are frequently used in cattle to induce and maintain anesthesia. The "triple drip" combination used in cattle, sheep,

Table 2.9.   Anesthetic induction regimens in cattle and small ruminants.

Drug	Dosage	Comments
Guaifenesin/ketamine	50–100 mg/kg IV in cattle and small ruminants	Guaifenesin is not approved for use in food animals.[35] Xylazine (0.1–0.2 mg/kg IM) may be used in unruly cattle to facilitate sedation prior to guaifenesin but is not typically necessary.
Triple drip: Guaifenesin/ ketamine/xylazine	Solution prepared as 1 g ketamine and 25–50 mg xylazine added to 1 L 5% guaifenesin. Administered IV initially at a 0.5–1.1 ml/kg to effect. May be maintained at 1.0–2.2 ml/kg/hr.[84]	This combination may be used without xylazine for nonpainful procedures or in debilitated patients to minimize cardiopulmonary side effects.
Ketamine/diazepam	Ketamine 2–5 mg/kg IV with diazepam (0.1–0.2 mg/kg) in cattle and small ruminants	In cattle, a tranquilizer or sedative may be necessary prior to administration of this combination. Butorphanol (0.01–0.05 mg/kg) may be administered just prior to injection to improve muscle relaxation. Onset is approximately 5 minutes and duration is 30–40 minutes. If anesthesia is maintained with an inhalant, low arterial blood pressure can be observed.[1]
Propofol	2 mg/kg IV in small ruminants	Rapid onset, short duration. May also be used with a benzodiazepine.
Tiletamine/zolazepam (Telazol®)	1–3 mg/kg IV or 3–5 mg/kg SC for induction of anesthesia in small ruminants	Longer duration of action and recovery duration when compared to ketamine and diazepam, but otherwise qualitatively similar. Does not provide analgesia.

and goats consists of a 5% guaifenesin solution, 1–1.5 mg/ml of ketamine, and 0.1 mg/ml of xylazine (0.5 mg/ml in horses) and has been found to be effective for maintaining general anesthesia. Hypoxemia, however, is a common side effect, and oxygen supplementation is highly recommended. Following anesthesia induction with a protocol that ideally doesn't require guaifenesin, 1–2 ml/kg/hr of this combined solution is administered for anesthetic maintenance. At these dose combinations, triple drip solutions should not be used for periods greater than one hour as toxicity may be observed at doses greater than 100 mg/kg of guaifenesin and recovery duration and quality are likely to be adversely influenced.

It is ideal if ruminants are maintained in sternal recumbency during anesthesia induction. A mouth speculum is then used to facilitate introduction of a cuffed endotracheal tube, which is recommended to protect the airway even if anesthesia is to be maintained by an intravenous agent. Endotracheal intubation in cattle is generally accomplished digitally or by blind passage of the tube into the pharynx coupled with external manipulation of the larynx.[32] In adult cattle, digital intubation can be performed by placing a speculum to hold the patient's mouth open and by directing the tube into the larynx with one's hand cupped over the end of the tube. Blind intubation can also be performed by extending the animal's head, elevating the larynx by external manipulation, and passing the tube into the trachea. In calves and smaller cattle, visual intubation with a laryngoscope is more commonly performed.

Although intubation can be performed after sedation with xylazine, the incidence of regurgitation is lower if surgical anesthesia is induced before endotracheal intubation is performed.[33] Regurgitation with an endotracheal tube in place is of minor concern, provided the pharynx is cleared and drained and the nasal cavity is flushed before extubation.[33]

Induction of anesthesia in young animals may be performed with an inhalant or using propofol or ketamine and a benzodiazepine.

Pigs (especially pot-bellied pigs) are challenging to anesthetize using injectable drugs due to difficulty in placing an IV catheter. However, if IV access is obtained, traditional anesthesia induction agents may be used and include combinations of ketamine or propofol and a benzodiazepine. Premedication is usually recommended. A solution of guaifenesin, ketamine, and xylazine (GKX) has also been described for induction and maintenance of anesthesia in mature swine.[34] Inhaled agents administered by face mask, may also be used to induce anesthesia in pigs.[35] Common agents and doses are included in Table 2.10.

Endotracheal intubation can be difficult in swine. The larynx in the pig is long and mobile, and there is a middle ventricle in the floor of the larynx near the base of the epiglottis. The arch of the cricoid cartilage is on an oblique angle with the trachea. Laryngeal spasm is easily induced. A laryngoscope is used for intubation of swine and topical anesthetic should be sprayed on the larynx to prevent laryngospasm. The endotracheal tube with a slight curve facilitates the maneuvers necessary to place the tube in the trachea. Initially the tube is placed in the larynx with the tip directed ventrally. It is then rotated 180 degrees to facilitate passage into the more dorsally located trachea.

Table 2.10. Anesthetic induction regimens in swine.

Drug	Dosage	Comments
Guaifenesin/ketamine/xylazine	5% guaifenesin solution in 5% dextrose, 1 mg/ml ketamine, and 1 mg/ml of xylazine IV at dose rate of 0.5–1.0 mg/kg[34]	May be used to induce and maintain anesthesia in swine. This combination of drugs is initially given rapidly at a dose of 0.5–1.0 mg/kg to induce anesthesia. This infusion may be continued at a rate of 2 ml/kg/hr to maintain anesthesia for up to 2.5 hours.[34] Recovery is rapid once the infusion is discontinued.
Ketamine	5–10 mg/kg IM with an alpha-2 agent, benzodiazepine, and/or opioid	The quality of ketamine anesthesia and recovery from the same is variable and dependent on adjunct drug usage. Often these combinations are used to provide heavy sedation to facilitate mask induction with an inhaled agent to allow for endotracheal intubation.
Tiletamine/zolazepam	5 mg/kg IM is administered following sedation with an alpha-2 agent and/or an opioid	Considerations are similar to those for ketamine combinations but a longer duration of action may result in more prolonged recovery.
Tiletamine/zolazepam (Telazol®/ ketamine/xylazine [TKX])	Add 4 ml ketamine (100 mg/ml) and 1 ml xylazine (100 mg/ml) to 5 ml Telazol® Administer 0.5–1 ml/20 kg IM	Duration of anesthesia of 10–30 minutes.

Due to difficulty intubating, anesthesia has been maintained using a face mask, but this technique does not prevent upper airway obstruction or protect the airway from foreign material.

Maintaining Anesthesia

Inhalation anesthesia is the preferred method of maintaining general anesthesia, especially when the procedure involves a total anesthetic time of longer than an hour. For the purpose of this text, details on inhalation anesthetic machines, equipment, techniques, and monitoring will not be described here but are available elsewhere.[4,16,35–37] Recall, however, that malignant hyperthermia is a syndrome of some pig species exposed to inhalation agents. Pigs should be carefully monitored for rises in body temperature. A rapid rise in temperature to 41°C (106°F) or above accompanied by tachypnea, hyperventilation, muscular rigidity, blotchy cyanosis, and tachycardia is seen.[38] Often, even if the inhaled agent is discontinued upon observation of early changes, this can result in fatality. Malignant hyperthermia is described on a very limited basis in horses.

In the US, halothane has been replaced by other inhaled anesthetic agents including isoflurane, sevoflurane, and desflurane. Isoflurane and sevoflurane have been evaluated in ruminants and all three have been assessed in horses.[39–43] While all three exhibit similar behavioral and cardiopulmonary characteristics, cost and unique aspects of the vaporizer (in the case of desflurane) have limited

the widespread use of sevoflurane and desflurane in non-equine species.[32,39,40] When inhaled agents are not feasible, repeat doses of induction agents may be used to prolong anesthesia or constant infusions of drug mixtures may be used. These can also be used as adjuncts to inhalation anesthesia (Table 2.11). Intravenously maintained anesthesia has the advantages of minimal equipment requirements, and may be more cost effective; however, lengthy maintenance on any of the injectable regimens is associated with a prolonged, and sometimes stormy, recovery. Because excretion of the anesthetic agent is slower than with an inhalation agent, the plane of anesthesia cannot be reduced quickly, which can be of further concern in debilitated or young animals. Therefore the general recommendation is that the anesthetic period not exceed one hour.

Intravenous maintenance of anesthesia in horses and ruminants is usually accomplished by a "triple drip" combination of guaifenesin, ketamine, and an alpha-2 antagonist (Table 2.11).[24,25,44] Alternate options in horses include alpha-2 and dissociative combinations, alpha-2 and propofol combinations, benzodiazepine and propofol or ketamine combinations.

Careful clinical monitoring of the patient—including assessment of anesthetic depth, reflex activity, and cardiovascular and respiratory system parameters during anesthesia—is important.[23] The invasiveness and degree to which this is performed should relate to the anesthetic risk assumed for a given patient. For performance of short procedures on generally healthy patients in "the field,"

Table 2.11.   Anesthetic maintenance in large animals.

Drug	Species	Dosage	Comments
Guaifenesin/ ketamine/ detomidine	Horses	Guaifenesin Ketamine: 2mg/ml Detomidine: 0.02mg/ml Initial infusion rate: 1–3ml/kg/hr[85]	Generally administered to effect. Recommended not to exceed 100mg/kg. 5–10% solutions of guaifenesin may be combined with any alpha–2 agent (xylazine, detomidine, dex/medetomidine, and romifidine). "Triple drip" can be used as an adjunct to inhalational anesthesia to reduce the concentration of inhalant required and potentially improve the quality of recovery from anesthesia, or it can be used to maintain anesthesia (total IV anesthesia).[86] When used solely for anesthesia maintenance, use should be limited to 1 hour. The user should be aware that reflex activity may be maintained.
Guaifenesin/ ketamine/ medetomidine	Horses	10% Guifenesin Ketamine: 2mg/ml Medetomidine: 0.002mg/ml Infusion rate: 1–3ml/kg/hr	
Guaifenesin/ ketamine/ romifidine	Horses	10% Guaifenesin Ketamine: 2mg/ml Romifidine: 0.05mg/ml Infusion rate: 1–3ml/kg/hr[85]	
Guaifenesin/ ketamine/ xylazine (GKX)	Cattle	5% Guaifenesin: 500ml Ketamine: 1mg/ml Xylazine: 0.05mg/ml Infusion rate: 0.5–2.2ml/kg[24,25]	
	Sheep and goats	10% Guaifenesin Ketamine: 2mg/ml Xylazine: 0.1mg/ml Infusion rate: 1–3ml/kg/hr	
	Horses	5% Guaifenesin: 500ml Ketamine: 1–2mg/ml Xylazine: 0.5mg/ml Infusion rate: 1–2ml/kg/hr	
Isoflurane	Cattle/Horse	Initial oxygen flow rate of 5–8L/min and vaporizer setting of 3–3.5% Maintain with oxygen flow rate of 3–5L/ min and 2–3% isoflurane for adult cattle and 1–2% in calves.[79]	Following injectable anesthesia induction and intubation guidelines based on use of a typical large animal anesthetic breathing circuit. Guidelines are as for small animals maintained on small animal anesthetic breathing circuit.
	Sheep, goats, and swine	Initial flow rate of 1–3L/min and vaporizer setting of 2–3% isoflurane, which is decreased based on clinical signs.	

monitoring equipment is typically minimal and one relies on the basic senses, such as palpation of the pulse, assessment of respiratory rate and character, and evaluation of ocular signs. For longer and more complex procedures in a hospital situation or in debilitated patients, additional monitoring, such as temperature, heart rate, and rhythm using an electrocardiogram, invasive or noninvasive blood pressure, capnography, pulse oximetry, and blood gas and electrolyte analysis may be warranted. In addition to administration of fluids to support vascular volume, inotropes and vasopressors may be required to ensure adequate blood pressure and tissue perfusion. Dopamine, dobutamine, and ephedrine are practical and effective drugs used to increase blood pressure.[23,45,46] Clinical experience in anesthetized horses indicates that dobutamine is more titratable to a desired response with fewer side effects than dopamine. However, dobutamine does require

administration by infusion, whereas ephedrine may be administered as an intravenous bolus.

Positioning of the patient is important during recumbency. Faulty positioning of the hind limbs can lead to peroneal or femoral nerve paresis.[47] The lower thoracic limb should be extended cranially to relieve pressure between the rib cage, brachial plexus, and vessels along the humerus; otherwise, radial nerve paresis may result. The upper thoracic and pelvic limb should be supported when the horse is in lateral recumbency to prevent venous occlusion and subsequent myopathies. The routine use of a waterbed, air mattress, or deep foam pad is recommended when placing anesthetized animals on an operating table for periods longer than 30–60 minutes. Hypotension during anesthesia is a significant contributor to postanesthetic myopathy in horses anesthetized with inhaled agents.[48]

Ventilatory compromise is of concern in anesthetized, recumbent horses and is more likely with the newer inhalation agents than with halothane. The causes include pharmacologic depression of the respiratory control center, decreased lung volume, inadequate thoracic expansion or diaphragmatic excursions, and mismatched distribution of ventilation and perfusion in recumbency.[36,42,49–52] Hypercarbia (and hypoxemia) may develop unless ventilation is assisted. Controlled ventilation is the most effective means of maintaining appropriate carbon dioxide tensions especially with newer inhaled agents; its detrimental cardiovascular effects can usually be managed. Permissive hypercapnia is sometimes used as a tool even in ventilated patients. Assisted ventilation allows adequate maintenance of oxygen levels, when compared to spontaneous ventilation, with less cardiovascular depression than during controlled ventilation; carbon dioxide levels may however continue to rise.[53] Hypoxemia may occur during anesthetic maintenance and is a potential problem in the recovery period.[51] While insufflation can be helpful, in critical hypoxemia an oxygen supplementation through a demand valve is a better way to maintain arterial blood gas tensions.[51]

Clinical monitoring during bovine anesthesia with inhalation anesthetics includes careful attention to the cardiovascular and respiratory parameters and to ocular signs.[32] Rotation of the eyeball is a reliable means of monitoring anesthetic depth, as well as progression of recovery from inhalation anesthesia.[34,54] As the anesthesia deepens, the eyeball rotates ventrally and medially. As depth of anesthesia further increases, the cornea is completely hidden by the lower eyelid (this is plane 2–3 of surgical anesthesia). A further increase in the depth of anesthesia causes the eye to rotate dorsally to a central position between the palpebral folds. This point denotes deep surgical anesthesia. Palpebral reflexes dull progressively, but the corneal reflex should remain strong. During recovery, eyeball rotation occurs in reverse order to that observed during induction of anesthesia. Cardiovascular monitoring is performed as with the horse, but it is common for cattle to remain hypertensive during inhalation anesthesia. The recovery of cattle from general anesthesia is usually smooth. As the animal recovers, it should be supported in sternal recumbency to reduce the chances of inhaling ruminal contents or developing bloat. The endotracheal tube is usually left in place until the animal is in sternal recumbency.

In sheep and goats, jaw tone may be used but some patients will maintain jaw tone even at an adequate plane of anesthesia. Swallowing signifies a lightening of anesthesia. Eye rotation is not a useful method of assessing anesthetic depth as it is in cattle.[8] Similarly, pupillary dilation is evident during light anesthetic planes and may also be evident during deep anesthesia, and so it is not typically used.

Ocular reflexes are usually of no value in monitoring anesthesia in pigs. The lack of superficial arteries makes it difficult to monitor anesthesia on the basis of pulse strength. Heart rate should be 80–150/minute in normal swine under anesthesia, and the respiratory rate should be 10–25/minute. The depth of anesthesia can also be judged by the degree of muscle relaxation including jaw tone and muscle fasciculation in response to the surgical stimulus.[35]

Fluid Therapy

The need for fluid therapy in the physiologically compromised patient is well recognized. The horse undergoing exploratory laparotomy for acute abdominal crisis is often in a state of shock. Similarly, the bovine patient with abomasal torsion often has major fluid volume and electrolyte deficits.

In the majority of the procedures described in this textbook, the patients are systemically healthy and do not have fluid imbalances prior to surgery; however, such animals do need attention with respect to intravenous fluid therapy while they are under anesthesia. The purposes of fluid therapy for a normal animal during anesthesia are to provide fluids for the patient's maintenance requirements, maintain adequate organ perfusion, maintain normal acid-base balance, and maintain an intravenous route for emergency medication if needed.[35]

Two basic approaches are available in fluid management of the surgical patient. The first approach is to adopt a standard protocol devised to meet likely or anticipated deficits; the second approach is to acquire clinical and laboratory data on an individual patient and to administer the appropriate fluids to meet the patient's specific requirements. The first approach is simple and particularly convenient for the practitioner in the field, where it is not possible to obtain laboratory data instantly. In addition, this approach is satisfactory for fluid administration during routine elective surgery. For the patient with a systemic illness, however, such as an acute abdominal crisis, it is desirable to obtain as accurate an assessment of the patient's fluid volume, acid-base balance, and electrolyte status as possible.

Diagnosis of Fluid Volume Deficits

The degree of dehydration or fluid volume deficit may be estimated by knowing the duration of the problem and evaluating various clinical signs including skin elasticity, pulse rate and character, character of the mucous membranes, temperature of the extremities, and nature and position of the eyes. These parameters are defined in Table 2.12. Skin elasticity is estimated by picking up skin on the side of the neck and pinching it. If the skin flattens out in 1–2 seconds, it has normal elasticity; if the skin takes longer than 8 seconds to flatten, severe dehydration is present. In dehydration, the mucous membranes change from moist and warm to sticky and dry, and then to cold

Table 2.12. Assessment of degrees of clinical dehydration.

	Mild	Moderate	Severe[a]
Skin	Elasticity	Decreased elasticity	No elasticity
Eyes	Slightly sunken, bright	Slightly sunken, duller than normal	Deeply sunken, dry cornea
Mouth	Moist, warm	Sticky or dry	Dry, cold, cyanotic
Body weight decrease estimated (%)	4–6	8	10
Fluid deficit (450-kg animal) (L)	18–27	36	45

[a] More dramatic clinical signs will be apparent in acute hypovolemic shock.

and cyanotic. Volume deficits also increase the capillary refill time from its normal 1–3 seconds.

A severe hypovolemic situation, such as fulminant endotoxic shock, presents a sequence of obvious clinical signs. These include a weak, irregular pulse and color changes in the mucous membranes (brick red in the vasodilatory phase of septic shock, progressing through to the cyanotic "muddy" appearance in very low cardiac output states). Capillary refill time is greater than 3 seconds, and the extremities are cold. Although these signs do not give a quantitative estimate of the volume deficit, they do indicate an urgent need for rapid infusion of intravenous fluids. The quantity of fluids given is based on the patient's response to therapy, rather than on any previous calculations.

It is possible to estimate the approximate fluid volume deficit by using clinical signs (Table 2.12). Under a state of moderate dehydration, the fluid deficit is considered to be 4–6% of the body weight. If signs of severe dehydration are observed, one generally considers that a fluid deficit is at least 10% of the body weight. This means that in a 450-kg animal, a fluid volume deficit of 45 L exists.

A simple laboratory estimate of the degree of hypovolemia may be obtained by simultaneous measurement of the packed cell volume (PCV) and total plasma protein (TPP). The use of PCV has been criticized because of its wide normal range (in the horse, the normal range is 32–52%) and its tendency to undergo changes associated with splenic contraction or hemorrhage, thus confusing attempts to estimate intravascular volume. When the PCV is considered in conjunction with the TPP, however, it is a valuable tool. The range of normal TPP values is more limited. Under certain conditions, such as peritonitis, protein loss can occur, and again, both PCV and TPP need to be evaluated simultaneously and serially.

The use of PCV and TPP estimations is particularly valuable as a monitoring aid during volume replacement. If TPP remains at a normal level while PCV decreases, or if TPP and PCV concurrently decrease, this generally signifies that volume replacement is proceeding satisfactorily. A continued increase in PCV and TPP despite intensive fluid therapy is a poor sign, signifying a continued decrease in intravascular volume, associated with persistent pooling of fluid peripherally. A decreasing TPP accompanied by an increasing PCV usually signifies that the intravascular volume is not increasing and that protein is being lost from the vascular system.

Admittedly, the aforementioned parameters initially reflect changes in the intravascular compartment, and acute loss from the interstitial or intracellular compartments may not be represented. Equilibration between compartments takes place, however; and with sequential monitoring, most disadvantages in the use of PCV and TPP are eliminated.

Other laboratory tests thought to have advantages in the evaluation of fluid deficits include the estimation of serum sodium, plasma osmolality, and serum creatinine.[55–57] Serum sodium estimation helps to characterize the nature of the fluid loss, but in most clinical situations, the clinician can decide whether the fluid loss is hypotonic, isotonic, or hypertonic based on the clinical problem. In addition, serum sodium estimation generally is not immediately available to the clinician. An accurate method of assessing volume deficits is through estimation of plasma osmolality.[58] Unfortunately, this test is not routinely available in clinical institutions, let alone in practice. Serum creatinine and urea concentrations are highly elevated in patients with acute dehydration and may be used to assess the degree of fluid replacement that is needed.

The practical methods available for assessing volume deficits in the surgical patient include the surgeon's clinical assessments and knowledge of the pathophysiology of the disease, estimation of the PCV and TPP, and probably most important, serial evaluation of the response to replacement therapy by both clinical examination and PCV and TPP estimation.

Diagnosis of Acid-Base Imbalance

Acid-base physiology is complex, and consequently, discussions on the cause, diagnosis, and treatment of acid-base imbalance are frequently confusing. The following is a simplified (and one hopes practical) summary of the identification of acid-base imbalance. Although some accuracy may be compromised because of simplification, it is of little significance to the animal.

Abnormalities of acid-base can be ascertained based upon clinical signs, serum biochemical profiles, or by

Table 2.13. Normal values used in the evaluation of fluid balance in large animals.

	Horse	Ox	Sheep	Swine
PCV (%)	32–52	24–46	24–50	32–50
Total protein (g/dL)	6–8	6–8	6.0–7.5	6–7
Electrolytes				
Sodium (mEq/L)	128–140	130–147	139–150	135–150
Potassium (mEq/L)	2.8–4.3	4.3–5.0	3.9–5.4	4.4–6.7
Chloride (mEq/L)	99–109	97–111	95–103	94–106
Blood gases and acid base values (venous)				
pH	7.32–7.44	7.31–7.53	7.32–7.53	
PCO_2 (mmHG)	38–46	35–44	36–40	
HCO_3 (mEq/L)	24–27	25–35	20–25	18–27
TCO_2 (mM/L)	24–32	21.2–32.2	21–28	

blood gas analysis. The advent of relatively inexpensive and portable blood gas analyzers has increased their practicality in the field and allows for quick and easy measurements of pH, PCO_2 and PO_2. An alternative method is to measure total carbon dioxide with a Harleco CO_2 apparatus.[55]

The pH represents the net effect of the influences of respiratory and metabolic mechanisms. The magnitude of the respiratory component is identified by the PCO_2. A PCO_2 greater than 45 mmHG generally indicates respiratory acidosis, whereas a PCO_2 less than 35 mmHG indicates respiratory alkalosis. The magnitude of the metabolic component is identified by either the bicarbonate concentration (HCO_3^-) or the base deficit/excess.[59]

The bicarbonate concentration can be misleading as a quantitative estimate of the metabolic component, because a primary change in carbon dioxide concentration directly causes a change in bicarbonate concentration that is not due to any change in the metabolic component. In addition, because of the presence of other buffer systems, the bicarbonate system is not responsible for buffering all of a given acid or base load. Base deficit/excess is a more accurate measure of quantitative changes in the metabolic component. Base deficit/excess is defined as the titratable acid or base, respectively, when titrating to a pH of 7.4 under standard conditions of PCO_2 (40 mmHG), temperature (38°C), and complete hemoglobin saturation.[56] The base deficit/excess is estimated by aligning the measured values of pH and PCO_2 on a normogram or is computed directly by the blood-gas machine. A base deficit less than −4 mEq/L indicates metabolic acidosis, whereas a base excess greater than +4 mEq/L indicates metabolic alkalosis.[59]

Despite the theoretic deficiencies in using bicarbonate levels as the measure of the metabolic component, the difference is negligible in most practical clinical situations. When PCO_2 is within normal range, the bicarbonate deficit (actual HCO_3^-–normal HCO_3^-) approximates the base deficit. It is commonly assumed in clinical practice that these two values are the same. If this approximation is accepted, then the bicarbonate may be read off a normogram in the same fashion as the base deficit.

To identify a respiratory-derived acid-base imbalance, arterial blood samples are necessary. In most presurgical and postsurgical patients, any acid-base problems have a primary metabolic component, and it is not usually necessary to obtain arterial samples. In large animals, most acid-base imbalances with a primary respiratory origin occur during anesthesia, when arterial blood samples may be conveniently obtained. Treatment of respiratory acidosis involves proper ventilation. Respiratory alkalosis is generally iatrogenic or compensatory.

In evaluating metabolically derived acid-base imbalance, venous blood samples are satisfactory. Normal values for venous blood gases are listed in Table 2.13. Severe metabolic acidosis is treated with an infusion of sodium bicarbonate. The following is an example of a calculation of the amount of bicarbonate needed using the blood-gas data from a patient with severe metabolic acidosis.

pH	7.113
P_{CO_2}	43.8 mmHG
HCO_3^-	11.9 mEq/L
TCO_2	12.9 mEq/L
Base deficit	13.6 mEq/L

Using the base deficit, the patient's bicarbonate deficit is calculated by the equation:

$$\frac{\text{Base deficit} \times \text{body weight (kg)} \times 0.3}{\text{Equivalent weight of } HCO_3^-}$$

$$= \frac{13.6 \times 450 \times 0.3}{12}$$

$$= 153 \text{ g bicarbonate}$$

The bicarbonate deficit may also be calculated from the bicarbonate level using the subsequent formula.

$$\frac{\left(\begin{array}{c}\text{Measured} \quad \text{normal} \\ \text{bicarbonate} - \text{bicarbonate} \\ \text{level} \qquad \text{level}\end{array}\right) \times BW \times 0.3}{12}$$

$$= \frac{(11.9 - 25) \times 450 \times 0.3}{12}$$

$$= \frac{13.1 \times 450 \times 0.3}{12}$$

$$= 147\ g\ \text{bicarbonate}$$

This example demonstrates the general approximation between using base deficit and bicarbonate levels. In both examples, if the denominator is eliminated from the equation the mMol or mEq of bicarbonate required to correct the base deficit will be obtained. It is usually recommended that bicarbonate only be administered after volume resuscitation and that initially only ⅓–½ of the calculated amount be given by infusion over a period of 20–30 minutes. This is because the factor 0.3 is an approximation of the volume of distribution of the bicarbonate, which is mostly accounted for by the extracellular fluid compartment into which the intravenously administered bicarbonate must distribute. Higher factors have been used by some (up to 0.6, which approximates the volume of distribution of total body water), especially in ruminant species.

If a blood-gas machine is not available, the measurement of total carbon dioxide determined by the Harleco CO_2 apparatus is a suitable alternative and gives a reliable measure of the bicarbonate excess or deficit.[55] The addition of acid to serum or plasma results in the liberation of free carbon dioxide, which is almost completely bicarbonate in origin:

$$\text{Total } CO_2 = \text{Dissolved } CO_2 \ (P_{CO_2} \times 0.03) + HCO_3^-\ \text{and}$$

$$\frac{HCO_3^-}{CO_2} = \frac{20}{1}$$

The bicarbonate, therefore, can be estimated by the following formula:

$$HCO_3^- = TCO_2 - \text{Dissolved } CO_2 = TCO_2 - 1.2\ \text{mEq/L}$$

This method is a convenient and economical way for the practitioner to plan and to monitor therapy for metabolic acidosis and to avoid overcorrection or undercorrection of the base deficit.

Although the situation of metabolic acidosis has been used to demonstrate the calculation of imbalances, clinical cases of metabolic alkalosis are identified in a similar manner. Typically, physiologic saline, which is considered an acidifying solution, is administered intravenously and the acid-base status monitored until it returns to normal.

Blood gases alone will not enable one to detect the presence or severity of metabolic acidosis in horses with previous alkalinizing therapy or mixed acid-base disturbances. An estimate of the serum or plasma concentration of unmeasured ions allows detection of these cases. The anion gap or the simplified strong ion gap calculation may be used:

$$\text{Anion gap} = (Na^+ + K^+) - (Cl^- + HCO_3^-)$$

$$\text{Strong ion gap} = \frac{2.24 \times \text{Total Protein (g/dL)}}{1 + 10^{(6.65 - pH)}} - \text{Anion gap}$$

The anion gap is a measurement of the difference between the concentration of unmeasured anions and unmeasured cations in serum. The strong ion gap measures the difference between only the unmeasured strong anions and cations.[60] In horses with normal serum protein levels, the anion gap will provide an accurate estimate of unmeasured strong ion concentrations. A high anion gap (>24 mmol/L) will occur when the concentration of unmeasured anions in plasma (i.e., lactate) is elevated and is a reflection of lactic acidosis. However, in cases of metabolic alkalosis, elevated levels of serum protein can mask the detection of unmeasured anions. The simplified strong ion gap calculation should be used in these cases and will provide the most accurate calculation in horses of varying age and concentrations of albumin, globulin, and phosphate.[60] An increased anion gap, even in the presence of a normal blood gas picture can occur in, for example, a horse with L-lactic acidosis previously administered sodium bicarbonate or in mixed acid-base disturbance, such as in a horse with anterior enteritis and metabolic acidosis due to L-lactic acidosis and metabolic alkalosis due to gastric reflux.[61]

Diagnosis of Electrolyte Abnormalities

The electrolytes of principal concern in the fluid management of surgical patients are sodium, potassium, and chloride ions. The levels of these electrolytes are not evaluated routinely in every patient in whom the need for fluid therapy is anticipated. In specific situations, however, evaluation of the status of these electrolytes is important. Sodium ion is an important electrolyte, and its concentration is intimately associated with fluid content in the body. Sodium and water are lost together (an isotonic loss) in surgical patients, and sodium ion is a routine component in replacement fluids; therefore, specific abnormalities in sodium are not of common concern unless there is a specific loss or gain of sodium. Hypernatremia may become a clinical problem in the patient that has received intensive fluid therapy and in which the addition of sodium bicarbonate to the balanced electrolyte solution has caused an excessive administration of sodium ion. This situation should be monitored in such patients.

A hyperkalemic state may occur during metabolic acidemia because of the redistribution of body potassium; intracellular potassium moves out of the cells into the extracellular fluid as the excess of hydrogen ions move into the cells. This scenario is reversed and may result in previously undiagnosed hypokalemia when the metabolic acidemia is corrected. Hyperkalemia may also be seen in certain disease states (e.g., urinary bladder rupture in foals or end stage renal failure) and if not addressed can lead to serious consequences that may be magnified in the anesthetized animal. Conversely hypokalemia may occur following correction of metabolic acidemia or as a result of inadequate intake (e.g., an anorexic patient) or excess loss (e.g., diarrhea or diuresis). Serum potassium levels under 3 mEq/L in the horse are indicative of significant hypokalemia.[62]

Calculation of the overall body deficit in potassium is difficult because the actual volume of distribution for the ion is uncertain. For convenience, an arbitrary volume of distribution of 40% of the body weight is used. In a 450-kg horse, for example, the potassium "space" may be considered $450 \times 0.4 = 180$ L. If a patient has a potassium level of 2.0 mEq/L, it is considered to have a deficiency of $180 \times (4 - 2) = 360$ mEq (normal potassium level is 4.0 mEq/L). The equivalent weight of potassium is 14. The patient is therefore deficient $360/14 = 26$ g potassium.

Decreases in chloride levels are observed in cattle with abomasal torsion. A significant correlation has been observed between postsurgical outcome and the presurgical serum chloride concentration.[63] Serum concentrations of sodium and potassium also decrease, but less dramatically.

Fluid Therapy in the Anesthetized Patient Undergoing Elective Surgery

In general, there are four essential principles of fluid therapy: the replacement of existing deficits, the fulfillment of maintenance requirements, the replacement of anticipated additional losses, and the monitoring of the patient's response to therapy. The routine surgical patient that has been fasted and held off water prior to anesthesia is likely to have a deficit at the time of anesthetic induction, but this can be challenging to quantitate. Hence fluid should be administered during anesthesia to compensate for this deficiency and in anticipation of maintenance requirements and ongoing losses (e.g., fluid evaporation from open tissues).

A polyionic, isotonic solution with a buffer should be administered during anesthesia. Lactated Ringer's solution, for example, is appropriate for this purpose (Table 2.3). In the uncompromised patient, metabolism of lactate by the liver yields a bicarbonate equivalent; the acetate and gluconate in Normosol-R are metabolized by the muscle to yield a bicarbonate equivalent.

Fluids should ideally be administered intravenously, using an indwelling catheter or needles at least 5 cm in length and properly threaded in the vein. If intravenous catheters are used, an aseptic preparation should be made before insertion, and every precaution should be taken to avoid phlebitis. A rate of administration of 4.4–6.6 ml/kg/hr is sufficient to maintain the patient's hydration in elective cases;[35] however, the patient should be monitored continually to ensure that such maintenance therapy is adequate.

If a patient becomes compromised during surgery, the fluid therapy regimen should be changed immediately to satisfy any specific requirements.

Fluid Therapy in the Compromised Patient, According to Requirements

Fluid therapy in the compromised patient should be directed specifically at the volume deficits, acid-base imbalances, and electrolyte changes. At the same time, intensive monitoring is required to ensure that the therapy is satisfactory and to recognize developing needs.

Volume replacement is usually the most important and urgent requirement in the compromised large animal patient. Polyionic replacement (isotonic) fluids with buffers (e.g., lactate and acetate) are used, except in the case of metabolic alkalosis. Because the rate of administration varies with the state of the animal, formulas for administration rate have little value in the compromised patient. Fluids are generally given rapidly, and the administration rate is dictated by changes in the clinical signs and the PCV and TPP. Rapid volume replacement to restore and maintain circulating blood volume is particularly urgent in patients exhibiting clinical signs of shock. Untoward sequelae of overzealous volume replacement are rare unless the animal is recumbent or has a low TPP or kidney failure. The usual error in volume replacement in large animals is the administration of an inadequate volume of fluids or slow administration of the volume.

When monitoring massive fluid replacement, a continued decrease in TPP without evidence that the volume deficit is being replaced indicates a vital protein loss. A TPP of less than 4 g/dL is an indication for plasma administration. In the absence of coagulopathies synthetic colloids such as hetastarch and dextran may be used to support colloid oncotic pressure.

The specific treatment of metabolic acidosis is not so straightforward. In the past, any base deficit was treated immediately with sodium bicarbonate (often in bolus form with priority over volume replacement), and it was generally considered better to give too much than too little. Based on more recent information, this practice requires modification for several reasons. The first is that metabolic acidosis in the large animal surgical patient usually occurs secondary to hypovolemia and inadequate peripheral tissue perfusion. Rectification of the primary problems usually corrects any accompanying acidosis

Table 2.14.   Composition of intravenous fluids (mEq/L).

Polyionic Replacement Solutions	Na⁺	K⁺	Ca⁺⁺	Mg⁺⁺	Cl⁻	Bicarbonate Precursor
Ringer's solution	147.5	4	4.5		156	
Lactated Ringer's solution	130.0	4	3.0		109	28 (lactate)
Normosol-R	140.0	5		3	98	50 (acetate, gluconate)
Polysol	140.0	10	5.0	3	103	55 (acetate)
Extracellular replacement fluid	140.0	5			115	30 (acetate)
Physiologic saline solution	154.0				154	
5% Bicarbonate	600.0					600
Lactated Ringer's solution +5 g/L NaHCO₃	190.0	4	3.0		109	87

(at least mild acidosis) and makes the specific administration of sodium bicarbonate unnecessary. In addition, as volume and tissue perfusion are restored, the acetate, gluconate, or lactate in the polyionic replacement fluids acts as a source of bicarbonate (Table 2.14).

Opinions vary on the value of the lactate in lactated Ringer's solution as a bicarbonate source in the compromised patient. The conversion of lactate to bicarbonate requires a functioning liver and adequate perfusion to provide oxygen; consequently, immediate provision of bicarbonate by lactate cannot be anticipated in the patient in shock. As perfusion is restored, exogenously administered lactate does not accumulate, but acts as a bicarbonate source. In addition, the liver can still metabolize lactate when the blood flow to the organ is 20% of normal and oxygen saturation is 50%.[64] The other criticism of giving lactated solutions for the treatment of patients in shock has been that lactic acidosis already exists in these patients. Although lactate will not be converted to bicarbonate in these patients while they are in shock, there is no evidence that its presence causes any harm. Exogenous lactate, given in lactated Ringer's solution, does not increase blood lactate levels in normal or shock patients.[65] Additionally, studies in humans have shown that administering lactate Ringer's solution to patients in hemorrhagic shock does not exacerbate the lactate acidosis that occurs secondary to hypoperfusion.[66] However, lactated Ringer's solution may be contraindicated for animals with severe septicemia, endotoxemia, or liver disorders because the liver's ability to uptake and metabolize lactate may be compromised in these animals.[66]

For more severely compromised patients in which conversion of the bicarbonate precursors to bicarbonate is not anticipated, specific administration of bicarbonate is appropriate. Bicarbonate is indicated to treat cases of metabolic acidosis caused by either hyponatremia or hypochloremia.[59] Its use in the treatment of lactic acidosis is still controversial. Bicarbonate supplementation is certainly indicated when the base deficit is 10 mEq/L or greater. The amount administered is based on calculation of the deficit, as described previously. It is important to avoid overadministration. In the past, practitioners considered sodium bicarbonate a benign drug because excess

bicarbonate could be excreted by the kidneys or converted to carbon dioxide and eliminated by the lungs.[67] Several potential hazards have been suggested, however: hypernatremia leading to hyperosmolality; iatrogenic alkalosis, which could interfere with neuromuscular function; and paradoxic acidosis of cerebrospinal fluid (CSF).[67] The last condition has been recognized in dogs and man.[68,69] The problem is best demonstrated by this equation:

$$HCO_3^- + H^+ \rightleftharpoons H_2CO_3 \rightleftharpoons H_2O + CO_2$$

Overadministration of sodium bicarbonate drives this reaction to the right, producing increased carbon dioxide. The carbon dioxide could potentially diffuse across the blood-brain barrier in preference to bicarbonate. The increased carbon dioxide in the CSF could cause the same reaction to be driven to the left, increasing hydrogen in the CSF and thereby leading to acidosis. The significance of this problem in large animals has yet to be substantiated, however.

Supplementary bicarbonate may be added to the polyionic replacement solution (if it does not contain calcium) or administered separately. If prolonged bicarbonate therapy is necessary, it may be desirable to give sodium bicarbonate in isotonic solution with sterile water or to substitute 5% dextrose solution for some of the sodium-containing replacement fluid to minimize the development of hypernatremia.

If a patient has metabolic alkalosis (typically a cow with an abomasal disorder), physiologic saline solution is administered. This will replace lost volume and restore depleted chloride levels, which are the cause of the alkalosis. At the same time, surgical correction of the abomasal problem with cessation of chloride sequestration is an equally important part of the therapy. In man, the use of sodium chloride is not satisfactory for the treatment of severe cases of metabolic alkalosis.[70] If kidney function is decreased, hypernatremia becomes a problem; dilute hydrochloric acid, administered until the base excess is corrected, improves this condition.[70] This treatment may be appropriate in severe cases in animals.

In the patient with a recognized potassium deficit, potassium may be added to the intravenous fluids at a rate of up to 10 mEq/L.[57] Depending on the rate of fluid administration this may be increased but it is generally recommended that the total amount administered prior to rechecking values not exceed 100 mEq.[71] Regardless of the amount a patient is to receive, a maximum infusion rate of 0.5 mEq/kg/hour should be strictly adhered to if one is to avoid complications.

The best indication of any fluid therapy protocol is the clinical response of the animal to the therapy. These observations should be accompanied by routine PCV and TPP estimations, acid-base status (blood gases or total carbon dioxide), and electrolyte assessment as appropriate. The animal's fluid status is dynamic, and the interval between measurements of these parameters depends on the individual clinical case. Because of the marked variability between cases and the need for continued monitoring, we have avoided quoting rates of administration.

Fluid Administration in the Compromised Patient without Preliminary Data

In certain field situations, the practitioner must initiate fluid therapy when the only preliminary data are those noted in the clinical examination. For most healthy patients the practitioner is best advised to use a balanced electrolyte solution and administer this based on clinical signs. In the compromised patient, fluid selection should be based on the changes most commonly observed with a given disease. For example, a horse with a suspected large colon lesion and is dehydrated should initially receive a balanced electrolyte solution. If the patient exhibits signs of shock, conservative bicarbonate administration may be considered after intravenous fluids have been administered. In cattle, many conditions necessitating surgery result in metabolic alkalosis. Hence physiologic saline solution or Ringer's solution may be most appropriate. If volume replacement therapy is prolonged, PCV and TPP, electrolytes and acid-base should be evaluated as soon as possible.

When performing volume replacement based on clinical examination alone, the clinician needs to have some concept of the volume of fluid necessary. Twelve to twenty L/hr of fluid have been given to horses in shock. In the absence of alpha-2 agonist drugs, if frequent or excessive urination occurs, the rate of the infusion should be decreased. After the initial rapid administration of fluids, the usual recommended flow rate is 3–5 L/hr.[62] A 450-kg horse needs 27 L of water per day for maintenance alone.[71]

References

1. Hall, L.W., Clarke, K.W., and Trim, C.M. Veterinary anesthesia. 10th Ed. New York, W.B. Saunders, 2000.
2. McGrath, C., and Richey, M. Large animal anesthesia. In Veterinary anesthesia and analgesia. Edited by D. McKelvey, K.W. Hollingshead. St. Louis, MO, Mosby, 2003, pp. 387–412.
3. Skarda, R.T. Local and regional anesthetic and analgesic techniques in ruminants and swine. In Lumb and Jones' Veterinary Anesthesia and Analgesia. 4th Ed. Edited by J.C. Thurmon, W.J. Tranquili, K.A. Grimm. Ames, IA, Blackwell Publishing, 2007, pp. 643–682.
4. Lumb, W.V., and Jones, E.W. Veterinary Anesthesia and Analgesia. 4th Ed. Edited by J.C. Thurmon, W.J. Tranquili, K.A. Grimm. Ames, IA, Blackwell Publishing, 2007.
5. Muir, W.W., and Hubbell, J.A. Equine Anesthesia Monitoring and Emergency Therapy. 2nd Ed. New York, Oxford University Press, 2009.
6. Bertone, J., and Horspool, L.J.I. Equine Clinical Pharmacology. W.B. Saunders, 2004.
7. Morishima, O.H., Pedersen, H., Finster, M., Sakuma, K., Bruce, S.L., Gutsche, B.B. Toxicity of lidocaine in adult, newborn, and fetal sheep. Anesthesiology, 55:7, 1981.
8. Gray, P.R., and McDonell, W.N. Anesthesia in goats and sheep. Part I. Local analgesia. Compend. Contin. Educ., 8:S33, 1986.
9. Moon, P.F., and Suter, C.M. Paravertebral thoracolumbar anesthesia in 10 horses. Equine Vet. J., 25(4):304–308, 1993.
10. Brock, K.A., and Heard, D.J. Field anesthesia techniques in small ruminants. Part 1. Local analgesia. Compend. Contin. Educ., 7:5407, 1985.
11. Cakala, S. A technique for the paravertebral lumbar block in cattle. Cornell Vet., 51:64, 1961.
12. Skarda, R.T. Local and regional anesthesia in ruminants and swine. Vet. Clin. Food Anim. Pract., 12:579–626, 1996.
13. Grubb, T.L., Riebold, T.W., Crismann, R.O., and Lamb, L.D. Comparison of lidocaine, xylazine, and lidocaine-xylazine for caudal epidural analgesia in cattle. Vet. Anaesth. Analg., 29:64–68, 2002.
14. Grubb, T.L., Riebold, T.W., and Huber, M.J. Comparison of lidocaine, xylazine, and xylazine/lidocaine for caudal epidural analgesia in horses. J. Am. Vet. Med. Assoc., 201:1187–1190, 1992.
15. Robinson, E.P., and Natalini, C.C. Epidural anesthesia and analgesia in horses. Vet. Clin. North Am. Equine Pract., 18:61–82, 2002.
16. Hall, L.W. Wright's Veterinary Anaesthesia and Analgesia. 7th Ed. Philadelphia, Lea & Febiger, 1971.
17. Green, E.M., and Cooper, R.C. Continuous caudal epidural anesthesia in the horse. J. Am. Vet. Med. Assoc., 184:971–974, 1984.
18. Martin, C.A., Kerr, C.L., Pearce, S.G., Lansdowne, J.L., and Boure, L.P. Outcome of epidural catheterization for delivery of analgesics in horses: 43 cases (1998–2001). J. Am. Vet. Med. Assoc, 222:1394–1398, 2003.
19. Goodrich, L.R., Nixon, L.R., Fubini, S.L., Ducharme, N.G., Fortier, L.A., Warnick, L.D., Ludders, J.W. Epidural morphine and detomidine decreases postoperative hindlimb lameness in horses after bilateral stifle arthroscopy. Vet. Surg., 31:232–239, 2002.
20. Benson, G.J., and Thurmon, J.C. Regional analgesia of food animals. In Current Veterinary Therapy: Food Animal Practice. Vol. 2. Edited by J.L. Howard. Philadelphia, W.B. Saunders, 1986, p. 71.
21. Weaver, A.D. Intravenous local anesthesia of the lower limbs in cattle. J. Am. Vet. Med. Assoc., 160:55, 1972.
22. Adams, O.R., and Stashak, T.S. Lameness in Horses. 6th Ed. Edited by G.M. Baxter. Ames, IA, Blackwell Publishing, 2011.

23. Hubbell, J.A.E., Robertson, J.T., Muir, W.W., and Gabel, A.A. Perianesthetic considerations in the horse. *Compend. Contin. Educ.*, 6:S401, 1984.

24. Carroll, G.L., and Hartsfield, S.M. General anesthetic techniques in ruminants. *Vet. Clin. Food Anim. Pract.*, 12:627–661, 1996.

25. Greene, S.A. Protocols for anesthesia of cattle. *Vet. Clin. Food Anim.*, 19:679–693, 2003.

26. Ames, K.N., and Reibold, T.W. Anesthesia in cattle. *In* Proceedings of the 11th Annual Convention of the American Association of Bovine Practitioners in 1978, p. 75, 1979.

27. Ducharme, N.G., and Fubini, S.L. Gastrointestinal complications associated with use of atropine in horses. *J. Am. Vet. Med. Assoc.*, 182:229, 1983.

28. Schatzmann, U., Tschudi, P., Held, J.P., Buhleback, B. An investigation of the action and haemolytic effect of glyceryl guaicolate in the horse. *Equine Vet. J.*, 10:224, 1978.

29. Geiser, D.R. Practical equine injectable anesthesia. *J. Am. Vet. Med. Assoc.*, 182:574, 1983.

30. Grandy, J.L., and McDonell, W.N. Evaluation of concentrated solutions of guaifenesin for equine anesthesia. *J. Am. Vet. Med. Assoc.*, 176:619, 1980.

31. Tranquilli, W.J., and Thurmon, J.C. Management of anesthesia in the foal. *Vet. Clin. North Am. Equine Pract.*, 6(3):651–663, 1990.

32. Hubbell, J.A.E., Hull, B.L., and Muir, W.W. Perianesthetic considerations in cattle. *Compend. Contin. Educ.*, 8:F92, 1986.

33. Trim, C.M. Sedation and general anesthesia in ruminants. *Calif. Vet.*, 4:29, 1981.

34. Thurmon, J.C., and Benson, G.J. Anesthesia in ruminants and swine. *In* Current Veterinary Therapy: Food Animal Practice. Vol. 2. Edited by J.L. Howard. Philadelphia, W.B. Saunders, 1986, p. 51.

35. Reibold, T.W., Goble, D.O., and Geiser, D.R. Principles and Techniques of Large Animal Anesthesia. 2nd Ed. Ames, IA, Iowa State University Press, 1995.

36. Soma, L.R. Equine anesthesia: Causes of reduced oxygen and increased carbon dioxide tensions. *Compend. Contin. Educ.*, 2:S57, 1980.

37. Soma, L.R. Textbook of Veterinary Anesthesia. Baltimore, Williams & Wilkins, 1971.

38. Anderson, I. Anaesthesia in the pig. *Aust. Vet. J.*, 49:474, 1973.

39. Auer, J.A., Garner, H.E., Amend, J.F., Hutcheson, D.P., Salem, C.A. Recovery from anaesthesia in ponies: A comparative study of the effects of isoflurane, enflurane, methoxyflurane and halothane. *Equine Vet. J.*, 10:18, 1978.

40. Grosenbaugh, D.A., and Muir, W.W. Cardiorespiratory effects of sevoflurane, isoflurane, and halothane anesthesia in horses. *Am. J. Vet. Res.*, 59:101–106, 1998.

41. Steffey, E.P. Enflurane and isoflurane anesthesia: A summary of laboratory and clinical investigations in horses. *J. Am. Vet. Med. Assoc.*, 172:367, 1978.

42. Steffey, E.P., Wheat, J.D., Meagher, D.M., Norrie, R.D., McKee, J., Brown, M., and Arnold, J. Body position and mode of ventilation influences arterial pH, oxygen, and carbon dioxide tensions in halothane-anesthetized horses. *Am. J. Vet. Res.*, 38:379, 1977.

43. Taylor, P.M., and Hall, L.W. Clinical anaesthesia in the horse: Comparison of enflurane and isoflurane. *Equine Vet. J.*, 17:51, 1985.

44. Muir, W.W. Inhalant anesthesia in horses. *In* 10th ACVA Vet Symp, pp. 110–111, Sept 2000.

45. Muir, W.W., and Bednarski, R.M. Equine cardiopulmonary resuscitation. Part II. *Compend. Contin. Educ.*, 5:S287, 1983.

46. Steffey, E.P., Howland, D., Jr., Giri, S., and Eger, E.I., 2nd. Enflurane, halothane, and isoflurane potency in horses. *Am. J. Vet. Res.*, 38:1037, 1977.

47. Heath, R.B., Redder, t., Stashak, T., and Shaw, R. Protecting and positioning the equine surgical patient. *Vet. Med. Small Anim. Clin.*, 67:1241, 1972.

48. Grandy, J.L., Steffey, E.P., Hodgson, D.S., and Woliner, M.J. Arterial hypotension and the development of postanesthetic myopathy in halothane-anesthetized horses. *Am. J. Vet. Res.*, 48:192, 1987.

49. Hall, L.W., Gillespie, J.R., and Tyler, W.S. Alveolar-arterial oxygen tension differences in anesthetized horses. *Br. J. Anaesth.*, 40:560, 1968.

50. Hornof, W.J., Dunlop, C.I., Prestage, R., Amis, T.C. Effects of lateral recumbency on regional lung function in anesthetized horses. *Am. J. Vet. Res.*, 47:277, 1986.

51. Mason, D.E., Muir, W.W., and Wade, A. Arterial blood gas tensions in the horse during recovery from anesthesia. *J. Am. Vet. Med. Assoc.*, 190:989, 1987.

52. McDonell, W.N., Hall, L.W., and Jeffcott, L.B. Radiographic evidence of impaired pulmonary function in laterally recumbent anesthetized horses. *Equine Vet. J.*, 11:24, 1979.

53. Hodgson, D.S., Steffey, Grandy, J.L., Woliner, M.J. Effects of spontaneous, assisted and controlled ventilatory modes in halothane-anesthetized geldings. *Am. J. Vet. Res.*, 47:992, 1986.

54. Thurmon, J.C., Romack, F.E., and Garner, H.E. Excursion of the bovine eyeball during gaseous anesthesia. *Vet. Med. Small Anim. Clin.*, 63:967, 1968.

55. Gentry, P.A., and Black, W.D. Evaluation of Harleco CO_2 apparatus: Comparison with the Van Slyke method. *J. Am. Vet. Med. Assoc.*, 167:156, 1975.

56. Siggaard-Anderson, O. Blood acid-base alignment nomogram: Scales for pH, pCO_2, base excess of whole blood of different hemoglobin concentrations, plasma bicarbonate, and plasma total CO_2. *Scand. J. Clin. Lab. Invest.*, 15:211, 1963.

57. Waterman, A. A review of the diagnosis and treatment of fluid and electrolyte disorders in the horse. *Equine Vet. J.*, 9:43, 1977.

58. Green, R.A. Perspectives in clinical osmometry. *Vet. Med. Small Anim. Clin.*, 8:287, 1978.

59. Haskins, S.C. An overview of acid-base physiology. *J. Am. Vet. Med. Assoc.*, 170:423, 1977.

60. Constable, P.D., Hinchcliff, K.W., and Muir, W.W.I.I.I. Comparison of anion gap and strong ion gap as predictors of unmeasured strong ion concentration in plasma and serum from horses. *Am. J. Vet. Res.*, 59:881–887, 1998.

61. Gossett, K.A., French, D.D., and Cleghorn, B. Laboratory evaluation of metabolic acidosis. *In* Proceedings of the Second Equine Colic Research Symposium. Athens, GA, University of Georgia, p. 161, 1986.

62. Carlson, G.P. Fluid therapy in horses with acute diarrhea. *Vet. Clin. North Am. Large Anim. Pract.*, 3:313, 1979.

63. Smith, D.F. Right-side torsion of the abomasum in dairy cows: Classification of severity and evaluation of outcome. *J. Am. Vet. Med. Assoc.*, 173:108, 1978.

64. Garner, H.E., et al. Postoperative care of equine abdominal crises. *Vet. Anesth.*, 4:40, 1977.

65. Brasmer, T.H. Fluid therapy in shock. *J. Am. Vet. Med. Assoc.*, 174:475, 1979.

66. Corely, K.T.T. Fluid therapy. *In* Equine clinical pharmacology. Edited by J.J. Bertone, L.J.I. Horspool. New York, Saunders, 2004, pp. 327–364.

67. Coffman, J. Acid:base balance. *Vet. Med. Small Anim. Clin.*, 75:489, 1980.

68. Berenyi, K.J., Wolk, M., and Killip, T. Cerebrospinal fluid acidosis complicating therapy of experimental cardiopulmonary arrest. *Circulation*, 52:319, 1975.

69. Bishop, R.L., and Weisfeldt, M.L. Sodium bicarbonate administration during cardiac arrest. *J. Am. Med. Assoc.*, 235:506, 1976.

70. Williams, D.B., and Lyons, J.H. Treatment of severe metabolic alkalosis with intravenous infusion of hydrochloric acid. *Surg. Gynecol. Obstet.*, 150:315, 1980.

71. Donawick, W.J. Metabolic management of the horse with acute abdominal crisis. *J. S. Afr. Vet. Assoc.*, 46:107, 1975.

72. St. Jean, G., Skarda, R.T., Muir, W.W., and Hoffsis, G.F. Caudal epidural analgesia induced by xylazine administration in cows. *Am. J. Vet. Res.*, 51:1232–1236, 1990.

73. Lin, H.C., Trachte, E.A., DeGraves, F.J., Rodgerson, D.H., Steiss, J.E., and Carson, R.L. Evaluation of analgesia induced by epidural administration of metdetomidine to cows. *Am. J. Vet. Res.*, 59:162–167, 1998.

74. Mpanduji, D.G., Bittegeko, S.B., Mgasa, M.N., and Batamuzi, E.K. Analgesic, behavioural, and cardiopulmonary effects of epidurally injected medetomidine (Domitor) in goats. *J. Vet. Med. A Physiol. Pathol. Clin. Med.*, 47:65–72, 2000.

75. Hendrickson, D.A., Kruse-Elliott, K.T., and Broadstone, R.V. A comparison of epidural saline, morphine, and bupivacaine for pain relief after abdominal surgery in goats. *Vet. Surg.*, 25:83–87, 1996.

76. Ko, J.C.H., Thurmon, J.C., Benson, G.J., et al. Evaluation of analgesia induced by epidural injection of detomidine or xylazine in swine. *J. Vet. Anaesth.*, 19:56–60, 1992.

77. Salonen, J.S., Vaha-Vahe, T., Vainio, O., and Vakkuri, O. Single-dose pharmacokinetics of detomidine in the horse and cow. *J. Vet. Pharmacol. Ther.*, 12:65–72, 1989.

78. Knight, A.P. Xylazine. *J. Am. Vet. Med. Assoc.*, 176:454, 1980.

79. Hoffman, P.E. Clinical evaluation of xylazine as a chemical restraint agent, sedative and analgesic in horses. *J. Am. Vet. Med. Assoc.*, 164:42, 1974.

80. Klein, L.V., and Baetjar, C. Preliminary report: Xylazine and morphine sedation in horses. *Vet. Anesth.*, 2:2–C, 1974.

81. Muir, W.W., Skarda, R.T., and Sheehan, W.C. Hemodynamic and respiratory effects of xylazine-morphine sulfate in horses. *Am. J. Vet. Res.*, 40:1417, 1979.

82. Mama, K.R. Traditional and non-traditional uses of anesthetic drugs- an update. *Vet. Clin. North Am. Equine Pract.*, 18:169–179, 2002.

83. Butera, T.S., Moore, J.N., Garner, H.E., Amend, J.F., Clarke, L.L., and Hatfield, D.G. Diazepam/xylazine/ketamine combination for short-term anesthesia in the horse. *Vet. Med. Small Anim. Clin.*, 74:490, 1978.

84. Tadmor, A., Marcus, S., and Eting, E. The use of ketamine hydrochloride for endotracheal intubation in cattle. *Aust. Vet. J.*, 55:537, 1979.

85. Muir, W.W. Total IV anesthesia in horses. *In* 10th ACVA Vet Symp, p. 109, Sept 2000.

86. Yamashita, K., Tsubakishita, S., Futaoka, S., Ueda, I., Hamaguchi, H., Seno, T., Katoh, S., Izumisawam Y., Kotani, T., and Muir, W.W. Cardiovascular effects of medetomidine, detomidine, and xylazine in horses. *J. Vet. Med. Sci.*, 62:1025–1032, 2000.

87. Funk, K.A. Glyceryl guaiacolate: Some effects and indications in horses. *Equine Vet. J.*, 5:15, 1973.

Chapter 3

SURGICAL INSTRUMENTS

Dean A. Hendrickson, DVM, MS, DACVS

Objectives

1. Familiarize the inexperienced surgeon with some general instruments commonly used in veterinary surgical practice.
2. Serve as a reference for the instrumentation used in various techniques that are discussed in this chapter.

Use of Surgical Instruments

The most important aspect of instrumentation is knowing which instrument to use at which time; this is essential to good surgical technique. It ensures that the particular surgical procedure is undertaken with minimal trauma to the tissues, is performed in the minimal amount of time, and ultimately results in the least harm to the patient. In learning about this wealth of instruments, it helps to handle them and to use them in situations such as laboratory work and practical sessions whenever possible.

Scalpel

The scalpel is used for the sharp division of tissue with minimal damage to nearby structures. Today, scalpels come with a variety of blade configurations, each designed for a specific purpose. The blades are disposable, thereby avoiding the need to be sharpened. Scalpel handles come in different sizes; no. 3 and no. 4 are generally adequate for most large animal surgical procedures. For work in deep cavities, such as rectovaginal fistula repair and urine-pooling operations, longer-handled scalpels are essential.

The scalpel must be held so that it is under complete control. It is grasped between the thumb and the third and fourth fingers, with the index finger placed over the back. To cut, make a smooth sweep with the rounded portion, or belly, of the blade, rather than with the point. The amount of pressure applied varies, but the aim is to produce a bold, single, full-thickness skin incision with a single sweep of the scalpel blade. Every time the blade contacts the tissue it creates another incision. Each of these incisions will need to heal. The skin of the bovine flank, for example, is tough, and the neophyte surgeon usually does not apply enough pressure when making an incision in this area; the skin in the inguinal area of the horse, on the other hand, is thin, and a light stroke over the tissues with the middle of the blade is adequate.

Figure 3.1A shows the stroke made with nos. 10, 20, 21, and 22 scalpel blades. The handle should be at an angle of 30° to 40° to the surface incised. Figure 3.1B depicts the pencil grip with nos. 10, 20, 21, and 22 scalpel blades. The pencil grip is used for nos. 11 and 15 blades when more precise incisions are required (Figure 3.2A). Figure 3.2B shows the incorrect use of a no. 15 blade. The bistoury blade (no. 12) has a hook shape and is used for lancing abscesses. The bayonet tip blade (no. 11) can also be used for lancing abscesses and for severing ligaments.

When the scalpel blade becomes dull, the blade is removed carefully by grasping the blade with a needle holder or hemostat (Figure 3.3). The proximal end of the blade is then bent slightly to clear the blade from the hub of the handle. Then the blade is pushed up and over the end of the scalpel handle. The reverse process is used to replace a scalpel blade. Although the blade may be too dull for a particular surgical procedure, the blade is still sharp enough to cause serious injury if care is not taken while removing it from the scalpel handle. The spent blade should be discarded appropriately.

To remove the new scalpel from its packet, the ends of the packet are grasped by the operating room nurse or nonscrubbed assistant and peeled open, exposing the end of the blade. The blade is carefully plucked out of the

Turner and McIlwraith's Techniques in Large Animal Surgery, 4th Edition. Dean A. Hendrickson and A. N. (Nickie) Baird.
© 2013 John Wiley & Sons, Inc. Published 2013 by John Wiley & Sons, Inc.

Fig. 3.1. Use of nos. 10, 20, 21, and 22 blades. **A.** Stroke. **B.** Pencil grip.

Fig. 3.2. **A.** Pencil grip for nos. 11 and 15 blades. **B.** Incorrect use of a no. 15 blade.

Fig. 3.3. Removing the used scalpel blade.

Fig. 3.4.   Aseptic technique for handling a new blade.

Fig. 3.5.   Correct way to hold scissors.

packet, contacting only the blade itself, to avoid a break in aseptic technique (Figure 3.4). Various types of scalpel blades and scalpel handles are illustrated later in this chapter. While many practitioners sterilize scalpel blades in their surgery packs so that they can be opened by the gloved surgeon, it should be noted that repeated sterilization has been shown to dull scalpel blades.

Scissors

A variety of scissors are available and are used for such procedures as cutting tissues or dissecting between tissue planes. Generally speaking, scissors used for tissue are light and are made with precision in mind. They must be kept sharp or they will crush tissues rather than cut them. Mayo or Metzenbaum scissors are used for most tissues. They are available with curved or straight blades. Straight scissors are used for working close to the surface of the wound, whereas the curved scissors are used for working deeper in the wound. Scissors are also classified according

to the shape of the tips, for example, sharp/sharp, sharp/blunt, and blunt/blunt. Some scissors are designed to cut wire. The heel of the wire-cutting scissors is used for this purpose. Various types of scissors are illustrated later in this chapter.

The scissors are grasped by placing the thumb and ring finger through the rings and setting the index finger against the blades. The index finger provides control of the tips of the scissors. The scissors must be kept near the last joint of the finger, and the fingers must not be allowed to slip through the rings of the handle (Figure 3.5). The end of the blade is used for cutting; however, when tough structures are encountered, the heel of the blade is used. The scissors should not be closed unless the surgeon can see the tips of the blades; otherwise, vital structures may be endangered. For blunt dissection, insert the closed tips of the scissors into the tissue, and then open the points. Scissors used for tissue work should not be used for cutting suture material; one of the various types of suture scissors should be used instead.

Fig. 3.6. **A.** Using rings to hold the needle holders. **B.** Palming the needle holder.

Bandage scissors are an essential part of large animal surgery instrumentation, especially in equine limb surgery, in which the areas to be treated are commonly under bandage, and much of one's day may be spent changing bandages on horses' limbs. Some bandage scissors have slightly angled blades, and the lower blade has a small *button tip* on it to protect structures under the bandage. If bandage scissors are used against soiled or contaminated wounds, they must be sterilized after use to prevent transfer of infection to another wound or another patient.

Needle Holders (Needle Drivers)

During a large portion of an operation, the surgeon uses needle holders. The type of needle holder depends on individual tastes. Some needle holders, such as Olsen-Hegar or Gillies, have suture-cutting scissors incorporated into the jaws to enable the surgeon to cut sutures

without reaching for suture-cutting scissors. These needle holders are useful in large animal practice where the surgeon is commonly working on their own. Care must be taken to avoid cutting the suture accidentally during the procedure. There are many variations of width and serrations in the heads of the needle holders.

There are two different ways to hold needle holders. The first is to hold the needle holder as the surgeon would hold scissors, that is, with the thumb and the ring finger in the rings of the handles (Figure 3.6A). The other option is to *palm* the needle holder. Palming generally provides the surgeon with better control over the tip of the needle holder. The needles used with needle holders are curved; straight needles are held by hand only and are usually reserved for the skin and bowel. With the needle holder, the needle should be driven through the tissues in an arclike motion, following the curve of the needle. The needle holder is then removed and is reapplied to the protruding point of the needle, which is extracted from

Fig. 3.8.   Passing hemostatic forceps.

Fig. 3.7.   Correct way to hold thumb forceps.

the tissue. The needle should be grasped by its thicker portion, rather than by the tip, because the tip may be easily bent or broken.

Some needle holders, such as the Mathieu, have a ratchet on the handle that releases when additional pressure is applied to the spring handles. These are time saving, but if the tissues resist passage of the needle, a firm grip cannot be applied to a needle without causing the needle holder to unsnap. Various types of needle holders are illustrated later in this chapter.

Thumb Forceps

Thumb forceps are used for grasping and holding tissues. They are held between the thumb and the middle and index fingers (Figure 3.7). It is common for the inexperienced surgeon to hold thumb forceps incorrectly, like a scalpel handle, especially toward the end of the operation when fatigue is setting in. Thumb forceps are usually held in the left hand while the right hand holds the scalpel or needle holder. Thumb forceps with teeth bite into tissue and prevent the instrument from slipping. Some surgeons consider these forceps too traumatic for use on hollow organs or blood vessels and reserve them for skin. Thumb forceps are illustrated later in this chapter.

Grasping Forceps

A variety of forceps used for larger portions of tissue maintain their hold with the use of a ratchet device on the handle. Allis tissue forceps have opposing edges with short teeth. They should be used sparingly and generally only on tissue that is going to be removed. They should not be used on skin edges or viscera. Vulsellum forceps are useful for grasping the uterine walls of the various

large animal species, to stabilize the walls during closure. Sponge forceps are used in the inguinal approach for cryptorchidism, to grasp the vaginal process. Towel-holding forceps (clamps) are useful for grasping skin edges, as well as for holding drapes in position.

Hemostatic Forceps

Hemostatic forceps are used to clamp the ends of blood vessels and thereby to establish hemostasis. They vary not only in size; they also vary in the shape and direction of the serrations. Halsted mosquito forceps are used for clamping small vessels.

When larger vessels are encountered, Kelly forceps may be more suitable. The amount of tissue crushed should be kept to a minimum. Hemostatic forceps are frequently used in conjunction with electrocautery. When ligating bleeding points, the tips of the instruments should be elevated to facilitate passage of the ligature. Curved hemostats should be affixed with the curved jaws pointing upward. If a scrubbed assistant is present during an operation, he or she should pass the instruments by slapping them, handles first, into the hands of the surgeon (Figure 3.8).

It is not within the scope of this chapter to describe the applications of more than a few forceps. A variety of the forceps used in large animal practice are shown later in this chapter.

Retractors

Retractors are used to maintain exposure at various surgical sites. Handheld retractors are held by an assistant. If the surgeon does not have the luxury of an assistant, as is often the case in large animal practice, self-retaining retractors can be used. Self-retaining retractors anchor themselves against the wound edges by maintaining fixed pressure on the retractor arms. When abdominal or thoracic retractors are used, moist sponges or towels are placed between the retractor blades and the tissues to minimize trauma to the wound edges. Examples of hand-held retractors are U.S. Army retractors, malleable retractors, Volkmann retractors, Jansen retractors, and Senn retractors. Among the self-retaining retractors, Weitlaner retractors and Gelpi retractors are useful for small incisions, such as laryngotomy and arthrotomy incisions in the horse. The large Balfour retractors are predominantly used in laparotomy incisions. Occasionally, if thoracotomy is indicated, Finochietto rib retractors are the instruments of choice. Retractors are illustrated later in this chapter.

General Surgery Pack

Listed below is a standard set of instruments routinely used by our hospital. Such a set of instruments suffices for most basic procedures. In the remainder of the text, these standard instruments are included as a general surgery pack, and any additional instruments required will be noted individually. Instruments in this standard set are

16 Towel forceps
4 Curved mosquito hemostats
4 Straight mosquito hemostats
2 Curved Kelly/Crile hemostatic forceps
2 Straight Kelly/Crile hemostatic forceps
2 Allis tissue forceps
1 Curved Mayo scissors
1 Straight Mayo scissors
1 S/S operating scissors (sharp/sharp)
1 Curved Metzenbaum scissors
1 Straight Metzenbaum scissors
2 Needle holders (1 Mayo-Hegar or Olsen-Hegar)
2 Right-angle forceps
1 Curved 6″ Ochsner forceps
1 Straight 6″ Ochsner forceps
1 No. 3 scalpel handle
1 No. 4 scalpel handle
3 3″ × 4″ thumb tissue forceps
2 1″ × 2″ Adson tissue forceps
1 Sponge forceps (curved or straight)

1 Saline bowl
4 Towels
Sponges in inverted bowl

Preparation of Instruments

The classification of the surgical procedure as clean, clean-contaminated, or contaminated-dirty may influence how the surgeon prepares the surgical instruments. To illustrate, we obviously do not advocate that the instruments used to castrate piglets all be individually wrapped and sterilized. Yet for some of the *clean* surgical procedures described in this book, the use of instruments that have been cold-sterilized may be construed as malpractice.

As part of overall planning, all the necessary instruments for the particular procedure should be obtained and prepared prior to the operation. In most cases, the surgeon must attend to his/her own needs for instruments and so must be able to anticipate the necessity for particular instruments.

Autoclaving, a sterilization technique using moist heat from steam, is the method of choice for preparing instruments for aseptic surgery. Once the packs are open, it is the surgeon's responsibility to be sure that the autoclaving process has reached all the instruments by observing the indicator system used to ensure sterility.

Gas sterilization, with ethylene oxide gas or hydrogen peroxide (Sterrad), is used for instruments that would be damaged by the heat of autoclaving. Materials that have been sterilized with ethylene oxide must be aerated for 1–7 days, depending on the material; otherwise, residual gas may diffuse from the goods and may irritate living tissues. Instruments sterilized with hydrogen peroxide can be used immediately.

Cold (chemical) sterilization is commonly used by large animal surgeons in practice for preparation of instruments. The instruments are soaked in one of the commercially available solutions for whatever time and at whatever concentration recommended by the manufacturer. Some of these solutions can be irritating to tissues, so care must be taken not to transfer excessive amounts of the solution into the surgical site. This method of instrument sterilization or disinfection is recommended for multiple surgical procedures, such as dehorning and castration.

General Surgical Instruments

Scalpel handles.

Mayo-Hegar needle holder.

Scalpel blades.

Olsen-Hegar combined needle holder and scissors.

Lister bandage scissors.

Littauer stitch scissors.

Mayo straight and curved dissecting scissors.

Operating scissors with blunt/blunt points.

Metzenbaum straight and curved scissors.

Operating scissors with sharp/sharp points.

Wire-cutting scissors.

Operating scissors with sharp/blunt points.

Backhaus towel clamp.

Roeder towel clamp.

Brown-Adson forceps.

Tissue forceps.

Adson forceps.

Allis tissue forceps.

Babcock intestinal forceps.

Michel clip applying-and-removing
forceps.

Doyen (Gillmann) compression
forceps.

Michel clips.

Crile straight and curved hemostatic forceps.

Kelly straight and curved forceps.

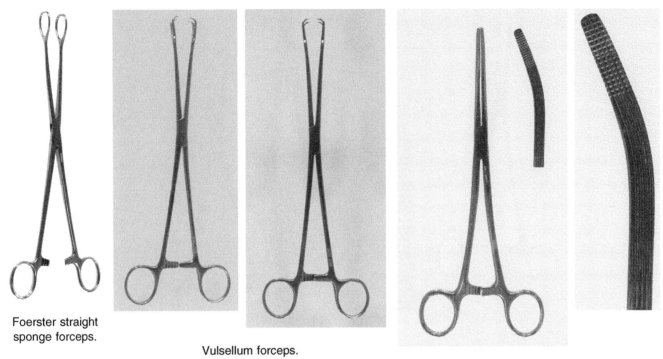

Foerster straight
sponge forceps.

Vulsellum forceps.

Rochester-Carmalt forceps.

Halsted mosquito straight and curved forceps.

Mixter curved
hemostatic forceps.

Ochsner straight and curved forceps.

Malleable retractor.

U.S. Army retractors.

Weitlaner self-retaining retractor.

Gelpi self-retaining retractor.

Senn retractor.

Volkmann retractor.

Balfour retractor.

Finochietto rib spreader.

Kern bone-holding forceps.

Putti double-ended bone rasp.

U.S. Army osteotome set.

U.S. Army chisel set.

Alexander chisel.

Mallet.

Volkmann double-ended curette.

Hibbs gouge.

U.S. Army gouge.

Alexander gouge.

Still-Luer bone rongeurs.

Pennyback rongeurs.

Bone rasp.

Dental elevator.

Periodontal probe.

Keyes skin punch.

Tenotomy knife.

Michel trephine.

Bulb syringe.

Gigli wire and handles.

Yankauer suction tip.

Instruments Used Specifically in Large Animal Surgery

Cattle leader.

Iowa pig snare.

Plain emasculator.

Easy twitch.

Serra emasculator.

Horse twitch.

Reimer emasculator.

Barnes-type dehorner.

Keystone dehorner.

Gouge dehorner.

Heavy-swine mouth speculum.

McPherson speculum.

Dental float.

Bayer mouth wedge.

Galt trephine.

Dental punches.

Closed, drop-jaw molar cutter.

Equine molar forceps.

Interchangeable steel handles for foregoing dental instruments.

Drop-jaw multiple molar cutter.

Half open, drop-jaw molar cutter.

Open, drop-jaw molar cutter.

Canine mouth gag (for llama tooth extraction).

Hoof nippers.

Thoroughbred vaginal speculum.

Hughes hoof groover.

German hoof knife.

Bennett's speculum.

Cow catheters.

Mare catheter.

Rumentomy board.

Stud catheter.

Hobday's roaring bur.

Jackson uterine biopsy forceps.

Obstetric chain handle.

Obstetric chains.

Strawberry roaring bur.

French-model roaring bur with hooks.

Modified Buhner
tape needle.

Udall teat bistoury.

Cornell teat curette.

Lichty teat knife with
blunt point.

Lichty teat knife with
sharp point.

Hugs teat-tumor extractor.

Teat slitter.

Wood-handle cattle trocar.

Udder infusion tube.

Corkscrew trocar.

Standard balling gun.

Teat cannula.

Endotracheal tube.

Stomach pump.

Tracheotomy tube.

Dose syringe.

Écraseur.

Chapter 4

SUTURE MATERIALS AND NEEDLES

Dean A. Hendrickson, DVM, MS, DACVS

Objectives

1. Discuss the features, indications, and limitations of the commonly used sutures in large animal surgery.
2. Describe the advantages and disadvantages to different types of needles and the indications for each.

Suture Materials

Sutures and ligatures are fundamental to any surgical technique because they maintain approximation of tissues as the wound heals. All sutures should maintain their strength until the wound has healed and as a general rule should be as strong as the healthy tissue through which they are placed. The ideal suture material should

- Elicit minimal tissue reaction
- Not create a situation favorable for bacterial growth
- Be nonelectrolytic, noncapillary, nonallergenic, and noncarcinogenic
- Be comfortable for the surgeon to handle
- Hold knots securely without cutting or fraying
- Disappear as soon as it is no longer needed
- Be economical to use

Needless to say, the ideal suture material has not been found and probably never will be; therefore, the surgeon must be familiar with the advantages and disadvantages of the various materials, and the selection of sutures should be based on suture-tissue interactions rather than habit or trade. A recent study suggested that there were 5269 different types of suture materials available.[1]

It is not the purpose of this chapter to present all the suture materials available, but rather to discuss the salient features of those commonly encountered in large animal practice. We have found that most surgeons, whether oriented to large or small animal practice, use a small variety of suture material. They learn the limitations, indications, and contraindications of these sutures, so they are able to adapt them to differing situations. However, good surgeons are always watching to see whether there is a better material available that will provide more benefits to their patients.

Clinical Application of Sutures

The selection of suture type and size is determined by the purpose of the suture, as well as by its biologic properties in the various tissues. Suture materials have traditionally been divided into two categories: absorbable and nonabsorbable sutures. Absorbable sutures begin to be digested or hydrolyzed by the patient during healing of the wound and continue to disappear when the wound has healed. Nonabsorbable sutures retain their tensile strength for longer than 60 days and may remain in situ indefinitely, even though they may be altered slightly. Due to their persistence within tissues, nonabsorbable sutures are more likely to cause suture sinus formation.

Suture materials can also be subdivided into multifilament and monofilament sutures. In general, synthetic monofilament sutures induce less tissue reaction and exhibit less capillarity than multifilament or braided sutures. Multifilament sutures may also harbor bacteria and thus potentiate infection and suture sinus formation. Indeed, the prevalence of suture sinus formation has been shown to be higher following implantation of multifilament sutures than for monofilament sutures.

The surgeon must take into account the rate of healing of the particular tissue because wounds of different tissues achieve maximal strength at different times. For example,

Turner and McIlwraith's Techniques in Large Animal Surgery, 4th Edition. Dean A. Hendrickson and A. N. (Nickie) Baird.
© 2013 John Wiley & Sons, Inc. Published 2013 by John Wiley & Sons, Inc.

visceral wounds heal rapidly, as do superficial wounds around the head. The surgeon must also consider whether infection or drainage will be likely. Chromic gut, for example, disappears more rapidly in the face of infection because of an increase in the local phagocytic activity. On the other hand, a braided or multifilament synthetic material may actually harbor bacteria when an infection occurs. If strength is required for a long period of time—for example, during the healing of a fascial wound—the use of a nonabsorbable synthetic suture material may be necessary. The presence of crystalloids is also a factor in choosing a suture material; for example, a nonabsorbable suture used in the bladder wall represents a foreign body conducive to urinary calculus formation. Absorbable sutures are the best choice for bladder surgery, and rapidly absorbing sutures provide even less likelihood of stone formation.[2,3] Other factors influencing the choice of suture are the surgeon's training, experience, judgment, and habits. However, habit is one of the poorest reasons to choose a suture material.

Once surgeons have chosen what they believe to be the suture material with the best characteristics, they must consider the size of the suture. The holding power of the tissue is the factor that usually determines the size of the suture material. Although all sutures enhance the development of infection, larger sutures retard wound healing and create a foreign-body reaction that is greater than the reaction caused by sutures with a smaller diameter. Consequently, the suture chosen should be just long enough to hold the tissue together.

The number of sutures placed in a wound is another consideration. As each new suture is placed in a wound, the stress on the other sutures decreases. In regard to wound healing, it is better to increase the number of sutures than to increase the size of the suture. Sutures that are placed too far apart lead to poor apposition of the wound edges and contribute to dehiscence, whereas sutures that are placed too close together can have a negative impact on the blood supply to the wound edge.[4] Generally speaking, sutures should be as far from each other as the sutures are wide (tension sutures for secondary support are an exception); however, in thicker-skinned areas, the spacing between the sutures may be increased.[4] The sutures must include the correct amount of tissue and should not be placed too tightly. Too much tension with sutures delays wound healing by causing ischemia at the wound edges. If the bite in the tissue is too small, the suture will cut through the tissues, and dehiscence may occur.

Knotting the suture is the next important consideration. The knot is the weakest point of a suture loop and actually decreases the strength of the suture material. Variations in knot type are more important than variations in suture type and size.[5] Good-quality knots are essential to any surgical procedure; unfortunately, a surgeon's performance decreases with time because of boredom or fatigue.[6] The reader is referred to Chapter 5, "Knots and Ligatures." Table 4.1 summarizes commonly used suture materials.

Absorbable Sutures

Surgical Gut

Gut is a natural absorbable suture that consists mainly of collagen obtained from the submucosa of sheep intestine or from the serosa of beef intestine. It is packaged in at least 85% alcohol, is sterilized with gamma irradiation, and cannot be resterilized once the package is open. Many of the synthetic sutures have essentially replaced gut as they cause significantly less tissue reaction, possess a greater tensile strength for the same diameter, and offer more consistent absorption profiles.

Gut may be plain or chromic. *Plain gut* loses its strength so rapidly that its use in certain regions may be contraindicated. *Chromic gut* is produced by exposure to basic chromium salts. This process increases the intermolecular bonding and results in greater strength, decreased reaction in tissues, and slower absorption. Gut is further classified according to the degree of chromicization: type A (plain) is untreated; type B has mild treatment; type C has medium treatment; and type D (extra chromic gut) has prolonged treatment. Because the absorption pattern of gut is quite variable, newer synthetic sutures are better choices for most procedures. The patient's reaction to gut is variable, but in general, plain gut loses its strength in 3–7 days. Gut is gradually digested by acid proteases from inflammatory cells and may be used when a suture is needed for only a week or two and absorption is desirable. The rate of absorption varies, depending on where the gut is implanted and, to some extent, on the size of the suture. It is rapidly absorbed if it is implanted in regions with a greater blood supply. Similarly, it is absorbed rapidly if exposed to gastric juices or other organ enzymes. Gut may be used in the presence of infection; however, the increased environment for enzyme digestion causes it to be absorbed rapidly.

Gut, in smaller sizes, handles well and possesses some elasticity. Larger diameter gut retains much of its memory and has poor handling characteristics. Three throws are required for knotting, and, when wet, the knot-holding ability decreases. The ends should be left slightly longer than other types of suture material to minimize the chances of untying. Despite the advent of synthetic absorbable sutures, gut is still used in large animal surgery for purely economic reasons, which is not generally a good reason for selecting a suture material.

Braided Absorbable Sutures

In our experience, the synthetic absorbable suture materials have, with few exceptions, replaced gut. Synthetic suture materials are advantageous for their good knot security, handling characteristics, consistent absorption patterns, and minimal tissue reaction.[7]

Table 4.1. Commonly used suture materials.

Suture	Material	Qualities	Advantages	Disadvantages
Surgical gut	Natural collagen from the submucosa of sheep intestine	Rapid absorption Digested enzymatically	Economical Good handling characteristics Some elasticity	Knot strength decreases when wet Loses strength within 3–7 days Tissue reaction
Polyglycolic acid (Dexon)	Polymer of glycolic acid	Synthetic Braided Absorbable Hydrolyzed into natural metabolites	Nonantigenic Does not swell when wet Minimal tissue reaction Good knot security Handling characteristics	Some tissue drag Capillary action
Polyglactin 910 (Vicryl)	Polymer of glycolic acid and lactic acid in a ration of 90:10	Synthetic Braided Absorbable Hydrolyzed into natural metabolites	Same as polyglycolic acid	Same as polyglycolic acid
Polyglactin 910 (Vicryl Rapide)	Same as polyglactin 910	Same as polyglactin 910	Same as polyglactin 910 Added benefit of more rapid absorption (50% strength retention at 5 days vs. 50% at 3 weeks for regular Vicryl)	Same as polyglactin 910 Should not be used in areas where extended strength retention is necessary
Polyglactin 910 antibiacterial (Vicryl Plus with Triclosan)	Same as polyglactin 910 plus Triclosan	Same as polyglactin 910 Plus antimicrobial characteristics	Same as polyglactin 910 Added benefit of providing local antimicrobial effects	Same as polyglactin 910
Braided 9-1 lactomer (Polysorb)	Polyester of glycolide and lactide (derivatives of glycolic and lactic acids)	Synthetic Braided Absorbable Coated	Excellent knot security and tensile strength Softer than Vicryl, better knot security	Braided material
Polydioxanone (PDS II)	Homopolymer of paradioxanone	Synthetic Monofilament Absorbable Hydrolyzed into natural metabolites	Less tissue drag Does not potentiate infection Persists longer in tissues High breaking strength	Brittle Tendency to break at knots
Polydioxanone antibacterial (PDS Plus Triclosan)	Same as polydioxanone	Same as polydioxanone	Same as polydioxanone Added benefit of providing local antimicrobial effects	Same as polydioxanone
Polyglyconate (Maxon)	Copolymer of trimethylene carbonate and glycolide	Synthetic Monofilament Absorbable Degrades via hydrolysis	Same as polydioxanone	Less breaking strength, greater stiffness, inferior mechanical force compared to PDS
Glycomer 631 (Biosyn)	Polyester of 60% glycolide, 14% doxanone, and 26% trimethylene carbonate	Synthetic Absorbable Monofilament	Less tissue reaction than braided suture More rapid absorption pattern Superior strength at implantation	More rapid absorption pattern

Continued

Table 4.1. Commonly used suture materials. *Continued.*

Suture	Material	Qualities	Advantages	Disadvantages
Poliglecapron 25 (Monocryl)	Segmented block copolymer of caprolactone and glycolide	Synthetic Monofilament Absorbable Degraded by hydolysis	Better handling characteristics than other monofilament absorbable sutures High initial tensile strength Increased pliability Good knot security Minimal tissue drag	Rapidly absorbed Maintains initial tensile strength for up to 2 weeks
Poliglecarpron 25 antimicrobial (Monocryl Plus Triclosan)	Same as polyglicaprone 25	Same as polyglicaprone 25	Same as polyglicaprone 25 Added benefit of providing local antimicrobial effects	Same as polyglicaprone 25
Polyglytone 6211 (Caprosyn)	Polyester of glycolide, caprolactone, trimethylene carbonate, and lactide.	Synthetic Absorbable Monofilament	Fast absorption Less tissue drag, better handling characteristics, and greater breaking strength than chromic gut	Very rapid absorption pattern. Should only be used in the bladder, uterus, and sub-cutaneous tissue
Silk	Protein filament from silkworms	Slow absorption by proteolytic degradation within 2 years Natural material	Excellent handling qualities Good knot holding properties	Potentially allergenic Capillary action
Cotton	Twisted yarn from cotton plant	Nonabsorbable	Good handling characteristics Economical for food animal use	Greater tissue reaction than silk Potentiates infection
Nylon (Dermalon, Ethilon, Supramid)	Long chain polymer	Nonabsorbable Synthetic Available as monofilament (most cotton) or multifilament	Inert Maintains most of its initial strength	High memory Poor knot security Bulky knot
Polypropylene (Prolene: Ethicon, Surgipro: Kendall)	Similar to nylon	Nonabsorbable Synthetic Monofilament	Similar to nylon	Similar to nylon
Polymerized caprolactam (Supramid, Vetafil)	Related to nylon	Nonabsorbable Synthetic Braided and coated	Coating minimizes capillarity High tensile strength Minimal tissue reaction Economical skin suture	Some knot slippage Potentiation of infection
Polyesters (coated: Dacron, Polydek, Ethibond) (uncoated: Mersilene, Dacron)	Polymer of ethylene glycol and terapthalic acid	Synthetic Nonabsorbable Coated or uncoated	Inert Prolonged strength	Uncoated forms create capillarity and tissue drag Coating reduces knot security Potentiation of infection
Stainless steel	Iron alloy (iron-nickel-chromium)	Nonabsorbable Multifilament of monofilament forms	Strongest suture material Good knot security Inert Can be repeatedly sterilized Does not potentiate infection like other braided sutures	Difficult to handle Bulky knots Can cut tissues and surgical gloves

These materials are polymers that are extruded as filaments and include polyglycolic acid (Dexon-Tyco), Polyglactin 910 (Vicryl-Ethicon), and lactomer 9-1 (Polysorb-Tyco). These compounds differ from gut in their reaction in tissues. They are invaded by macrophages, yet their disappearance is independent of the local cellular reaction. These compounds are hydrolyzed into natural body metabolites, rather than absorbed by an enzymatic process. The breaking strength of these synthetic sutures diminishes more or less in a straight line, when compared to the almost exponential decline of the strength of gut in tissues. This characteristic absorption pattern was the main reason for the introduction of these synthetic materials, because they are more consistent and reliable in this regard than gut. Unlike gut, synthetic sutures do not swell when wet. These materials have a low coefficient of friction, and it is necessary to use a surgeon's knot with multiple throws to prevent slippage or untying of the knots.

Early braided sutures were coated to reduce tissue drag. Polyglactin 910 was coated with equal parts of a copolymer of glycolide and lactide (polyglactin 370) and calcium stereate (coated Vicryl). Polyglycolic acid is now constructed of filaments finer than the original suture to provide better handling and smoother passage through the tissues (Dexon-S). The coatings reduced the knot security as the sutures became more "slippery." Braided 9-1 lactomer (Polysorb) reduced tissue drag by incorporating softer filaments and consequently had better knot security than either Vicryl or Dexon-S.[8] The newer designs of the suture materials have not altered their reactivity or other biologic properties. However, Vicryl is now available as a more rapidly absorbing suture (Vicryl-Rapide) and as an antimicrobial impregnated suture (Vicryl-Plus with Triclosan). The more rapidly absorbing suture is best suited for surgical sites that have rapid tissue healing such as the bladder and the uterus. The use of a rapidly absorbing suture in these structures should limit the formation of uroliths and adhesions to the uterus. The tricolosan coating reduces bacterial attachment to the suture material,[9] and has been shown to reduce pain postoperatively in pediatric use likely due to a reduction in subclinical infections.[10] Antimicrobial sutures have also been shown to inhibit bacterial colonization using in-vivo models.[11,12] In a study involving 2088 operations in people undergoing open abdominal surgery, the infection rate decreased from 10.8% (PDS II loop suture) to 4.9% (Vicryl plus) with the only change being the use of an antimicrobial impregnated suture for abdominal closure.[13] While the use of antimicrobial sutures has created a lot of discussion, both negative and positive, it should be remembered that attention to correct surgical technique is the most important step in reducing surgical site infections. However, when correct surgical technique is combined with antimicrobial impregnated sutures, even fewer surgical site infections may be seen by the practitioner, and their use should be carefully considered.

Absorbable Monofilament Sutures

Absorbable monofilament sutures minimize the tissue drag that occurs with braided sutures, and monofilament nature of the suture is believed to reduce the potentiation of infection and the harboring of bacteria. Polydioxanone (PDS), a homopolymer of paradioxanone, and polyglyconate (Maxon), a copolymer of trimethylene carbonate and glycolide, are two synthetic monofilament sutures with similar properties. Like polyglycolic acid and polyglactin 910, both are degraded by hydrolysis in a predictable manner, although more slowly. Studies show that polydioxanone has a superior breaking strength, longer-lasting mechanical performance over 28 days, and less stiffness compared to polyglactin.[14] Similarly, polyglyconate can withstand high immediate loads for up to 21 days before weakening due to absorption. Polyglyconate surpasses polydioxanone in strength up to 4 weeks after implantation and knot security.[7] When comparing immediate strength and knot security in an in-vitro model, polyglyconate was stronger than polydioxanoe.[8] Glycomer 631 (Biosyn) is a newer synthetic monofilament absorbable suture material that is similar to polyglyconate. It is stronger when implanted but loses its strength more rapidly. It is indicated in bowel surgery, uterine surgery, subcutaneous closure, and skin closure where suture removal will be difficult to achieve.

Poliglecaprone 25 (Monocryl), a segmented block copolymer of caprolactone and glycolide, is a more recently developed absorbable monofilament suture designed to have the favorable properties of other monofilament sutures but with superior handling characteristics.[7] Poliglecaprone 25 has been shown to have the advantages of a greater initial tensile strength than polydioxanone, chromic gut, or polyglactin 910; increased pliability compared to polyglyconate, polydioxanone, or gut; less tissue drag than gut; and good knot security.[7,15] However, poliglecaprone 25 is absorbed faster than polyglactin 910 and polydioxanone, maintaining only 20 30% of its initial tensile strength 2 weeks after implantation.[15] Poliglecaprone 25 (Monocryl Plus) is also available as an antimicrobial impregnated suture material. It has been shown to inhibit bacterial colonization after direct invivo challenge with *Staphylococcus aureus* and *Escherichia coli* in animal models.[11] Polyglytone 6211 (Caprosyn) is another synthetic monofilament absorbable suture material with a rapid absorption pattern. These sutures should be limited to use in the bladder or uterus of large animals. They have been designed to replace gut suture materials.

Nonabsorbable Sutures

Silk

Silk, a continuous protein filament produced by silkworms, has traditionally been considered a nonabsorbable suture. However, the consensus in recent literature is that silk is indeed slowly absorbed in vivo at a rate dependent upon the type and condition of the tissue in which it is implanted, the physiological status of the patient, and characteristics of the silk (virgin vs. extracted black braided fibrion and the diameter of the silk fiber).[16] Research shows that silk fibers in vivo are susceptible to proteolytic degradation, lose tensile strength within a year of implantation, and are undetectable within 2 years.[16]

Silk fibrion fibers are usually braided, dyed, and coated with wax or silicone for use as sutures, which are referred to as *black braided silk*. Virgin silk is not commonly used due to its potential allergenic nature in some patients, although it is still commercially available. Silk suture has been widely used in human surgery although its use has declined with the availability of synthetic sutures. A similar trend has been seen in veterinary surgery. It is popular with some veterinary surgeons, however, and its superb handling quality is the standard for the producers of the synthetic suture materials. It has excellent knot-holding properties as well. Silk possesses capillary action, which means it should not be used in the presence of infection because it will provide a refuge for bacteria and will result in a nidus of infection. Silk is still used for vascular surgery, although the newer synthetic sutures are better for this purpose.

Cotton

The most common application of cotton in large animal practice is as umbilical tape. *Cotton* is the twisted yarn from the filament of the cotton plant. It handles well, but it produces more tissue reaction than silk. Cotton can potentiate infection because it can harbor bacteria, and the fistulation that may result resolves only when the offending suture material has been removed. Nevertheless, cotton is a useful, economical suture material in a variety of situations, especially those involving food animals. It has been used as a suture in the perineal region for prolapses of the uterus, vagina, and rectum, where the suture will be removed.

Nylon

Nylon (Dermalon, Ethilon, Supramid) is a long-chain polymer available in monofilament and multifilament forms. It is most commonly used in the monofilament form. Nylon is a stiff suture that should be stretched out following its removal from the manufacturer's packet. It has significant *memory,* which is defined as the suture's ability to resist bending forces and to return to its original configuration. The new varieties of nylon are more pliable and provide very good knot security. Similar to other monofilament materials, plastic deformation occurs during knot tightening, locking the suture in place. Nylon is relatively inert when implanted in tissues; a thin connective tissue capsule is produced around the suture, and this characteristic is one of its major advantages when it is used as a buried suture. Nylon loses a slight amount of strength initially, after which no appreciable diminution

in strength is noted. Because there are no interstices to harbor bacteria, the monofilament form of nylon fares better than multifilament sutures in the presence of infection.

Nylon is available in multifilament forms (Nurolon). Braiding this suture gives it some better handling characteristics than the monofilament form, but increases the possibility of harboring bacteria.

Polypropylene and Polyethylene

Polypropylene (Prolene and Surgilene) and *polyethylene* are polyolefins that are usually available in monofilament form. These sutures are relatively biologically inert and lose little strength in situ over a 2-year period. However, knot security has been shown to be inversely proportional to the memory and size of the suture, and because these sutures have very high memory, their knot retention is poor compared to the smaller monofilament alternatives. It is very important to securely tighten each throw as the knot is tied. Multiple loosely tied knots should be avoided. The first throw of a knot with polypropylene tends to slip unless tension is maintained. Both these suture materials are more suitable for use in infected wounds than the braided synthetic materials. Polypropylene has been recommended for closure of abdominal incisions in patients that are predisposed to developing postoperative infection because of its high tensile strength. However, due to its mechanical properties and persistence in the tissues, polypropylene has been associated with suture sinus formation following equine abdominal wall closure.[17] The amount of tissue incorporated in the suture loops, the suture tension, and the knot volume should be minimized to reduce the risk of sinus formation.[18] The slower-degrading, synthetic, monofilament sutures, such as polyglyconate and polydioxanone, may be better options for equine abdominal wall closure.

Polymerized Caprolactam

Polymerized caprolactam (Supramid, Vetafil) is a synthetic suture material used extensively in large animal practice, especially livestock practice. It is available for veterinary use only. The twisted fibers are made from a material related to nylon and coated to minimize capillarity.[19] Compared to gut or silk, the material has a high tensile strength and causes little cellular reaction in tissues. Polymerized caprolactam is packaged in plastic dispenser bottles in which it is chemically sterilized; in this form, it is suitable for use in skin closure. Because of its smoothness, some knot slippage occurs with this material, and at least three knots are required for a safe knot.[4] In general, the material behaves like the other braided synthetics. The suture should not be used in the presence of infection, nor should the suture material be buried. Either of these events can lead to the formation of a chronic draining tract that will not resolve until the suture is removed. For this reason, this material should only be used for skin suture. From the standpoint of economics, polymerized caprolactam has a useful place in large animal practice. Surprisingly, little has been written about its behavior in the tissues of domestic animals.

Polyesters

Polyesters consist of Dacron, a polymer of ethlylene glycol and terapthalic acid, that has been coated or impregnated with various finishes. Tevdek and Ethiflex are Teflon-impregnated Dacron, whereas Polydek is Teflon-coated Dacron. Ethibond is Dacron coated with polybutylate, and Ticron is silicone-impregnated Dacron. The suture is also available in uncoated forms (Mersilene and Dacron), but these sutures naturally have more tissue drag than the coated forms.[20] Coating or impregnating the suture decreases capillary action and tissue drag, but also reduces the knot-holding ability. These materials need four throws, all squared, or five throws, two slip and three squared.

The polyesters are strong sutures and are used when prolonged strength is required. Because of the multifilament nature of this material, bacteria and tissue fluids can penetrate the interstices of the polyester sutures. This can produce a nidus of infection, converting contamination to infection. Immobile bacteria have been transported inside the suture material; this is more significant than the spread of infection on the surface of the suture material.[9,21] Consequently, these suture materials must be used under aseptic circumstances, circumstances that unfortunately may not always exist in large animal practice.

Stainless Steel

Stainless steel is an alloy of iron (iron-nickel-chromium) and is available in multi- or monofilament forms. It is difficult to handle because it is easily kinked; yet it is the strongest of all suture materials. Stainless steel holds knots well, but the knots tend to be bulky. It is one of the most unreactive suture materials and can be repeatedly sterilized, but it has a tendency to cut tissues, as well as surgeons' gloves. Unlike the braided synthetics, stainless steel does not harbor bacteria and can be used in the presence of infection. Its use in large animal practice is infrequent.

Skin Stapling Devices

Disposable *skin stapling devices* have become available for use in surgery. They are commonly used for closing the skin of horses following laparotomy for the surgical correction of colic. One advantage of the device is its speed: the instrument closes skin incisions that are up to 2 feet long in a minute or so. This factor is important when the survival of the animal could be adversely affected by a longer anesthetic time. One study showed that the use of staples saved an average of 15.5 minutes of closing time per incision.[22] In a meta-analysis, if staples were used in

human orthopedic surgery, it was noted that there was a significantly higher risk of developing a wound infection when using staples compared to sutures.[23] The review is based upon 6 papers and included 683 wounds and 332 patients. In hip replacement alone, the patients were four times more likely to have an infection after staple closure then after suture closure. There was no significant difference in the development of inflammation, discharge, the dehiscence, necrosis, or allergic reaction. Although staples are well tolerated by horses and can remain in the skin almost indefinitely, it is best to remove them in 2–3 weeks before the hair grows back.

Early research indicated that skin staples might be very effective in contaminated wounds as they are inert and unlikely to potentiate bacterial infection.[24] Skin staples have been used commonly after abnormal surgery without any untoward effects. The complications seen in human orthopedic surgery have not been evaluated in horses. It is possible that larger, longer-term studies might show similar problems in horses. The surgeon should pay particular attention to incisional infections when using staples. A small pair of forceps is available for removal of the staples once the wound has healed. We have used staples in a variety of other skin incisions in horses and found them equally acceptable. The only limitation of staples is cost, although we have used them in situations such as colic surgery, in which the cost of the staples is only a small part of the total bill. We have also used skin staples in calves, other small ruminants, and llamas, although economy is a limiting factor in these species. Staples are particularly useful in wound closure where there is no tension. They can be applied with the use of a twitch in show horses where sedation of local anesthesia cannot be used.

Tissue Adhesives

Cyanoacrylate

The tissue adhesive *2-Octylcyanoacrylate* has been shown in people to provide more rapid closure of wound edges than sutures and staples.[25] Tissue adhesives have also been shown to be at least equivalent in cosmetic outcomes.[26] Similar studies have not been done in large animals; however, it is possible that using tissue adhesives over suture lines may improve the overall cosmetics and strength of the incision closure.

Needles

Surgical needles are essential for the placement of sutures in tissues. They must be designed to penetrate the tissue with a minimum of resistance and trauma; they should be rigid enough to prevent bending, yet flexible enough to prevent breaking. Naturally, they must be clean and resistant to corrosion. The selection of the needle is determined by the type of tissue to be sutured, its location and accessibility, and the size of the suture material.

Surgical needles have three basic components: the eye, the body (or shaft), and the point. The eye is usually of two types—*closed eye* or *swaged (eyeless)*. The closed eye is similar to a household sewing needle, and the eye itself is available in a variety of shapes. Swaged-on needles are permanently attached to the suture (Figure 4.1). The suture and needle are of approximately the same diameter. The outstanding advantage of a swaged-on needle is that tissues are subjected to less trauma, because only a single strand, rather than a double strand, of suture is pulled through the tissue. In addition, handling of the suture and needle is minimal, and it is ready for immediate use. At the end of surgery, the needle and the remaining piece of suture are discarded, and dull needles are continually culled. Tying the suture to the eye of the needle lessens the possibility of separation, but further increases the trauma as the suture material is drawn through the tissue.

Needles are usually curved, although some surgeons prefer to use straight needles, especially when suturing skin or bowel. Needles have a variable curvature, and they may be 1/4-, 3/8-, 1/2-, or 5/8-circle or half-curved (Figure 4.2). Selection of a needle depends on the depth of the region to be sutured. When suturing deep in a wound, for example, the needle will have to "turn a sharp corner." In this case, a 1/2-circle or 5/8-circle needle would be most suitable. Curved needles must be used with needle holders.

The body of the needle is available in a number of different shapes: round, oval, flat, or triangular. Flat and triangular bodies have cutting edges; round and oval-bodied needles usually taper from the small diameter at the point to a larger diameter at the eye.

Needles are also available with varying types of points (Figure 4.3). Cutting needles are designed to cut through dense, thick, connective tissue, such as bovine skin. Cutting needles can be reverse cutting, where the cutting edge is provided along the convex side of the needle, rather than on the concave surface. The purpose of a reverse-cutting needle is to minimize the excessive cutting of transfixed tissue. Another modification of the cutting needle combines the cutting point with a round needle shaft so that the needle will readily penetrate the dense tissue but not cut through it; this has been called a *taper cut needle*. One company manufactures a needle of similar concept that is useful in tough, dense tissues such as cartilage (K-point needle). This needle readily penetrates the cartilage of the equine larynx.

Noncutting needles, or round needles, have no edges and are less likely to cut through tissues (Figure 4.3). They are used for abdominal viscera, connective tissue, vessels, and other fragile tissues. Round (atraumatic) needles are actually round behind the tip, but the remaining portion of the shaft is oval. This design prevents angular or rotational displacement of the needle within the jaws of the needle holder.

Fig. 4.1. A swaged-on needle. The suture and needle have approximately the same diameters.

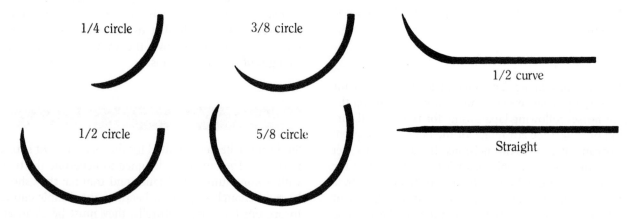

Fig. 4.2. Various needle shapes.

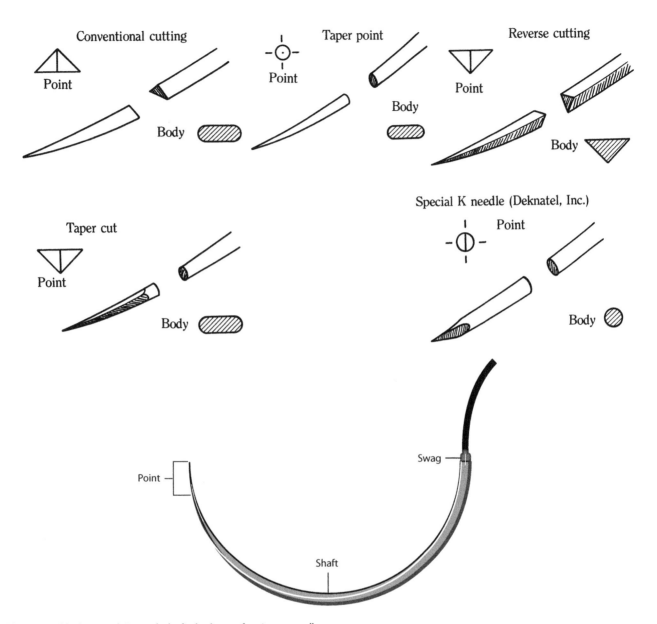

Fig. 4.3. Various points and shaft designs of suture needles.

Long-stemmed needles are also used in food animal practice. They are useful for placing heavy suture materials into the tissues, such as in vaginal prolapse in cattle.

References

1. Hochberg, J., Meyer, K.M., and Marion, M.D. Suture choice and other methods of skin closure. *Surg. Clin. North Am.*, 89:627–641, 2009.
2. Appel, S.L., Lefebvre, S.L., Houston, D.M., Homberg, D.L., Arnold Stone, J.E., Moore, A.E., and Weese, J.S. Evaluation of risk factors associated with suture-nidus cystolitys in dogs and cats; 176 cases (1999–2006). *J. Am. Vet. Med. Assoc.*, 233:1889–1895, 2008.
3. Kosan, M., Gonulanlan, U., Ozturk, B., Kulacoglu, S., Erguder, I., Akdemir, O., and Cetinkaya, M. Tissue reactions of suture materials (polyglactine 910, chromed catgut and polydioxanone) on rat bladder wall and their role in bladder stone formation. *Urol. Res.*, 36:43–49, 2008.
4. Swaim, S. Surgery of Traumatized Skin: Management and Reconstruction in the Dog and Cat. Philadelphia, W.B. Saunders, 1980.
5. Kim, J.C., Lee, Y.K., Lim, B.S., Rhee, S.H., and Yang, H.C. Comparison of tensile and know security properties of surgical sutures. *J. Mater. Sci. Mater. Med.*, 18:2363–2369, 2007.
6. Magilligan, D.J., and DeWeese, J.A. Knot security and synthetic suture materials. *Am. J. Surg.*, 127:355, 1974.
7. Kawcak, C.E., and Baxter, G.M. Surgical materials and wound closure techniques. *Vet. Clin. Equine*, 12:195–205, 1996.
8. Shettko, D.L., Frisbie, D.D., and Hendrickson, D.A. A comparison of knot security of commonly used hand-tied laparoscopic slipknots. *Vet. Surg.*, 33:521–524, 2004.
9. Edminston, C.E., Seabrook, G.R., Goheen, M.P., Krepel, C.J., Johnson, C.P., Lewis, B.D., Brown, K.R., and Towne, H.B.

Bacterial adherence to surgical sutures: can antibacterial-coated sutures reduce the risk of microbial contamination? *J. Am. Coll. Surg.*, *203*:481, 489, 2006.

10. Ford, H.R., Jones, P., Gaines, B., Reblock, K., and Simpkins, D.L. Intraoperative handling and wound healing: controlled clinical trial comparing coated VICRYL Plus antibacterial suture (coated polyglactin 910 suture with triclosan) with coated VICRYL suture (coated polyglactin 910 suture). *Surg. Infect.*, *6*:313–321, 2005.

11. Ming, X., Nichols, M., and Rothenburger, S. In vivo antibacterial efficacy of MONOCRYL plus antibacterial suture (poliglecaprone 25 with triclosan). *Surg. Infect.*, *8*:209–213, 2007.

12. Storch, M.L., Rothenburger, S.J., and Jacinto, G. Experimental efficacy study of coated VICRYL plus antibacterial suture in guinea pigs challenged with *Staphylococcus aureus*. *Surg. Infect.*, *5*:281–288, 2004.

13. Justinger, C., Moussavian, M.R., Schlueter, C., Kopp, B., Kollmar, O., and Schilling, M.D. Antibiotic coating of abdominal closure sutures and wound infection. *Surgery*, *145*:330–334, 2009.

14. Fierheller, E.E., and Wilson, D.G. An in vitro biomechanical comparison of the breaking strength and stiffness of polydioxanone (sizes 2,7) and polyglactin 910 (sizes 3,6) in the equine linea alba. *Vet. Surg.*, *34*:18–23, 2005.

15. Bezwada, R.S., Jamiolkowski, D.D., Lee, I.Y., Agarwal, V., Persivale, J., Trenka-Benthin, S., Erneta, M., Suryadevara, J., Yang, A., and Liu, S. Monocryl suture, a new ultra-pliable absorbable monofilament suture. *Biomaterials*, *16*:1141–1148, 1995.

16. Altman, G.H., Diaz, F., Jakuba, C., Calabro, T., Horan, R.L, Chen, J., Lu, H., Richmond, J., and Kaplan, D.L. Silk-based biomaterials. *Biomaterials*, *24*:401–416, 2003.

17. Trostle, S.S., and Hendrickson, D.A. Suture sinus formation following closure of ventral midline incisions with polypropylene in three horses. *J. Am. Vet. Med. Assoc.*, *207*:742–746, 1995.

18. Trostle, S.S., Wilson, D.G., Stone, M.C., and Markel, M.D. A study of the biomechanical properties of the adult equine linea alba: a relationship of tissue bite size and suture material to breaking strength. *Vet. Surg.*, *23*:435–441, 1994.

19. Stashak, T.S., and Yturraspe, D.J. Considerations for selection of suture materials. *Vet. Surg.*, *7*:48, 1978.

20. Edlich, R.F., Gubler, K., Wallis, A.G., Clark, J.J., Dahlstrom, J.J., and Long, W.B., 3rd. Wound closure sutures and needles: a new perspective. *J. Environ. Pathol. Toxicol.*, *29*:339–361, 2010.

21. Masini, B.D., Stinner, M.D., Waterman, S.M., and Wenke, J.C. Bacterial adherence to suture materials. *J. Surg. Educ.*, *68*: 101–104, 2011.

22. Ramey, D.W., and Rooks, R.L. Consider the use of skin stapling equipment to expedite equine surgery. *Vet. Med.*, *80*:66, 1985.

23. Smith, T.O., Sexton, D., Mann, C., and Donell, S. Sutures versus staples for skin closure in orthopaedic surgery: meta-analysis. *BMJ*, *340*:1199, 2006.

24. Stillman, R.M., Marino, C.A., and Seligman, S.J. Skin staples in potentially contaminated wounds. *Arch. Surg.*, *119*:138, 1984.

25. Pearl, M. Choosing abdominal incision and closure techniques. *J. Reprod. Med.*, *49*:662–670, 2004.

26. Quinn, J., Wells, G., and Sutcliffe, T. Tissue adhesive versus suture wound repair at 1 year: randomize clinical trial correlating early, 3-month, and 1-year cosmetic outcome. *Ann. Emerg. Med.*, *32*:1–9, 1998.

Chapter 5

KNOTS AND LIGATURES

Dean A. Hendrickson, DVM, MS, DACVS

> ## Objectives
> 1. Learn basic knotting techniques for the square knot, granny knot, and surgeon's knot.
> 2. Describe the applications of ligatures and two ligature techniques—the transfixation ligature and the three-forceps method of tissue ligation.

Principles of Knot Tying

The following are several important principles of knots and ligatures that the surgeon should consider:

- The amount of friction between the strands of suture determines knot security.
- Suture size and type impact the amount of friction between strands and thus knot security; the smallest size suture and knot that will not jeopardize wound strength should be used.
- Monofilaments create less friction against one another and the tissue. They have been designed to deform when tied to provide increased knot security.
- The length to which the suture ends should be cut depends on the security of the knot. For example, catgut suture tends to swell and untie when exposed to moisture, so the surgeon should leave the suture ends slightly longer than other sutures.
- Studies show that regardless of suture type, maximum knot security is reached at a maximum of two additional throws to the starting square knot (four throws total). Additional throws will exacerbate tissue irritation and impede healing. They should be used when a surgeon's knot or slipknot is used.[1-3]

- If instruments such as clamps are to be applied to the suture, as in herniorrhaphy in foals and calves, they should not be applied to those parts of the suture material that will remain in situ.

Knotting Techniques

The *square knot* is the knot used most in surgery (Figure 5.1). The knot is usually tied with needle holders, which should remain parallel to the wound, whereas all movements are made perpendicular to the wound. Uniform tension to the ends of the suture ensures that the knot ends up as a square and not as two half-hitches (slipknot). Two half-hitches result from unequal tension on the two ends during tying (Figure 5.1).

The *granny knot* is a slipknot that will not hold, especially if the strain on the ends is unequal; its use is not recommended (Figure 5.1).[4] Knots that tighten when the second throw is pressed home, as well as knots that end a continuous suture in which two strands are tied to one, are also prone to slippage.[3]

Knots stay tied because of the friction of one component against another. At least three separate throws are required to achieve the minimum amount of friction with the square knot. Monofilament suture materials, such as nylon, polypropylene, and braided synthetics, especially those that are Teflon coated, have poor knot security. With these materials, the first throw may loosen before the next throw is applied. Knotting technique warrants careful attention when using such suture materials. However, newer monofilament suture materials are designed to deform when the knot is tightened to improve knot security beyond that of braided suture. The surgeon can ensure knot security with braided synthetics with four throws, all squared (a double square knot) or with a knot with five throws, two slip and three squared.[3] Care must be taken with steel because it also is prone to slippage if the knots are poorly placed. The reader is referred to Chapter 4, "Suture Materials and Needles."

Turner and McIlwraith's Techniques in Large Animal Surgery, 4th Edition. Dean A. Hendrickson and A. N. (Nickie) Baird.
© 2013 John Wiley & Sons, Inc. Published 2013 by John Wiley & Sons, Inc.

Two half-hitches knot.

Granny knot.

Miller's knot.

Reinforced knot.

Square knot.

Surgeon's knot.

Fig. 5.1. Surgical knots.

4-S modified Roeder knot

Fig. 5.1. *Continued.*

A *surgeon's knot* is used when the first throw of a square knot cannot be held in position because of excessive tension on the wound edge (Figure 5.1). The surgeon's knot is basically the same as a square knot, except the first part of the knot consists of two wraps. The surgeon's knot should be further reinforced by four additional throws (Figure 5.1). The *Miller's knot* is very useful for ligating pedicles. There are two encircling wraps of suture to increase friction between the suture and pedicle (Figure 5.1). The knot should be finished with four throws, all squared. In locations where tying knots is difficult, such as deep in the abdomen, or in laparoscopy, a 4-S modified Roeder knot can be very helpful (Figure 5.1). It is essentially a slipknot that uses friction to keep from loosening. The knot is tied, the loop placed over the structure to ligate, and the knot is pushed down with a knot pusher to tighten.

Tying with the Needle Holder

In most instances, knots are tied with the aid of a needle holder (Figure 5.2A to F). The instrument tie is recommended for most surgery because of its adaptability and because it is economical, when compared with the one-hand or two-hand tie. It is possible to use short pieces of suture material and still grasp the suture firmly.

The technique for an instrument tie is as follows: a loop of the long end of the suture is made around the end of the instrument with the instrument in front of the suture (Figure 5.2A). The short end of the suture is grasped by the needle holder, which is then pulled through the loop, setting the knot down securely (Figure 5.2B and C). Traction must be applied in the same plane as the knot (Figure 5.2D) while keeping the instrument and hand with suture close to the tissue. The second throw is begun by wrapping the long end of the suture around the instrument, but in the opposite direction (Figure 5.2E). It is important to not lift the suture ends or the first throw will loosen. The short end of the suture is grasped and pulled through the loop (Figure 5.2F). The surgeon's knot is made using essentially the same procedure, except the first loop is doubled by placing a double loop around the needle holder.

Knots should be tied with the correct tension. Excessive tension results in strangulation of the tissues, which leads to necrosis and delayed wound healing. Similarly, the wound should not be allowed to gape, because of either too few sutures or lack of tension. To relieve the tension on individual sutures, the number of sutures used to close the incision should be increased; the underlying principle is that when sutures are uniformly spaced, the tension is distributed equally among the sutures.

Ligatures

A *ligature* is a loop of suture used for occluding a blood vessel either before or after it is severed. Ligature loops are frequently used in laparoscopy for structures within the abdominal cavity. Laparoscopic ligatures, such as the 4-S modified Roeder knot, are usually formed using a knot pushing device and a slipknot. These techniques are covered in depth elsewhere.[5,6]

To prevent slipping, a ligature can be converted to a *transfixation ligature* by passing it through the middle of the vessel. It is tied around half the vessel and then around the entire vessel. Transfixation ligatures can be used to ligate several blood vessels within tissues (Figure 5.3). As little tissue as possible should be left distal to the ligature because the stump so created will become necrotic and will have to be absorbed by the animal. Care must be taken not to cut the stump too short or the ligature may slip over the end and result in the loss of fixation. Double loops are stronger than single loops because of the distribution of friction and tensile forces. In addition, the bursting strength of a loop is inversely proportional to the volume that it encloses. In other words, the tension on the suture is proportional to the volume. Practically speaking, mass ligation of tissue is more apt to break than are ligatures around small bleeding points or isolated vessels. Furthermore, vessels can recannulize within a large mass of ligated tissue.

When large amounts of tissues must be ligated, the *three-forceps method* can be used. The forceps are placed on the pedicle, as shown in Figure 5.4. Forceps A are distal and forceps C are proximal. The pedicle is divided between

Fig. 5.2. **A–F.** Tying with a needle holder.

Fig. 5.3. Transfixation ligature.

Fig. 5.4. Three-forceps method of tissue ligation.

forceps A and B, and the ligature is placed proximal to forceps C. The first throw on the ligature is made; and, as forceps C are removed, the ligature is tied into the crease left by forceps C. Further throws are then placed on the ligature, and forceps B are loosened to check for hemorrhage. The main drawback of this technique is that the tissue in the crease has been crushed and could allow hemorrhage on the proximal side of the ligature. A better option in this instance is a Miller's knot without the use of a crushing forceps technique.

References

1. Brown, R.P. Knotting techniques and suture materials. *Br. J. Surg.*, *79*:399–400, 1992.

2. Magilligan, D.J., and DeWeese, J.A. Knot security and synthetic suture materials. *Am. J. Surg.*, *127*:355, 1974.

3. Swaim, S. Surgery of Traumatized Skin: Management and Reconstruction in the Dog and Cat. Philadelphia, W.B. Saunders, 1980, p. 269.

4. Shettko, D.L., Frisbie, D.D., and Hendrickson, D.A. A comparison of knot security of commonly used hand-tied laparoscopic slipknots. *Vet. Surg.*, *33*:521–524, 2004.

5. Carpenter, E.M., Hendrickson, D.A., James, S., Franke, C., Frisbie, D.,Trostle, S., and Wilson, D. A mechanical study of ligature security of commercially available pre-tied ligatures versus hand tied ligatures for use in equine laparoscopy. *Vet. Surg.*, *35*:55–59, 2006.

6. Price, P.B. Stress, strain and sutures. *Ann. Surg.*, *128*:408, 1948.

Chapter 6

SUTURE PATTERNS

Dean A. Hendrickson, DVM, MS, DACVS

Objectives

1. Provide an overview of the indications for and uses of different suture patterns.
2. Detail the technique for the following basic suture patterns:
   - Simple interrupted
   - Simple continuous
   - Interrupted horizontal mattress
   - Continuous horizontal mattress
   - Vertical mattress suture
   - Near-far-far-near suture
   - Subcuticular suture
   - Cruciate (cross mattress) suture
   - Continuous lock stitch (Ford interlocking suture)
3. Describe suture techniques that are most advantageous for the closure of hollow organs, for tendon repair, and for the closure of wounds under high tension.

Basic Suture Patterns

A wide variety of suture patterns for use under different circumstances is available to the surgeon. Each pattern will have some good features and some detrimental features. It is important to choose the appropriate combination of suture pattern, suture type, suture size, and knot type to provide the best outcome for the patient. If one pattern does not produce optimum results, a new technique must be mastered. Suture patterns are divided into interrupted or continuous patterns, and the following patterns are often used by the large animal surgeon.

Simple Interrupted Suture

The simple interrupted suture is the oldest and most widely used suture pattern. It is easy and relatively rapid to perform. However, because each suture must be tied individually it often takes longer to close an incision when using a simple interrupted pattern. The technique of insertion depends on the thickness of the tissue apposed. The needle and suture are inserted at a variable distance from one side of the incision, across the incision at right angles, and through the tissue on the other side. For a right-handed surgeon, this would be accomplished from right to left, and the reverse would apply for a left-handed surgeon (Figure 6.1). The knot should be offset, so as not to rest against the incision. If this suture is used for skin closure, the point of insertion will vary, depending on the thickness of the skin. This may be 1 cm in bovine skin or 2–3 mm for the thin skin on the inguinal area of a foal. The simple interrupted suture should appose the wound margins, but it may invert them if it is pulled too tightly or if the insertion and exit points are too far from the cut edge. The spacing between the sutures depends on the tension on the wound edges and the distance the suture is placed from the wound edge. In general, the sutures should form squares where the distance between sutures is equal to twice the distance between the suture insertion and the wound edge. Gaping of the wound edges should be avoided. While the simple interrupted pattern is often considered the "Gold Standard" in intestinal anastomosis, it is rarely used as the continuous patterns have become more popular. There is some concern that simple interrupted patterns will lead to greater adhesion formation.

Simple Continuous Suture

This continuous suture is made up of a variable number of simple bites and is tied only at the ends (Figure 6.2 and Figure 6.3). It is used in tissues that are elastic and will

Turner and McIlwraith's Techniques in Large Animal Surgery, 4th Edition. Dean A. Hendrickson and A. N. (Nickie) Baird.
© 2013 John Wiley & Sons, Inc. Published 2013 by John Wiley & Sons, Inc.

Fig. 6.1. Simple interrupted suture with cross section of suture bite.

Fig. 6.3. Simple continuous suture with cross section of suture bite (swaged-on needle).

Fig. 6.2. Simple continuous suture with cross section of suture bite (eyed needle).

not be subjected to a lot of tension. The bites in the edges of the wound are made at right angles to the edges of the wound, but the exposed part of the suture passes diagonally across the incision. This suture pattern can be applied rapidly. Ending the suture depends on whether a swaged-on needle or a needle with an eye is used. To end the suture with an eyed needle, the needle is advanced through the tissues, and the short end of the suture is held on the proximal end of the needle passage. A loop of suture is pulled through with the needle, and the loop is tied to the single end on the opposite side (Figure 6.2). When a swaged-on needle is used, the needle end of the suture is tied to the last available loop of suture material that is exterior to the tissues (Figure 6.3). If any one of the sutures in a continuous suture pattern fails, the strength of the suture line will be lost. If one suture fails in an interrupted suture pattern, the remaining sutures have a better chance of maintaining the strength of the suture line. Continuous suture patterns are generally chosen for bowel anastomosis as there is less foreign material at the anastomosis site and they are more rapidly applied. Consequently, there is less contamination of the peritoneum.

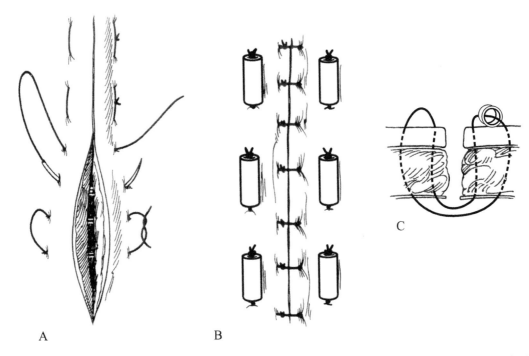

Fig. 6.4. **A.** Interrupted horizontal mattress suture. **B.** Interrupted horizontal mattress sutures as tension-relieving sutures, using pieces of rubber. **C.** Cross section of horizontal mattress.

Interrupted Horizontal Mattress Suture

The interrupted horizontal mattress suture is illustrated in Figure 6.4A. The external parts of the suture lie parallel to the wound edges. To limit eversion, the needle should be angled through the skin, and the wound edges should oppose each other gently. This suture can be used in conjunction with pieces of rubber tubing or with buttons to act as a tension suture (Figure 6.4B). In this situation, the suture is placed some distance from the skin edges. Another pattern of sutures, such as the simple interrupted suture, is used to align the edges of the incision more precisely. The horizontal mattress suture probably provides the best tension relief of all of the suture patterns, but because of the geometry of the horizontal mattress suture, the sutures have a tendency to reduce the blood supply to the wound edges (Figure 6.4C). The horizontal mattress suture is probably best reserved for muscle belly reapposition.

Continuous Horizontal Mattress Suture

The continuous horizontal mattress suture, illustrated in Figure 6.5, is similar to the horizontal mattress pattern, except it is continuous. Its main advantage is speed, and it is not often used in large animal surgery.

Vertical Mattress Suture

Initially, the suture and needle make a bite close to the wound edge and then pass across the incision to take a small bite on the opposite side (Figure 6.6A). The needle

Fig. 6.5. Continuous horizontal mattress suture.

is then reversed in the jaws of the needle holder and is returned to the opposite side, where it takes a larger bite. The suture bites should be placed an adequate distance from the wound edge and from each of the ipsilateral bites so that the suture does not pull through the skin. If this suture is used as the sole method of skin closure, a partial skin-thickness "near" bite of the suture pattern will ensure adequate approximation of the wound edges; if used as

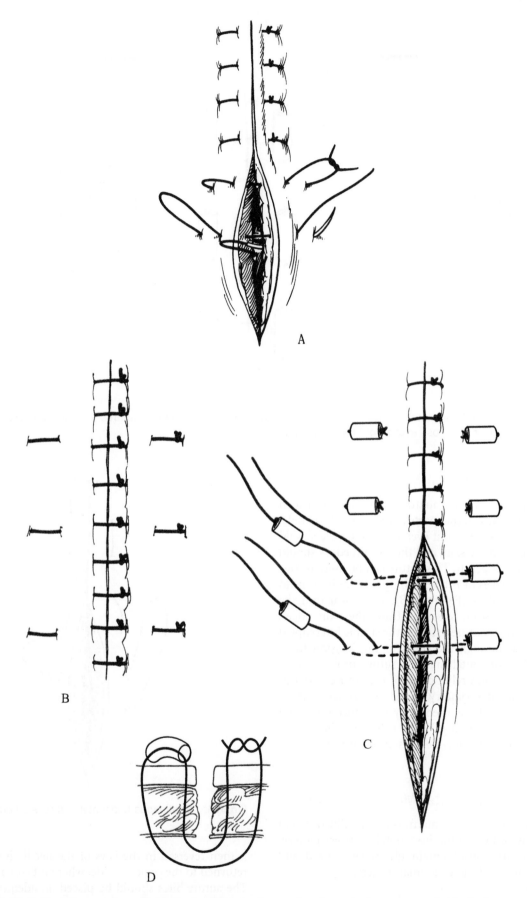

Fig. 6.6. **A.** Vertical mattress suture. **B.** Vertical mattress suture as tension-relieving sutures. **C.** Vertical mattress suture using pieces of rubber. **D.** Cross section of vertical mattress.

tension-relieving sutures some distance from the wound, simple interrupted sutures can accurately align the wound edges (Figure 6.6B).

Compared with the horizontal mattress pattern, the geometry of this suture allows better blood circulation to the wound edges and thereby decreases the chances of necrosis of the margins of the wound. A disadvantage of this suture compared to the horizontal mattress pattern is that it uses slightly more suture material and may take longer to insert.

The vertical mattress suture is popular in repairing traumatic lacerations of the skin of equine limbs, where the blood supply may already be compromised. Like the horizontal mattress suture, it can also be used as a tension suture in conjunction with stents, such as pieces of rubber tubing, or with buttons. Pieces of rubber or buttons minimize tissue cutting by the suture material by spreading out the tension over a greater area (Figure 6.6C and D). The vertical mattress suture provides the second most tension relief of the tension-relieving suture patterns.

Near-Far-Far-Near Suture

This suture, illustrated in Figure 6.7, is a tension suture often used in large animal surgery. It provides slightly less tension relief than the vertical mattress suture pattern. As the name suggests, the first bite is made close to the wound and then passes under the wound across its edges at right angles to emerge at a greater distance from the wound edge on the second side of the wound. The next part of the

Fig. 6.7. **A** and **B**. Near-far-far-near suture.

suture consists of crossing over the wound to the original side and inserting the needle and suture at a distance farther from the edge than the original entry point, similar to the distance achieved on the first bite on the second side of the wound. The suture is then directed into the wound perpendicular to the edges of the wound, crosses the wound, and emerges close to the wound edge on the second side, similar in distance from the wound edge as the first bite. Then the suture ends are tied. This suture is less time consuming to insert than the vertical mattress suture and is an excellent tension suture. This suture has been used to close the linea alba of horses whenever tension on the wound edges is excessive. One of the main benefits of this tension-relieving suture is that the needle is always placed "forehand" and never needs to be reversed.

Subcuticular Suture

This suture is used to eliminate the small scars produced around the suture holes of suture patterns that penetrate the epidermis. The first part of the suture is placed by directing the needle, from deep to superficial into the apex of the incision in the opposite direction of the incision (Figure 6.8). The needle is then reversed and is directed along the incision from superficial to deep. The knot is tied and, in this way, will be pulled into the deeper tissues. The remainder of the suture pattern is placed like a horizontal mattress suture, with the needle crossing the incision at right angles, but advancing underneath the dermis parallel to the incision. A knot similar to the one used in the simple continuous pattern finishes the suture. The needle is then reversed and is directed back along the incision; the knot at this end should also be subcutaneous. The suture material used for this pattern should be synthetic and absorbable and should be relatively unreactive and sterile. The suture bites are taken parallel to the incision, where there is little dead space (Figure 6.8C), and perpendicular to the incision where there is more dead space (Figure 6.8D).

Cruciate (Cross Mattress) Suture

The cruciate suture, illustrated in Figure 6.9, is commenced by inserting the needle from one side to the next, as one would place a simple interrupted suture. The needle is then advanced without penetrating the tissue, and a second passage is made parallel to the first. The suture ends are then on opposite sides of the wound and form an "x" on the surface of the wound. This suture pattern is used by some surgeons if the skin edges are under mild tension.

The cruciate suture has been used to close the small hole made by a hypodermic needle that is used for deflating a gas-distended bowel and as a skin-closure technique after arthroscopy or laparoscopy. It has some tension-relieving properties and takes almost half the time to place when compared to a simple interrupted pattern in an incision.

Fig. 6.8. **A** and **B**. Subcuticular suture.
C. Cross section showing parallel suture
bites. **D**. Cross section showing
perpendicular suture bites.

Fig. 6.9. Cruciate (cross mattress) suture with cross section
of suture bite.

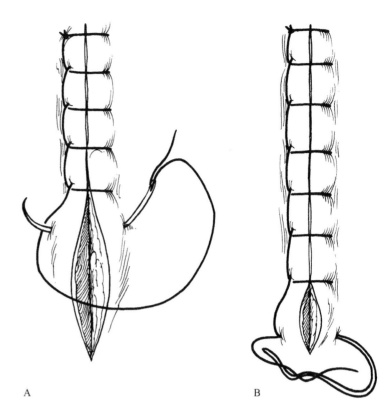

Fig. 6.10. **A** and **B.** Continuous lock stitch (Ford interlocking suture).

A   B

Continuous Lock Stitch (Ford Interlocking Suture)

The continuous lock stitch is a modification of the simple continuous suture (Figure 6.10). In this continuous pattern, the needle is passed perpendicularly through the tissues in the same direction. Once the needle is passed through the tissues, it is drawn through the preformed loop and is tightened. Each subsequent stitch is locked until the end of the incision is reached. To end the lock stitch, the needle should be introduced from a direction opposite the insertion of the previous sutures, and the end should be held on that side. The loop of suture is formed, and the loop is tied to the long end of the suture. The interlocking suture is commonly used in the skin of cattle following a laparotomy. Good approximation of the skin edges can be obtained, especially with the thick skin on the flanks of cattle.

Suture Patterns Used for Closure of Hollow Organs

A suture pattern used for a hollow organ must be placed meticulously because of the disastrous consequences possible if infectious material should leak. In the intestinal tract, for example, gas, solid, and liquid feces propelled by peristalsis place strain on the suture line. Fortunately, the walls of the healthy gastrointestinal tract are tough, pliable, and easy to manipulate. On the other hand, the friable uterus of a cesarean patient with a decomposing

fetus may be difficult to suture. Another advantage of surgery of hollow organs is that the organs generally heal quickly and are remarkably secure in as little as 1 week to 10 days after surgery.

A watertight closure was once thought to be mandatory when suturing a hollow organ; however, any technique that opposes the wound edges well is satisfactory because a fibrin clot provides an almost immediate seal. Eversion of the mucosa, however, is detrimental and can lead to the leakage of septic contents, resulting in peritonitis.

Classically, suture patterns used on hollow organs have been inverting sutures or opposing sutures. When suturing the intestinal tract, the strength of a suture depends on the inclusion of the submucosal or fibromuscular layer. Absorbable or nonabsorbable sutures may be used to close the gastrointestinal tract; however, with current absorbable suture varieties, absorbable suture materials are considered the standard of care. Needles used for hollow-organ surgery should be round-bodied (noncutting), with the suture material swaged on to reduce the size of the hole made on the organ wall. The needle size should approximate the diameter of the suture as closely as possible to allow the bowel to close around the suture as completely as possible. Noncutting needles are less likely to lacerate suture material that may have been placed in a deeper layer.

Interrupted or continuous sutures can be used in hollow-organ surgery. Interrupted sutures have been thought to be safer because, if one knot becomes untied, the integrity of the entire suture line will not be jeopardized. By using interrupted sutures, the tension on each suture can be adjusted, thereby ensuring an optimum blood supply to the wound edges. However, the use of interrupted sutures requires more knots and consequently more suture material, leaving more foreign material and creating a greater inflammatory response. In most instances, two to three runs of a continuous pattern are used for bowel closure.

Interrupted Lembert Suture (Inverting)

The Lembert suture is a commonly used suture in gastro-intestinal surgery (Figure 6.11). The suture is directed through the tissue from the outside, toward the cut edge of the incision. It penetrates the serosa, muscular, and submucosal layers, but not the mucosa. The suture exits on the same side and emerges close to the edge of the incision. It is reinserted on the opposite side of the incision, close to the incision edge, passes laterad through the serosa, muscular, and submucosal layer and is brought up again through the muscular and serosal layers. The wall of the viscus automatically inverts as the knot is tied. The knot should not be so tight as to strangulate the tissues. At no stage does the suture penetrate the lumen of the viscus; it is considered a safe and useful stitch in gastro-intestinal surgery, especially the stomach, and can be used as a one-layer closure. It is also suitable for use in the uterus and the rumen of large animals. The main draw-back of the Lembert suture pattern is the amount of inversion. It should not be used where lumen diameter is already compromised.

Continuous Lembert Suture (Inverting)

The Lembert suture can be performed in a continuous pattern (Figure 6.12). The same spacing is used as in the interrupted suture, and the continuous suture is tied to itself at its proximal end and again at its distal end. The

Fig. 6.11. **A.** Interrupted Lembert suture. **B.** Lembert suture before tightening. **C.** Lembert suture after tightening.

Fig. 6.12. Continuous Lembert suture.

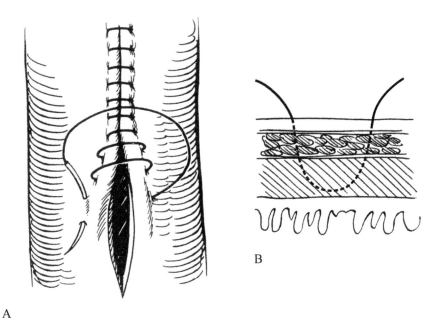

Fig. 6.13. **A.** Cushing suture. **B.** Cross section of Cushing suture.

A

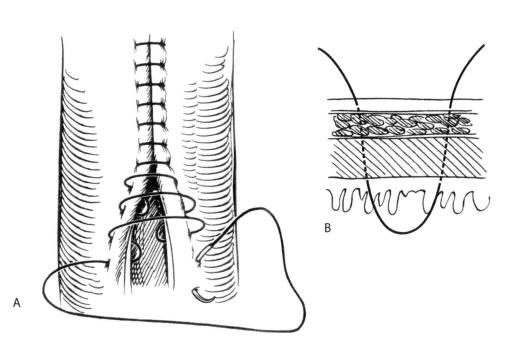

Fig. 6.14. **A.** Connell suture. **B.** Cross section of Connell suture.

suture is commonly used in both intestinal and uterine closures and requires less time than the interrupted suture.

Cushing Suture (Inverting)

This is a method of continuous suturing in which the bites are made parallel to the edges of the wound (Figure 6.13). As the suture is placed, it penetrates the serosa, muscular, and submucosal layers, but does not pass through the mucosa; hence, it does not enter the lumen of the viscus. The suture crosses the incision at right

angles and is tied to itself at the proximal end and at the distal end. It is generally used as the outer tier on a double-layer closure and can be executed rapidly. The main benefit is that it is a minimally inverting pattern. The main disadvantage is that the suture run is perpendicular to the blood supply.

Connell Suture (Inverting)

The Connell suture resembles the Cushing suture, but the suture material penetrates all layers of the bowel (Figure 6.14). The suture is tied when the first stitch has been

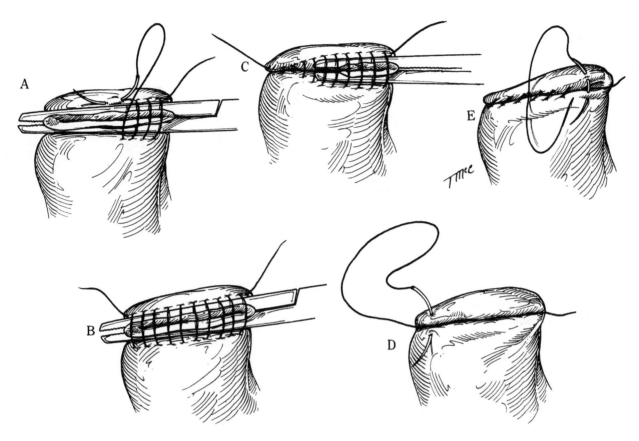

Fig. 6.15.   A–E. Parker-Kerr oversew.

taken and is tied again at the far end of the incision. Once outside the serosal surface, the needle and suture cross the incision and are reinserted in the serosa of the opposite side at a point that corresponds to the preceding exit site. The directions of the Connell and Cushing suture are the same, and both sutures invert tissue. The Connell pattern is rarely used due to the concerns with bacterial "wicking" along the suture that has penetrated the lumen of the bowel.

Parker-Kerr Oversew (Inverting)

This suture pattern is a combination of the Lembert and Cushing patterns, and it is used to close the stump of a hollow viscus (Figure 6.15). It is essentially a Cushing pattern oversewn by a Lembert pattern. The first layer of the suture pattern, which is a Cushing pattern, is performed over a pair of forceps placed on the end of the stump (Figure 6.15A and B). The forceps are withdrawn slowly as the suture is pulled in both directions; this inverts the wound edges without opening the lumen, which would result in contamination (Figure 6.15C). A continuous Lembert suture is then used as an oversew using the same suture (Figure 6.15D). The needle end of the suture is brought back as the second layer to be tied at the origin of the first layer (Figure 6.15E). The suture

patterns can be reversed in this technique, using a Lembert for the pattern directly over the forceps and oversewing this with the Cushing, when the forceps have been withdrawn. The most common application of this suture pattern in large animal surgery is in the jejunocecal anastomosis in the horse.[1,2] This suture pattern is used in the stump of the terminal ileum. This pattern has largely been replaced by stapling equipment.

Purse-String Suture (Inverting)

This pattern comprises a continuous suture placed in a circle around an opening; however, the suture is tied when the entire circumference of the circle has been followed (Figure 6.16). To aid inversion of the suture, an assistant should grasp that part of the purse string that is exactly opposite the knot and should exert upward traction. The purse string is then tightened following the release of the tissue forceps. Like the Cushing suture, the suture does not penetrate the lumen. Another layer of sutures may be used over the purse string, either in the form of another purse string or in a series of Lembert sutures. The purse-string suture is used to oversew an opening that evacuates gas in the gastrointestinal tract that is made by a needle or trocar puncture. It can also be used to stabilize permanent indwelling fistulae or cannulae.

Simple Interrupted Suture (Appositional)

The simple interrupted suture can be used successfully to close the intestinal tract. It should be used to gently oppose the wound edges, thereby causing minimal interference to the blood supply. In Figure 6.17, the suture is placed through all the layers approximately 3–4 mm from the wound edges. The suture is then tightened. Generally, the suture is placed through all layers except the mucosa. This pattern is best reserved for end-to-end anastomosis of bowel with significant differences in lumen diameter. Interrupted patterns leave more foreign material and take longer to place than continuous patterns.

Simple Continuous Suture (Appositional)

The simple continuous suture is the most commonly used suture pattern in the intestinal tract. Similar to the simple interrupted pattern, it should be used to gently oppose the wound edges, thereby causing minimal interference to the blood supply. The suture is placed through all layers except the mucosa. This suture pattern allows rapid apposition of the bowel wall while minimizing the amount of suture material used. In horses, a simple continuous pattern is often followed by a minimally inverting pattern such as a Cushing Pattern.

Gambee Suture (Combination Inverting and Appositional)

The Gambee suture pattern is used for intestinal anastomosis as a single-layer closure (Figure 6.18). The suture and needle are introduced like a simple interrupted suture and pass from the serosa, through all layers, except the mucosa. The needle is then directed back through the submucosa. The suture crosses the incision, passes through the submucosa and out through the submucosa, muscular, and serosal layers. The suture is tied firmly, so that the tissue compresses on itself. Although it takes longer than a simple interrupted pattern, the Gambee pattern is useful in equine gastrointestinal surgery because it inverts the mucosa into the lumen. When this technique was evaluated experimentally in horses, it caused minimal adhesion formation and stenosis.[3]

Double-Layer Inverting Patterns

A two-layer inverting pattern (using Cushing, Connell, or Lembert) produces an anastomosis with higher initial tensile and bursting strength.[4] The incidence of adhesions is lower, but internal cuff formation may potentially produce intraluminal obstruction.

For end-to-end anastomosis of the small intestine, a double-layer anastomosis composed of a simple continuous mucosal layer and a continuous Lembert seromuscular layer has been advocated.[3,4] This technique inverts only

Fig. 6.16. **A** and **B**. Purse-string suture.

Fig. 6.17. Simple interrupted suture used in bowel.

T. serosa

T. muscularis

T. submucosa
T. mucosa

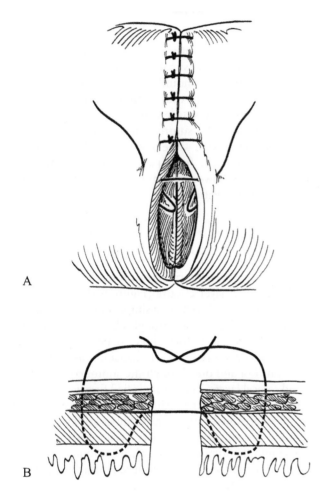

Fig. 6.18. **A** and **B.** Gambee suture.

Fig. 6.19. Stent bandage.

one layer and results in a minimum reduction of lumen diameter. The incidence of fibrosis and suture tract inflammation is higher with this technique than with Gambee and crushing patterns; however, adhesions were not present in six horses when this technique was used, as compared to a 50% adhesion incidence with the other two techniques.[3,4] The author prefers a simple continuous appositional pattern followed by a minimally inverting Cushing pattern. Further details of intestinal resection, anastomosis, and gastrointestinal stapling are available in *McIlwraith's and Turner's Equine Surgery: Advanced Techniques.*[5]

Stent Bandages (Tie-Over Dressings)

These dressings are used over areas such as the proximal regions of the limbs and the torso where it is difficult to apply a pressure dressing. As well as applying some localized pressure and minimizing postoperative swelling, this bandage helps keep dirt and bedding away from the skin incision. These dressings also can assist in the elimination of dead space, such as the throatlatch region following

modified Forssell's operation for cribbing. They have been used to cover skin incisions following the closure of the linea alba for celiotomy.

For smaller incisions, a sterile gauze bandage is used. For larger incisions, a rolled hand towel is used. The bandage material should be long enough that the ends slightly overlap the ends of the incision. Following closure of the skin incision, an assistant holds the rolled dressing firmly in position. Using synthetic monofilament suture material, a continuous horizontal mattress suture or interrupted horizontal mattress sutures are placed (Figure 6.19). As the sutures are tied, slight tenting of the skin may occur. This will disappear when these sutures are removed. The stent is usually removed 4–7 days after surgery, depending on the procedure. The bandage helps keep the incision dry because of its wicking effect, but it should not become moist enough to allow excessive fluid to gain access to the incision. The stent should be removed if excessive moisture persists.

Suture Patterns for Severed Tendons

Frequently, the large animal surgeon is presented with a traumatic wound involving severed tendons. If the tendon ends are not in approximate alignment, suturing may be indicated.

One has to weigh the advantages and disadvantages of suturing tendons. To appose the tendon ends properly with suture material, the tendon must be subjected to additional trauma. Nonabsorbable materials are generally used because of their ability to maintain strength during the protracted course of tendon healing. In the face of infection or contamination, these materials may potentiate infection, or a chronic draining tract may form. Nevertheless, tendon repair can be indicated to approximate the ends and to facilitate healing. This is especially true in horses, where traumatic laceration of the flexor tendons occurs frequently. Research suggests that when possible, performing tenorrhaphy greatly increases the prognosis of the horse returning to riding status. If a tendon is sutured, some form of external support will be necessary to minimize extreme forces placed on the repair. However too rigid of coaptation can lead to adhesion formation. Adhesion formation is one of the reasons that horses with flexor tendon injury do not return to their previous level of use.[6–8] Gap formation has been implicated as leading to more adhesions. When the tendon ends are held in close proximity, primary intention healing occurs; when there is a gap between the tendon ends, second intention healing takes place. Gap formation occurs when the surgical technique is poor or when the "pull" on the tendon is greater than the strength of the repair. Reviews of tendon repair techniques in people concluded that the repair strength is dependent upon the number of suture lines that cross the tendon gap and that sutures placed in the epitendon increase the repair strength by 10–50%.[9]

Locking-Loop Tendon Suture

A commonly used pattern is the locking-loop tendon suture (modified Kessler pattern) shown in Figure 6.20. This suture is strong, causes minimal interference with tendon blood supply, and exposes little of the suture material.[10]

The needle is inserted into the severed end of the tendon and emerges from the surface of the tendon (Figure 6.20A). The needle is then passed transversely through the tendon just superficial to the longitudinal part of the suture (Figure 6.20B). This results in a loop of suture locking around a small bundle of tendon fibers. When more tension is applied to the repair site, the grip of the suture loop on these fiber bundles becomes tighter. The needle is then reinserted in a longitudinal direction and passes under the transverse portion of suture material (Figure 6.20C); this process is repeated on the other piece of tendon (Figure 6.20D). After placement of the suture,

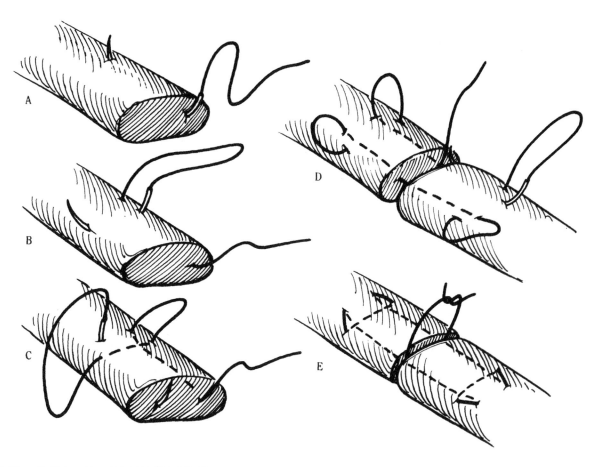

Fig. 6.20. **A–E.** Locking-loop tendon suture.

Fig. 6.21. **A–G.** 3-loop pulley suture.

Cross section of tendon

Fig. 6.22.   Six strand Savage repair.

all the loops should be tightened in turn and the suture tied snugly, so slight "bunching" occurs at the junction (Figure 6.20E).

Monofilament nylon or polypropylene is the recommended suture material for this pattern. The largest-diameter monofilament nonabsorbable suture should be used. At this time, the largest commercially available suture material of this type is no. 2 nylon. A single locking-loop suture pattern with this material in equine tendon is insufficient to prevent gap formation during weight bearing, even when the area is immobilized with a cast. In-vitro biomechanical studies have shown that a double locking-loop pattern should be used because it is twice as resistant to gap formation and failure as a single locking-loop pattern. Three locking-loop patterns can be used, but they may be technically difficult and time consuming to apply.[11]

Another good tendon repair suture pattern is the three-loop pulley pattern (Figure 6.21). The suture is inserted across the diameter of the severed tendon (Figure 6.21A) and then moved to the other portion of the tendon and inserted in the same plane (Figure 6.21B). This is repeated two more times, dividing the tendon into three planes (Figure 6.21C). The sutures are then tightened and the knot tied (Figure 6.21D). Similar suture materials and external coaptation as for the locking loop pattern should be used.

Other patterns include the Savage Technique.[12] (New Figure 6.22) In a recent study, the 10-strand modified Savage technique provided approximately 3 times the tensile strength in a cadaver model than did the three-loop pulley.[11]

References

1. Donawick, W.J., Christie, B.A., and Stewart, J.V. Resection of diseased ileum in the horse. *J. Am. Vet. Med. Assoc.*, *159*:1146, 1971.
2. Owen, R.R., Physick-Sheard, P.W., Hilbert, B.J., Horney, F.D., and Butler, D.G. Jejuno or ileocecal anastomosis performed in seven horses exhibiting colic. *Can. Vet. J.*, *16*:164, 1975.
3. Auletta, L., Lamagna, F., Uccello, V., Lamagna, B., and Pasolini, M.P. In vitro comparison of three suture techniques for anastomosis of the equine small intestine. *Equine Vet. J.*, *40*:46–50, 2011.
4. Sherlock, C., Lee, W., Mueller, P.O., Eggleston, R., and Epstein, K. Ex vivo comparison of three hand sewn end-to-end anastomoses in normal equine jejunum. *Equine Vet. J.*, *39*:76–80, 2011.
5. McIlwraith, C.W., and Robertson, J.T. McIlwraith's and Turner's Equine Surgery: Advanced Techniques, 2nd edn. Baltimore, Williams & Wilkins, 1998.
6. Belknap, J.K., Baxter, G.M., and Nickels, F.A. Extensor tendon lacerations in horses: 50 cases (1982–1988). *J. Am. Vet. Med. Assoc.*, *203*:428–431, 1993.
7. Foland, J.W., Trotter, G.W., Stashak, T.S., McIlwraith, C.W., Turner, A.S., and Aanes, W.A. Traumatic injuries involving tendons of the distal limbs in horses: A retrospective study of 55 cases. *Equine Vet. J.*, *23*:422–425, 1991.
8. Mespoulhes-Riviere, C., Martens, A., Bogaert, L., and Wilderjans, H. Factors affecting outcome of extensor tendon lacerations in the distal limb of horses. A retrospective study of 156 cases (1994–2003). *Vet. Comp. Orthop. Tramatol.*, *21*:358–364, 2008.
9. Boyer, M.I., Strickland, J.W., Engles, D., Sachar, K., and Leversedge, F.J. Flexor tendon repair and rehabilitation: State of the art in 2002. *Instr. Course Lect.*, *52*:137–161, 2003.
10. Tang, J.B., Pan, C.Z., Xie, R.G., and Chen, F. A biomechanical study of Tang's multiple locking techniques for flexor tendon repair. *Chir. Main.*, *18*:254–260, 1999.
11. Smith, R.L., Murphy, D.J., Day, R.E., and Lester, G.D. An ex-vivo biomechanical study comparing strength characteristics of a new technique with the three-loop pulley for equine tenorrhaphy. *Vet. Surg.*, *40*:768–773, 2011.
12. Savage, R., and Risitano, G. Flexor tendon repair using a "six strand" method of repair and early active mobilization. *J. Hand Surg.*, *14*:396–399, 1989.

Chapter 7

PRINCIPLES OF WOUND MANAGEMENT AND THE USE OF DRAINS

Dean A. Hendrickson, DVM, MS, DACVS

Objectives

1. Describe the fundamental principles of wound management and healing in large animals.
2. Discuss factors that impact wound healing and how they may be used to predict the wound environment.
3. Describe techniques for wound exploration and debridement.
4. Describe the indications for antimicrobial therapy in wound management.
5. Describe basic principles and appropriate wounds for primary closure, second-intention healing, and delayed primary closure.
6. Provide indications and applications for the use of drains in wound management.

Wound Management

There are three main methods of wound management and healing: primary closure, delayed primary closure, and second-intention healing. Primary closure describes the initial closure of wounds. Delayed primary closure entails a period of open wound management to establish a healthy wound bed until the wound edges can be approximated. Second-intention healing describes wounds that are left to heal without surgical correction via wound contraction and epithelialization. Wound contraction is an active process characterized by the centripetal movement of the whole thickness of the surrounding skin, which results in diminished wound size. It is the major process for reestablishment of skin continuity in wound healing by second-

ary intention, with the exception of the distal limbs. In the distal limbs, epithelialization plays the major role in skin closure, and the resulting fragile epithelium is devoid of hair follicles and sweat glands. An understanding of the basic physiological processes involved in wound healing will aid the practitioner in developing the best treatment regimen for traumatic wounds.

Most of the discussion in this chapter is directed at horses because the incidence of traumatic wounds is highest in this species, but the basic principles are the same for ruminants and swine. Emphasis is placed on wounds of the distal limbs, where wound healing can be a difficult and frustrating process.

Assessment of Traumatic Wounds

The initial assessment of a traumatic wound enables the practitioner to evaluate the blood supply to the wound, viability of surrounding tissues, and any other factors that may inhibit or retard wound healing or increase the wound's susceptibility to infection. The characteristics of the wound—including the type, degree of contamination, location, size, and surrounding vascular supply—can be readily evaluated upon presentation. The type of wound—e.g., laceration, abrasion, puncture—is a good indication of the wound's blood supply and contamination, as well as the viability of the surrounding tissue. Wounds can also be categorized by their degrees of contamination; clean, clean-contaminated, contaminated, or infected. Clean and clean-contaminated wounds are suitable for primary or delayed primary closure. Traumatic wounds are generally contaminated or infected wounds, which are not suitable for primary closure. Contaminated and infected wounds can be converted to clean wounds and closed primarily through debridement and lavage, or they can be healed via secondary or tertiary intention.

The location of the wound is important to take into account because certain areas have physiological advantages or disadvantages that affect wound healing as well

---

Turner and McIlwraith's Techniques in Large Animal Surgery, 4th Edition. Dean A. Hendrickson and A. N. (Nickie) Baird.
© 2013 John Wiley & Sons, Inc. Published 2013 by John Wiley & Sons, Inc.

as anatomical structures. In horses, wounds on the body heal well via second intention, whereas wounds on the distal limb are prone to developing exuberant granulation tissue, hypertrophic scarring, and cell transformations.[1] Research has shown that the distal limb wound environment is very different from that of wounds on the body; profibrotic growth factor expression and fibroblast proliferation is prolonged, collagen synthesis is increased, myofibroblasts fail to organize as they do in bodily wounds, and collagen degradation is decreased.[2-7] These studies coincide with the in-vivo observations that wounds of the distal limbs exhibit persistent inflammation, increased retraction, retarded epithelialization, and decreased contraction, making healing difficult and frustrating in many cases.[5,8] The distal limb lacks the underlying musculature and vascular supply that the trunk has, which undoubtedly accounts for many of these physiological limitations of wound healing. Other anatomical considerations associated with the location of the wound include structure involvement, cosmetic importance, movement (wounds over joints vs. the trunk), and underlying bony prominences. All of these have implications for the wound's vascular supply; physiological factors associated with wound healing; and, subsequently, the best method of management for the wound.

Information from the client, such as the mechanism and time of injury and any prior treatment that may have been administered, is beneficial in determining the wound environment and identifying any underlying factors that might compromise healing. For example, many topical ointments and systemic treatments inhibit or retard wound healing. Shearing injuries, as opposed to crushing injuries, generally have a better surrounding vascular supply and are more amenable to closure. The initial care of traumatic wounds has a large impact on the outcome; therefore, it is beneficial to familiarize clients with first aid and the use of nonirritating cleansing solutions, sterile dressings, and pressure bandaging.

Wound Preparation

Because of the environment in which large animals reside, contamination may be so extensive that some trauma patients will require a complete hosing down, especially in the winter and spring when barnyards are muddy. In these cases, tap water is the only practical answer, although its application directly onto the wound should be minimized.

To prepare the wound itself, the edges of the wound should be clipped and, in most instances, shaved. An ample area around the wound should be clipped in case additional exposure to deeper parts of the wound is required. To prevent the introduction of hair into the wound, a sterile water-soluble lubricating gel such as K–Y can be used to protect the wound. Once the wound is clipped, the gel can be rinsed off with sterile saline or water.

Wound cleaning should be minimally traumatic, and the agents used should be relatively noncytotoxic. The cleansing agent can be delivered by gravity or by low pressure with the aid of a bulb syringe. Wounds can be cleaned by scrubbing with woven or nonwoven gauze, or by lavage. Scrubbing causes significant mechanical trauma to the wound, so it is important to weigh the benefits of this method against the trauma it causes to the wound bed. High-pressure lavage units are more effective in removing bacteria than conventional techniques; they do not, as it was once believed, force bacteria deeper into the wound or cause significant tissue injury.[9] They can be equally traumatic, though, if caution is not used to maintain the pressure below 15 pounds per square inch (psi). To attain pressure below 15 psi, it has been shown that a 35-ml syringe can be used with a 25-, 21-, and 19-gauge needle. When the size of the syringe is decreased to 6 or 12 ml, the pressure exceeds 15 psi. Low-pressure lavages can be achieved by punching holes in the top of a saline bottle with a 16-gauge needle. Normal or isotonic saline is an effective agent for mildly contaminated wounds and can be used in a lavage or as a cleaner. Tap water will suffice for grossly contaminated wounds, although it is hypotonic and causes edema of the tissues. The wound microenvironment is usually acidic, so a final rinse with physiological sodium bicarbonate following wound cleaning has been recommended in an effort to restore the tissue to normal pH.[10] This may help ensure the maximal efficacy of topical antibiotics and the host's local immune responses.

Antiseptic agents are used for skin preparation, wound cleaning, and lavage, but they are not effective against bacteria deep in the wound tissue and most are cytotoxic. Their use is best reserved for skin surrounding the wound; and, in some cases, antiseptic agents are indicated to remove necrotic debris or tissue from the wound. Povidone-iodine scrub and chlorhexidine can be used on periwound tissue, whereas strong antiseptics such as hydrogen peroxide, acetic acid, and Dakin's solution are reserved only for grossly contaminated wounds. A 0.05% solution of chlorhexidine gluconate and a 1% povidone-iodine solution are recommended because they have been shown to be less cytotoxic than other.[10,11] Hydrogen peroxide (3% solution) can be useful for its effervescent action, which can lift debris from the wound, but is not very bactericidal and is relatively cytotoxic.[10] Soap solutions should also be avoided because they are irritating to the tissues. If contamination of the wound is massive, however, the advantages gained by the action of the soap may outweigh the disadvantage of irritated tissues. Newer surfactant-based wound cleansers have been shown to be very effective in mildly contaminated wounds.

Wound Exploration

Traumatic wounds should always be thoroughly explored to rule out the possibility of a foreign body. A foreign body left undetected in a wound reduces the number of organisms needed for infection to start, inhibits or prolongs wound healing, and can result in a poor cosmetic outcome. Depending on the temperament of the horse, chemical restraint may be necessary. For most traumatic wounds where there may be significant blood loss, tranquilizers should be avoided because of their vasodilation effects, which may enhance hypovolemia or produce shock.[12] Xylazine and detomidine are recommended to allow basic evaluation of the wound. Morphine or butorphanol may be added to the injection if increased analgesia is required.[12] Direct infiltration of the wound with a local anesthetic along its edges should be avoided if possible. This method of desensitizing the wound drives contamination deeper into the wound and may even open up new tissue planes; therefore, the use of regional analgesia is preferable. General anesthesia is indicated if the injury is so extensive that a local anesthetic is impractical or if the animal is too fractious. It is also indicated if extensive debridement and cast application are to be performed. The reader is referred to Chapter 2, "Anesthesia and Fluid Therapy," for details on anesthesia and restraint.

Wound exploration can be accomplished via manual palpation of the area, surgical exploration, ultrasound, and radiography. Contrast agents can be useful for identifying and following draining tracts to their source. When exploring wounds that might involve synovial structures, thorax, or abdomen, it is crucial that the practitioner use strict aseptic technique. If it is suspected that the wound may communicate with a synovial structure, a needle may be inserted into the synovial cavity at a distant site and fluid withdrawn for cytology and culture and sensitivity testing. Sterile saline should be injected into the cavity to see whether it communicates with the wound and determine whether the joint capsule or tendon sheath has indeed been penetrated.

Excision and Debridement of the Wound

In some instances, contaminated and infected traumatic wounds can be converted to clean wounds through debridement of the wound. Debridement promotes contraction and epithelialization in a wound and is used to remove necrotic tissue and foreign material, reduce bacterial numbers that potentiate infection, and excise excess granulation tissue to facilitate closure. Horses are particularly susceptible to developing exuberant granulation tissue in wounds of the distal limb. Debridement can be accomplished by a number of ways, including mechanical, chemical, and natural methods. Mechanical methods such as sharp excision, application of wet-to-dry and dry-to-dry dressings, hydrotherapy, and scrubbing of the wound are common in equine practice. They should be used sparingly as the tissue that is left behind is generally traumatized and often leads to more necrotic tissue. Sharp excision using either a scalpel or tissue scissors is the least traumatic to the tissue that is left behind and should be used most frequently. Dead tissue (fascia, adipose tissue,

muscle) should be selectively excised from the wound, as well as small, detached fragments of bone, contaminated skin edges, and edematous tissue. If possible, nerves, blood vessels, and tendons that appear viable should be left. If the wound is heavily contaminated, an initial preparation and debridement may be followed by a second preparation and debridement, with a change of gloves and instruments.

Antimicrobial Therapy

Antimicrobial therapy is indicated to reduce the bacterial load in traumatic wounds, especially those on the distal limb where the degree of contamination is usually high and anatomical factors impede local immune defenses. Disadvantages to their use, however, include superinfection, adverse reactions in the patient, and bacterial resistance. The practitioner should consider the location and type of wound, tissue involved, and level of structure involvement when determining whether antimicrobial therapy is necessary for a wound and the most appropriate regime.[10] Tetanus prophylaxis is always indicated in the horse.

The use of topical antibiotics or antibacterial agents has been controversial. Exudate on the wound can prevent effective contact of the agent with the microorganisms, and many topical antibacterial agents can inhibit wound healing. However, there is evidence that topical antibiotics, when used correctly, can be effective at reducing bacterial numbers in wounds. Topical antibiotics should not be applied longer than 2 weeks.

A wound culture and sensitivity test will establish which organism(s) are infecting the wound and, in conjunction with the appearance of the wound and response from the horse, will allow the practitioner to ascertain whether antimicrobial therapy is necessary. Gram-negative aerobic enteric species, anaerobic bacteria, *Staphylococcus aureus*, and *Streptococcus pyogenes* are the most common organisms found in traumatic wounds.[10] Quantitative bacteriology can also be used to determine the necessity of antimicrobial therapy. Wound healing may not be adversely affected by bacteria if there are fewer than 10^5 organisms per gram of tissue. If a foreign body exists in the wound, the level of bacteria is decreased to 10^4 organisms per gram of tissue.

Systemic antibiotics are used often during the treatment of grossly contaminated traumatic wounds in large animals. To be effective, antibiotic administration needs to be initiated as soon as possible, and adequate dosage levels need to be maintained. Systemic antibiotics should not be applied topically to reduce the risk of bacterial resistance.

Other Therapies

Other than antibiotics and tetanus prophylaxis, the judicious use of nonsteroidal, antiinflammatory drugs should be considered. Drugs such as phenylbutazone are often indicated, especially for horses. Unlike high dosages of corticosteroids, these drugs have little to no effect on the course of wound healing. They diminish pain from inflammation, improve the overall well being of the horse, encourage ambulation, and thereby stimulate circulation, especially in the limbs. Corticosteroids are not usually used in the treatment of traumatic wounds unless the surgeon is treating a separate problem.

Methods of Closure and Healing

Primary Closure

Appropriate Wounds

Primary wound closure is suitable only for wounds with sufficient surrounding tissue so that the skin edges can be approximated with minimal tension. Wounds that are grossly contaminated or infected or that contain foreign material should not be closed primarily. Factors to consider are those discussed previously: the vascular supply to the wound, anatomical considerations, wound characteristics, and degree of contamination. For example, a wound on the head may heal with first intention even after a 24-hour delay, whereas a wound on the distal limb may not respond to primary closure after several hours.

Suturing Traumatic Wounds

An important factor relating to whether a wound can be closed primarily is the tension that is created by approximating the skin edges. The wound needs to be closed without undue tension. It is preferable to leave some of the wound edges apart rather than to apply sutures under tension, because those sutures will produce ischemia of the wound edges and a larger defect than before. Tension-relieving suture patterns, such as the vertical and horizontal mattress patterns, may be used in combination with stents to minimize local ischemia in the wound edges. In the skin edges themselves, the author prefers to use the near-far-far-near pattern (see Chapter 6, "Suture Patterns").

Dead space should be closed whenever possible; this can be accomplished by deep closure with absorbable suture material or by using a pattern that will pull the skin down onto the defect. Braided, nonabsorbable synthetic materials should be avoided in the deeper layers. If used in the face of contamination, they can become infected and harbor this infection until they are removed by the surgeon or extruded by the animal. Synthetic absorbables, such as polyglyconate (Maxon), glycomer 631 (Caprosyn), and lactomer 9-1 (Polysorb) (see Chapter 4, "Suture Materials and Needles"), are useful for this purpose; if infection does result, they will maintain tensile strength longer than a material such as chromic gut. Noncapillary, nonreactive synthetic material, such as nylon or polypropylene, should be used for tension-relieving sutures that

can be applied to the wound edges. Use sutures that are just large enough to hold the tissue together to reduce the amount of foreign material in the wound.

Drains are indicated in the treatment of traumatic wounds in which unobliterated dead space or the likelihood of fluid accumulation exists. The use of drains is detailed later in this chapter.

Delayed Primary Closure

Appropriate Wounds

Delayed primary closure is used for wounds that cannot be closed immediately due to excessive swelling or contamination. It is often appropriate for distal limb wounds in the horse to reduce the healing time and achieve a greater cosmetic outcome. The wound is allowed to heal to a certain point by secondary intention. Excess granulation tissue may be allowed to form so that the skin expands over the defect. Following sharp excision of the granulation tissue, there is adequate skin to close the wound without excessive tension.

Secondary-Intention Healing

Appropriate Wounds

Wounds that are grossly contaminated, have extensive tissue loss, or contain a significant amount of debris or necrotic tissue should be treated via second intention. Wounds that are on the body heal well and are cosmetically satisfactory, by secondary intention. However, distal limb wounds in horses are not always suitable for second-intention healing because they are particularly prone to developing excessive granulation tissue, hypertrophic scarring, and cell transformations.

Moist Wound Healing

A moist wound environment is now known to produce the most optimal environment for wound healing. Moist wound healing allows the exudate to remain in contact with the wound to enhance the host's immune response and speed healing. Wound fluid contains enzymes, growth factors, and various chemokines and cytokines that promote the influx of phagocytic cells and leukocytes to the wound for natural debridement of necrotic tissue and debris. Growth factors and cytokines also stimulate fibroblasts, epithelial cells, and angiogenesis, promoting the growth of new tissue.[13]

During second-intention healing, the goal is to maintain a moist wound environment without letting the wound exudate become so abundant that the periwound tissue is macerated. Recent advances in veterinary wound care products have made it possible to adapt the dressing and bandage regime to best suit the needs of the wound at various stages in the healing process.

Wound healing by this process needs constant attention if one wants to obtain the best functional and cosmetic results. Although the wound is "granulating in," it should receive regular cleansing with a minimally toxic surfactant-based wound cleanser. The intact skin that is ventral to the wound should be protected from serum scald with a bland ointment, such as petroleum jelly. Parenteral antibiotics are used only in the initial stages of healing, unless signs of diffuse infection develop.

Other Considerations

For wounds on the distal limb that are healed by secondary intention, excessive granulation tissue ("proud flesh") can become a major problem. Prevention consists of avoiding irritating and oil-based ointments, minimizing movement, and maintaining the wound under a pressure bandage or cast. If excess granulation tissue exists, it must be removed until it approximates the level of the surrounding skin; otherwise, the migration of epithelium will be severely retarded. Excision of granulation tissue with a sharp scalpel, while being careful not to disrupt the advancing epithelium at the wound edge, is the treatment of choice. Caustics and astringents are still popular, but their action is not selective, and they remove the delicate epithelium along with the granulation tissue.

If bone or tendon is exposed, as it often is in traumatic wounds of large animals, it must be covered by granulation tissue before epithelium covers the defect. Sequestration of bone usually results if the periosteum has become dried or if the initial injury has chipped off a piece of bone. As soon as it is identified, the sequestrum should be removed; this may mean incising through the already-formed bed of granulation tissue. Exposed bone should be covered with moist soft tissues or a moistened calcium alginate dressing as soon as possible.[13] Skin grafting is indicated in wounds in which a large defect exists or slow skin healing is anticipated. This is discussed in detail in Chapter 8, "Reconstructive Surgery of Wounds."

Wound Care and Closure Techniques

Prior to closure, the wound is managed as described in the previous section on second-intention healing. The wound should be cleansed, debrided if necessary, and managed with appropriate dressings. After a healthy wound bed has been established and if the edges may be approximated without undue tension, the wound is prepared to be sutured. The wound edges should be sharply excised to freshen the wound and should be undermined to facilitate closure. Debridement of the most superficial layers of granulation tissue covering the wound is always indicated because it dramatically reduces the bacterial load and the risk of infection. However, overzealous debridement and undermining will compromise the blood supply to the wound, potentially causing local ischemic necrosis, and can lead to incisional dehiscence. The

wound is sutured the same as by primary intention. Dead space and tension should be minimized as much as possible, and drains may be indicated.

Use of Drains

Indications

The basic purpose of drainage is to facilitate healing by obliterating dead space or by removing unwanted material from a particular location. The simplest method of wound drainage is the open technique, in which the skin is left unsutured. This technique is commonly used in large animal surgery when a primary closure cannot be performed.

When a primary closure is performed and drainage remote from the incision is desired, some form of artificial drainage is necessary. Artificial drains may be classified as either *passive* or *active*. Passive drains, such as the Penrose drain, rely on gravity and capillary action to remove fluid, whereas active drains are closed-suction systems that remove fluid by negative pressure.

The indications for drainage cannot be sharply defined and indeed are controversial. Drains are beneficial in postoperative situations in which seroma formation is a potential problem or when the complete obliteration of dead space is not possible, which can occur after the internal fixation of fractures, for example. Contaminated wounds, especially those involving the thoracic and peritoneal cavities, or instances where infection or contamination of these cavities is a potential problem, are common indications for drainage as well. However, the previous philosophy of "when in doubt put a drain in" has yielded to a more cautious approach, with a careful analysis of the benefits and disadvantages. Drains should never be used to make up for poor surgical technique.

The widespread use of drains has given rise to complications in both human and veterinary patients. In a recent review of abdominal drains post laparoscopic cholecystectomy, elective use of drains increased wound infection rates and delayed hospital discharge.[14] Both latex (Penrose) and Silastic drains potentiate infection as foreign material. Many valid indications for the use of drains still exist, but one should be more critical of the type of drain used, the number of times it is used, the duration of use, and how it is used. With regard to any drain, one should pay careful attention to aseptic technique at the time of placement and the postoperative management of the drains. Drainage should not be used as a substitute for meticulous debridement or careful closure of a wound.

Passive Drains

Passive drains, such as Penrose and bandage drains, are indicated for wounds that cannot be closed without creating subcutaneous dead space. At present, the latex Penrose drains and the perforated tube drains of plastic or Silastic (Redi-Vacette Perforated Tubing) are the most commonly used drains in large animal surgery. The Penrose drain is a thin, latex tube usually 7–12 mm in diameter (2.5-cm diameter drains are also available); it functions by capillary action and gravity flow, with drainage occurring around the drain rather than through the lumen. Fenestration of these drains for passive drainage is contraindicated, because it decreases the surface area of the drain and increases the chance of tearing the drain during removal.

The advantages to using Penrose drains are their ease of insertion and their need for less maintenance than suction drains. In many cases, the use of a Penrose drain in a wound is sufficient to minimize the postoperative accumulation of blood or fluid. Penrose drains become walled off from the wound rapidly, however, with a decrease in their efficacy; and they also predispose the depths of the wound to retrograde infection from airborne and skin contamination. Additionally, Penrose drains are not indicated for drainage of the peritoneal cavity because they may potentiate infection and should be restricted to wounds and the obliteration of subcutaneous dead space.

In a typical wound closure, the drain is inserted with the end exiting in the most dependent location remote from the incision, and the incision is sutured. The dependent end of the drain is sutured to the skin. The stab incision through which the drain exits should be of sufficient size to allow drainage to occur around it. The drain should be inserted so that only one end emerges from the wound, and the deep end of the drain is retained within the wound by a suture that can be removed later (Figure 7.1). A dependent region for the emergence of at least one end of the drain should be selected. The drain should not be brought out through the primary incision, because it encourages drainage through the incision. Daily cleansing of the drain, and bandage covering if possible, should be performed to minimize the occurrence of retrograde infection. In addition, retrograde infection is time related, and the drain should be removed as soon as it is considered nonfunctional. The drain itself acts as a foreign body, and a daily drainage of fewer than 50 ml/day may be purely drain induced.[15]

Use of Penrose Drains to Treat Hygromas

Penrose drains can be used effectively in the treatment of hygromas in which fluid removal by drains can facilitate obliteration of the cavity by granulation tissue. It is also believed that the foreign-body effect of the drains may be advantageous in stimulating a granulation response in these cases. Stab incisions are made dorsally and ventrally into the hygroma, using aseptic technique. Fibrin and debris within the cavity are removed, and the drains are inserted (Figure 7.2). The drains may be left in place 10 days to 2 weeks.

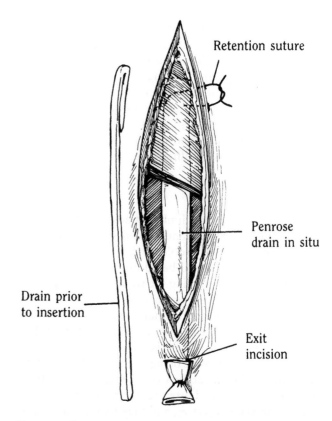

Fig. 7.1.   Penrose drain with one end emerging from wound. The retention suture can be removed later and the drain extracted from the exit incision.

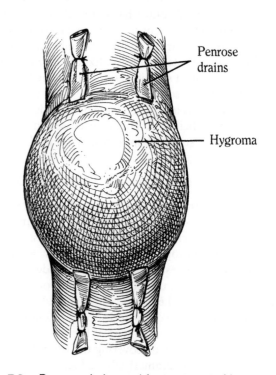

Fig. 7.2.   Penrose drain used for treatment of hygroma.

Active Drains

Active drains are usually indicated only for deep traumatic wounds when more than overflow drainage is necessary. When these drains can be managed appropriately and it is possible to maintain the negative pressure apparatus on the animal, the use of sealed, continuous suction drainage is definitely superior to the use of Penrose drains.[16,17] These drains should not be used as substitutes for hemostatic control and atraumatic technique during surgery, however.

Fenestrated Tube Drain

A fenestrated tube drain is laid in the wound and exited through the skin by using a trocar (Figure 7.3A) to form a tight seal around the drain. Constant suction can then be applied externally, and fluid can be evacuated from a deep tissue space (Figure 7.3B). It is important that wound closure be airtight. Various evacuators are available commercially, but a simple and economical technique is the use of a syringe, as illustrated in Figure 7.3. The three-way stopcock is used to reduce further the possibility of retrograde infection when the syringe is emptied and suction is reapplied. The drains are heparinized prior to insertion; however, the suction pulls tissue into the holes in the drain, and clogging eventually results. The drains are generally effective long enough to eliminate the acute accumulation of serum following orthopedic surgery and for other procedures in which the dead space cannot be completely obliterated.[16]

Peritoneal Drainage

Peritoneal drainage following laparotomy in large animals can be indicated in instances such as peritonitis, intra-abdominal abscesses, and hemorrhage and to remove leakage from anastomosis or lavage fluid following equine abdominal surgery.[18,19] Active abdominal drainage and lavage has been successfully used in horses to treat peritonitis and to prevent septic peritonitis and abdominal adhesions following intestinal surgery or abdominal contamination.[18,19] When used in conjunction with lavage, abdominal drainage may reduce the incidence of abdominal adhesions by removing excess fibrin and inflammatory cells and may facilitate the mechanical separation of bowels.[18,19]

The authors perform peritoneal drainage for a few hours after equine abdominal surgery if any amount of lavage fluid has been left in the abdomen at closure. In this case, a centrally fenestrated tube drain is placed with the nonfenestrated ends and exits cranially and caudally. The drain is removed within 12 hours. With peritoneal drainage of longer duration, the fenestrations of a tube drain will become clogged by fibrin, adhering omentum, or viscera. The ideal method for peritoneal drainage is the use of a sump-Penrose combination. A sump drain is a double-lumen, fenestrated tube drain that incorporates a smaller air vent. The air vent allows air to enter the drained region with the object of displacing fluid into the drain. (An example of this is the Shirley wound drain.) By placing such a drain within a Penrose drain (Figure 7.4), occlusion of the fenestrations of the central tube drain is delayed, and drainage efficiency is increased.

Sophisticated, intra-abdominal sump drains, which also allow sterile irrigation, have been developed for man. Whenever air or fluid ingress systems are used, careful technique is mandatory to prevent the introduction of infection. Bacterial filters should be used with the air channel of sump drains. If any ingress flushing system is to be combined with drainage, it is recommended that the flushing or irrigation be performed through a separate tube positioned through a separate entry site.

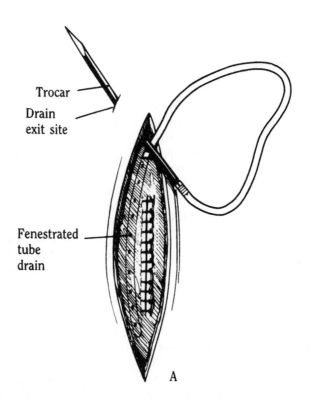

Trocar

Drain
exit site

Fenestrated
tube
drain

A

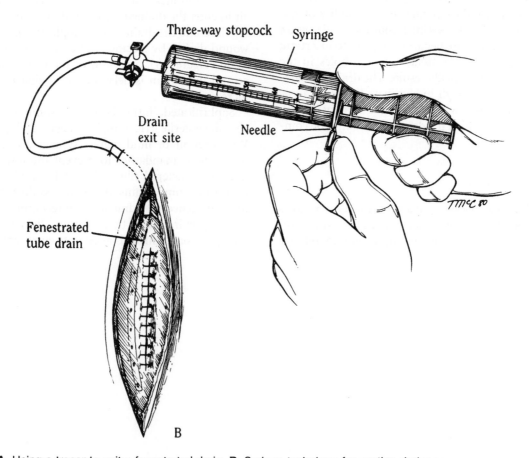

Three-way stopcock   Syringe

Drain
exit site

Needle

Fenestrated
tube drain

B

Fig. 7.3.   **A.** Using a trocar to exit a fenestrated drain. **B.** Syringe technique for suction drainage.

Fig. 7.4.   Sump-Penrose drain combination.

References

1. Knottenbelt, D.C. Equine wound management: Are there significant differences in healing at different sites on the body? *Vet. Dermatol.*, 8:273–290, 1997.

2. Schwartz, A.J., Wilson, D.A., Keegan, K.G., Ganjam, V.K., Sun, Y., Weber, K.T., and Zhang, J. Factors regulating collagen synthesis and degradation during second-intention healing of wounds in the thoracic region and the distal aspect of the forelimb of horses. *Am. J. Vet. Res.*, 63:1564–1570, 2002.

3. Theoret, C.L., Barber, S.M., Moyana, T.N., and Gordon, J.R. Expression of transforming growth factor beta (1), beta (2), beta (3), and basic fibroblast growth factor in full-thickness skin wounds of equine limbs and thorax. *Vet. Surg.*, 30:269–277, 2001.

4. Wilmink, J.M., Nederbragt, H., Van Weeren, P.R., Stolk, P.W.T., and Barneveld, A. Differences in wound contraction between

horses and ponies: The in vitro contraction capacity of fibroblasts. *Eq. Vet. J.*, 33:499–505, 2001.

5. Wilmink, J.M., Stolk, P.W.T., Van Weeren, P.R., and Barneveld, A. Differences in second intention wound healing between horses and ponies: Macroscopic aspects. *Eq. Vet. J.*, 31:53–60, 1999.

6. Wilmink, J.M., Van Weeren, P.R., Stolk, P.W.T., Van Mil, F.N., and Barneveld, A. Differences in second intention wound healing between horses and ponies: Histological aspects. *Eq. Vet. J.*, 31:61–67, 1999.

7. Wilmink, J.M., and Van Weeren, P.R. Second-intention repair in the horse and pony and management of exuberant granulation tissue. *Vet. Clin. Eq.*, 21:15–32, 2005.

8. Cochrane, C.A., Pain, R., and Knottenbelt, D.C. In-vitro wound contraction in the horse: Differences between body and limb wounds. *Wounds*, 15:175–181, 2003.

9. Bahrs, C., Schnabel, M., Frank, T., Zapf, C., Mutters, R., and von Garrel, T. Lavage of contaminated surfaces: An in vitro evaluation of the effectiveness of different systems. *J Surg. Res.*, 112:26–30, 2003.

10. Brumbaugh, G.W. Use of antimicrobials in wound management. *Vet. Clin. Eq.*, 21:63–75, 2005.

11. Van den Boom, R., Wilmink, J.M., O'Kane, S., Wood, J., and Ferguson, M.W. Transforming growth factor-β levels during second intention healing are related to the different course of wound contraction in horses and ponies. *Wound Rep. Regen.*, 10:188–194, 2002.

12. Wilson, D.A. Principles of early wound management. *Vet. Clin. Eq.*, 21:45–62, 2005.

13. Hendrickson, D.A. Second intention wound healing. *In* Wound Care Management for the Equine Practitioner. Jackson, WY, Teton NewMedia, 2004, pp. 100–139.

14. Gurusamy, K.S., Samraj, K., Mullerat, P., and Davidson, B.R. Routine abdominal drainage for uncomplicated laparoscopic cholecystectomy. *Cochrane Database Syst. Rev.*, (17):CD006004, 2007.

15. Golovsky, D., and Connolly, W.B. Observations on wound drainage with a review of the literature. *Med. J. Aust.*, 1:289, 1976.

16. Parker, M.J., Livingstone, V., Clifton, R., and McKee, A. Closed suction surgical wound drainage after orthopaedic surgery. *Cochrane Database Syst. Rev.*, (18):CD001825, 2007.

17. Reid, R.R., and Dumanian, G.A. A minimalist approach to the care of the indwelling closed suction drain: A prospective analysis of local wound complications. *Ann Plast. Surg.*, 51:575–578, 2003.

18. Hague, B.A., Honnas, C.M., Berridge, B.R., and Easter, J.L. Evaluation of postoperative peritoneal lavage in standing horses for prevention of experimentally induced abdominal adhesions. *Vet. Surg.*, 27:122–126, 1998.

19. Nieto, J.E., Snyder, J.R., Vatistas, N.J., Spier, S.J., and Hoogmoed, L.V. Use of an active intra-abdominal drain in 67 horses. *Vet. Surg.*, 32:1–7, 2003.

Chapter 8

RECONSTRUCTIVE SURGERY OF WOUNDS

Dean A. Hendrickson, DVM, MS, DACVS

Objectives

1. Provide an overview of some reconstructive procedures that are used to alleviate tension in large wounds, facilitate primary closure, or increase the cosmetic outcome of the wound.
2. Describe how to use undermining and tension relief incisions to close large wounds that cannot be closed primarily without creating excessive tension.
3. Describe the indications for Z-plasty and its application as a relaxation procedure for elliptical defects and as a scar revision procedure.
4. Describe techniques of skin grafting and full-thickness sliding skin flap procedures.

Elliptical Excision Undermining for Repair of an Elongated Defect

In some cases an elongated defect will be too wide for its edges to be sutured without excess tension. Using scissors, the surgeon undermines the adjacent skin in an elliptical fashion using a combination of sharp and blunt dissection (Figure 8.1A). Blunt dissection is best as it maintains the most blood supply to the edge of the incision. The mobilized skin flaps can then be moved toward each other to allow a primary closure (Figure 8.1B). The use of tension sutures in addition to the row of simple interrupted sutures may be indicated.

Wound Closure Using Tension-Relieving Incisions

Also known as the *mesh expansion technique*, this procedure utilizes small, tension-relieving skin incisions made adjacent to the wound to facilitate wound closure or, at least, to decrease the healing time for the primary defect.[1,2].

The skin adjacent to the defect is undermined to a depth according to the vascular supply of the location of the wound.[1] Wounds on the trunk should be undermined to the panniculus muscle to retain the cutaneous vasculature, whereas wounds on the distal limb should be undermined along the plane between the subcutaneous tissue and deep fascia.[1] Following undermining, a series of stab incisions is made parallel to and approximately 1 cm from the skin edge (Figure 8.2A). Three rows of stab incisions are made on each side of the wound in a staggered fashion, with the adjacent rows approximately 1 cm apart (Figure 8.2A). The size of the stab incisions varies. In the initial description of the technique, the use of 10-mm stab incisions allowed sufficient expansion in fresh wounds and resulted in more rapid healing than when 7-mm tension-relieving incisions were used. In older wounds, however, with fibrosis and thickening of the surrounding skin, longer incisions (approximately 15 mm) are recommended. When the stab incisions have been made, the original wound edges are drawn into apposition and are sutured (Figure 8.2B). Tension relieving sutures such as the near-far-far-near pattern using large-diameter sutures have been recommended for closure.[1] It can be helpful to approximate the wound edges first to ensure that the relief incisions are made where the most tension is present.

Wounds are managed postoperatively with bandaging or casting, depending on the individual case. The need for adequate postoperative support of the suture line should be recognized. Based on previous work, undermining can be performed for at least 4 cm on either side of the wound,

Turner and McIlwraith's Techniques in Large Animal Surgery, 4th Edition. Dean A. Hendrickson and A. N. (Nickie) Baird.
© 2013 John Wiley & Sons, Inc. Published 2013 by John Wiley & Sons, Inc.

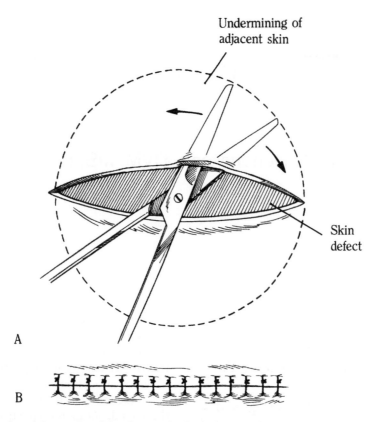

Undermining of adjacent skin

Skin defect

A

B

Fig. 8.1. **A** and **B.** Elliptical excision undermining for repair of an elongated defect.

A

B

Fig. 8.2. **A** and **B.** Use of tension-relieving incisions to facilitate wound closure.

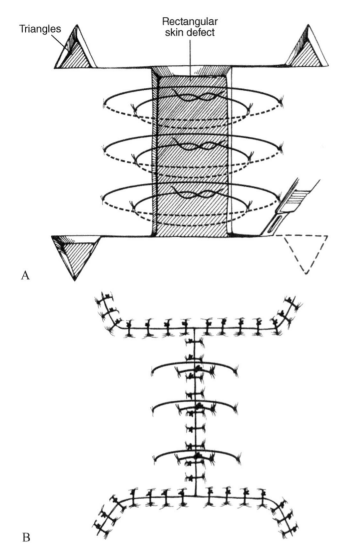

Fig. 8.3. **A** and **B.** Sliding H-flap.

without detrimental effects.[3] The release of blood and exudate through the stab incisions may facilitate the success of the technique by aiding revascularization and preventing hematoma and seroma formation.

Sliding H-Flap

This technique is used for the repair of rectangular or square defects. As illustrated in Figure 8.3A, two flaps are generally created; however, if skin is not available on both sides, half of the H-plasty may be used.[4] The actual defect serves as the crossbridge of the letter *H*, and two arms are created (Figure 8.3A). Triangles are cut at either end of each arm to prevent puckering of the skin when the flaps within the H are undermined and are slid together (Figure 8.3A). Near-far-far-near, or *vertical mattress sutures*, are preplaced in the undermined flaps to act as tension sutures. The two flaps are then brought together and are sutured in a simple interrupted pattern (Figure 8.3B). When performed correctly, sliding the flaps together

closes the triangular defects. These incision lines are also sutured in a simple interrupted pattern (Figure 8.3B).

Z-Plasty

Z-plasty has two major indications. It may be used as a relaxation procedure for elliptical defects, and it may be used for scar revision of the palpebra when scar formation has produced acquired ectropion. It is helpful to draw the "Z" using a sterile pen prior to the beginning of the procedure to confirm the correct area of relaxation.[5]

The use of Z-plasty as a relaxation procedure for elliptical incisions is illustrated in Figure 8.4. A Z-incision is made adjacent to the elliptical defect (Figure 8.4A). The central incision of the Z (AB) should be perpendicular to the elliptical defect and centered over the area of greatest tension. The two triangles created by the incision should be equilateral, that is, having angles of 60°. The triangles are undermined to create two skin flaps. These skin flaps are then interchanged (Figure 8.4B), and they are sutured in place (Figure 8.4C). The principle behind this technique is that the interchange of the two flaps lengthens the original line (AB) by 50%.

In the second situation, illustrated in Figure 8.5, a linear scar (AB) has excessive tension along its longitudinal axis, which results in an acquired ectropion of the upper eyelid (Figure 8.5A). If a Z-plasty is performed in the previous manner, with AB as the central arm of the Z, tension will be relieved, and the upper eyelid will be relaxed (Figure 8.5B).

Removal of Excessive Scar Tissue

A cross section of a typical situation in which exuberant granulation tissue of scar tissue coexists with incomplete skin closure is illustrated in Figure 8.6A. A dotted line indicates the incision for removal of the excess tissue, which is removed with sharp dissection (Figure 8.6B); this allows the primary closure of the skin over the dead space (Figure 8.6C). Placement of a subcutaneous drain is appropriate in this situation.

Skin Grafting

Skin grafting is indicated for wounds that are not amenable to closure or will not yield satisfactory healing via secondary intention. In equine practice, skin grafting is most beneficial in healing wounds with extensive tissue loss or in areas of cosmetic importance, locations where wound healing is impaired such as the distal limb, or where wound contracture could interfere with function, such as near the eye.

Several methods of free-skin grafting are available, including full- and split-thickness mesh grafts and sheet grafts.[6-9] Full-thickness grafts are comprised of the epidermis and dermis, whereas split-thickness grafts include only a portion of the dermis. Split-thickness grafts tend

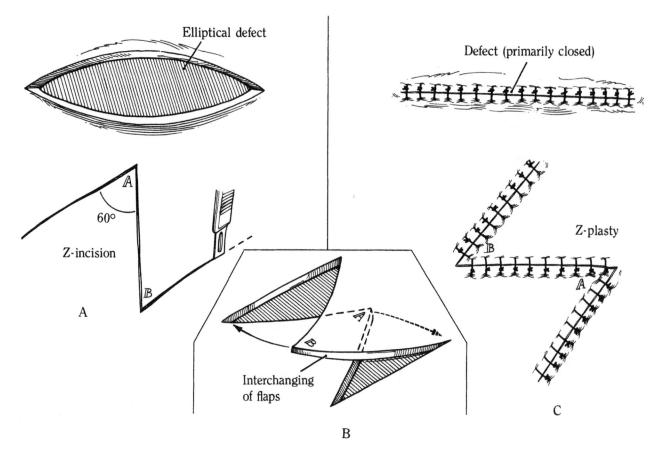

Fig. 8.4. **A–C.** Z-plasty as a relaxation procedure.

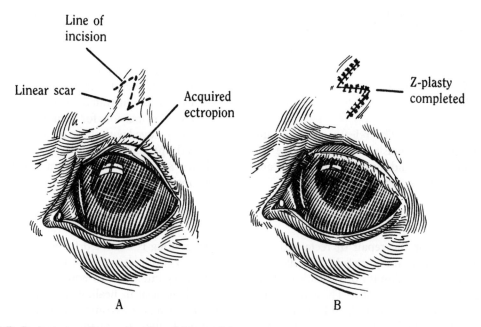

Fig. 8.5. **A** and **B.** Z-plasty to relieve ectropion of the eyelid.

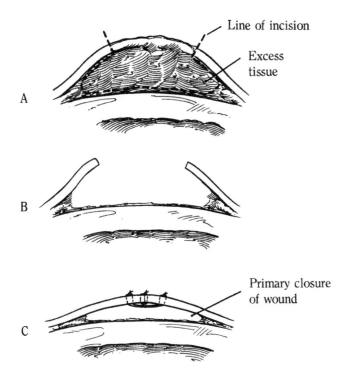

Line of incision

Excess tissue

A

B

Primary closure of wound

C

Fig. 8.6. Removal of excessive scar tissue (debulking) to allow primary closure of a wound.

to have better success than full-thickness grafts, but the procedure is complicated and requires additional equipment, such as a dermatone, and will not be discussed here. Meshed grafts, especially "Meek" grafts are considered superior to sheet grafts because of their higher tolerance for motion and less incidence of seroma formation.[9] Non-meshed grafts are rarely used in equine procedures, although sheet grafts can be effective on fresh wounds with no granulation tissue.[8] Pedicle grafting is not commonly used in the horse.

Split-thickness and full-thickness mesh expansion grafts have been shown to yield the most cosmetic healing and the quickest epithelialization rates in equine limb wounds. However, these procedures are often not practical for use in the field, require specialized tools and general anesthesia, and are limited to certain wounds. Pinch grafts, followed by punch grafts, have the slowest epithelialization rates and result in significantly less cosmetic healing than the mesh expansion grafts.[6,10] These wounds tend to heal with a cobblestone-like appearance and may have random hair growth patterns. However, the pinch- and punch-grafting techniques described here are the most economical options for the equine patient because they do not require anesthesia, can be performed in the field, and do not require special equipment. Even if the graft does not take, its presence seems to stimulate epithelialization from the periphery. However, prior to performing a pinch- or punch-grafting procedure, it is important to inform the client of the cosmetic outcome of these procedures, which may not be satisfactory for a show horse.

The last grafting procedure discussed in this section is the tunnel graft. It can be used in areas of high mobility, such as the limb, where other grafts may not take due to excessive movement. This procedure can be performed using strips of either full-thickness or split-thickness grafts. For the purpose of this book, the use of full-thickness grafts is described because they can be harvested in the field and do not require additional equipment.

Recipient Bed Preparation

To ensure acceptance of the graft, it is imperative that the recipient bed has a good blood supply and healthy tissue and that the area can be effectively immobilized. A splint may be indicated for wounds located near or on joints and can be incorporated into the bandage following the grafting procedure. Debridement of the recipient site prior to graft placement may also be necessary. Ideally, the granulation bed should be healthy, free of infection, and level with edges of the skin prior to the skin graft. If the bed is not ready to accept the graft, additional wound therapy should be performed prior to placing the graft. The most common reason for graft failure is an inappropriate bed of granulation tissue.

Pinch-Skin Grafting

Skin grafts may be harvested from multiple locations on the horse; however, for cosmetic reasons, they are usually taken from the ventral abdomen or beneath the mane on the neck. In the standing sedated horse, the graft donor site is usually the neck. The area is anesthetized by the subcutaneous administration of local analgesic solution in the shape of an inverted *L*. Because granulation tissue is devoid of nerves, analgesic infiltration of the recipient site is unnecessary. The recipient site is prepared without the use of antiseptic agents to minimize trauma to the granulation tissue bed. Lavage with saline or a surfactant-based wound cleanser followed by saline is most appropriate. The donor site is clipped and prepared as for aseptic surgery.

When both the wound and the donor site have been prepared, the author prefers to harvest the grafts from the donor site first by elevating small pinches of skin (7 mm × 7 mm) with a needle or forceps and excising the pinches of skin with a scalpel blade (Figure 8.7A). The excised pinches of skin are transferred to a gauze moistened with saline solution or preferably blood. The recipient bed is prepared by making a series of small, shallow "pockets" in the granulation tissue bed with a number 15 or 11 scalpel blade. The openings of the pockets should point proximally while the deepest end of the pocket is most distal. The pockets should be made in parallel rows 1–2 mm below the surface of the wound (Figure 8.7B), with approximately 1 cm between each pocket over the whole granulation bed (Figure 8.7C). When all the pockets have been made, it is beneficial to apply pressure to the

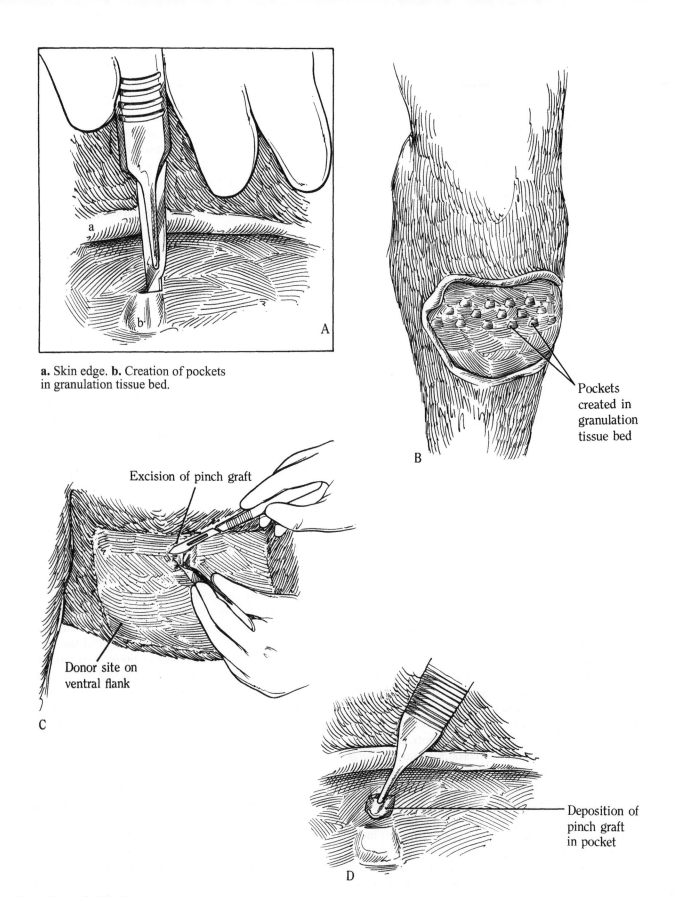

a. Skin edge. **b.** Creation of pockets in granulation tissue bed.

Pockets created in granulation tissue bed

Excision of pinch graft

Donor site on ventral flank

Deposition of pinch graft in pocket

Fig. 8.7. **A–D.** Pinch-skin grafting.

wound for 3–4 minutes to reduce the hemorrhage from the newly created pockets in the granulation bed.

The pinches of skin are flattened as necessary and are inserted in each pocket of the granulation bed, just as one would insert a coin into a watch pocket (Figure 8.7D).[10] The graft is inserted with the epithelial side facing out. This procedure is repeated until all pockets have been filled. The wound is carefully dressed with a nonadherent foam dressing, ensuring that the grafts are not extruded from their pockets, and bandaged.

Punch-Skin Grafting

Punch-skin grafting is similar to pinch-skin grafting, except cylindrical plugs of skin are inserted into cylindrical holes in the granulation tissue.[11] The advantages to punch grafting parallel those of pinch grafting. Punch-skin grafting is preferred by some clinicians. The technique can be applied to a thinner granulation tissue bed than pinch grafts, which require a certain depth to create tissue pockets.[11] It is also believed that a more cosmetic result may be obtained.

The general principles of recipient and donor site preparation are the same as in pinch grafting. When the recipient site has been aseptically prepared, small circular holes are made in the granulating bed using a 6-mm biopsy punch (Figure 8.8A). These recipient holes are spaced about 7 mm apart in every direction over the entire surface of the wound. Blood clots forming in the recipient areas are removed prior to placement of the grafts or are prevented by filling the recipient holes with cotton swabs.[11]

Donor grafts are taken from beneath the mane or the ventrolateral abdominal area using an 8-mm biopsy punch (Figure 8.8B). The donor grafts are then placed one at a time into the recipient site (Figure 8.8C). The 8-mm donor grafts have a tendency to contract and therefore fit snugly into the 6-mm diameter recipient holes. The subcutaneous tissue should be removed from the plugs prior to insertion. A sterile nonadherent foam dressing is placed on the wound after surgery, and a bandage is applied.

Tunnel Grafting

In this procedure, strips of full-thickness grafts are placed inside tunnels that are created in the granulation tissue of the recipient bed (Figure 8.9). The strips can be excised by making parallel incisions into the subcutaneous tissue of the donor site, or they can be cut from a full-thickness sheet that is already harvested from the donor site, which is closed primarily following graft removal. The strips are generally 2–3 mm wide and should be slightly longer than the wound to facilitate suturing of the grafts at the end of each tunnel. A simple interrupted suture is used for securing the grafts in place. The granulation tissue of the recipient bed can be allowed to extend slightly over the level of the surrounding skin so that when the grafts are placed through the tunnels, which are excised approximately

5 mm below the surface of the granulation tissue surface, they are flush with surrounding skin. A cutting needle, flattened Kirschner wire with trocar point, a straight teat blade, or malleable alligator forceps can be used to form the tunnel in the granulation bed.[12] The tunnels should be formed 1–2 cm apart from each other to avoid potential disruption from adjacent tunnels where the graft may fail. Small forceps are used to pull the graft through the tunnel. An alternative method has been described that uses adhesive tape attached to the haired side of the graft to facilitate placement of the strip in the tunnel. The strip of graft and tape are threaded through the eye of a half-curved or straight cutting needle (10–2 cm), which is used to guide the strip through the tunnel with the haired side of the graft facing outward.[12] With this technique, multiple passes of the needle through the tunnel or smaller graft strips can be used when the wound exceeds the length of the needle. After 6–10 days, the granulation tissue should be excised from over the top of and between the grafts. Compared to pinch and punch grafting, tunnel grafting places a greater volume of skin into the wound without requiring additional specialized equipment.

Bandaging and Postgrafting Care

The author prefers to cover the grafted area with a semi-occlusive foam dressing secured by antimicrobial gauze. An elastic adhesive dressing can be used to maintain pressure over the graft site, although care must be taken to not impede blood supply to the area. A cast or pressure bandage is also applied to minimize movement. It is also recommended that the horse be confined to a box stall to ensure minimal movement at the surgical site. The first bandage should be left on for 1 week, and subsequent bandage changes should be performed as needed. Minimizing the amount of bandage changes will reduce displacement of the grafts and the amount of new bacteria introduced into the graft site. During bandage changes, any exudates on the graft site should be carefully wiped off with sterile, saline-soaked sponges, or preferably by using a surfactant based wound cleanser. The grafts can usually be identified in 2–3 weeks; failure to identify grafts at this time does not necessarily imply an unsuccessful result. As noted before, the procedure typically enhances the rate of epithelialization at the periphery of the wound and reduces healing time.

Random Pattern Flaps

In equine practice, random pattern flaps are used more commonly than axial patterns due to their superior skin perfusion and response to tension.[6,13] The suggested method of flap elevation is sharp dissection because research indicates that although it is more time consuming than other modalities, it yields the most satisfactory closure of the defect. Sharply dissected flaps are reported to have greater bursting strengths, less drainage

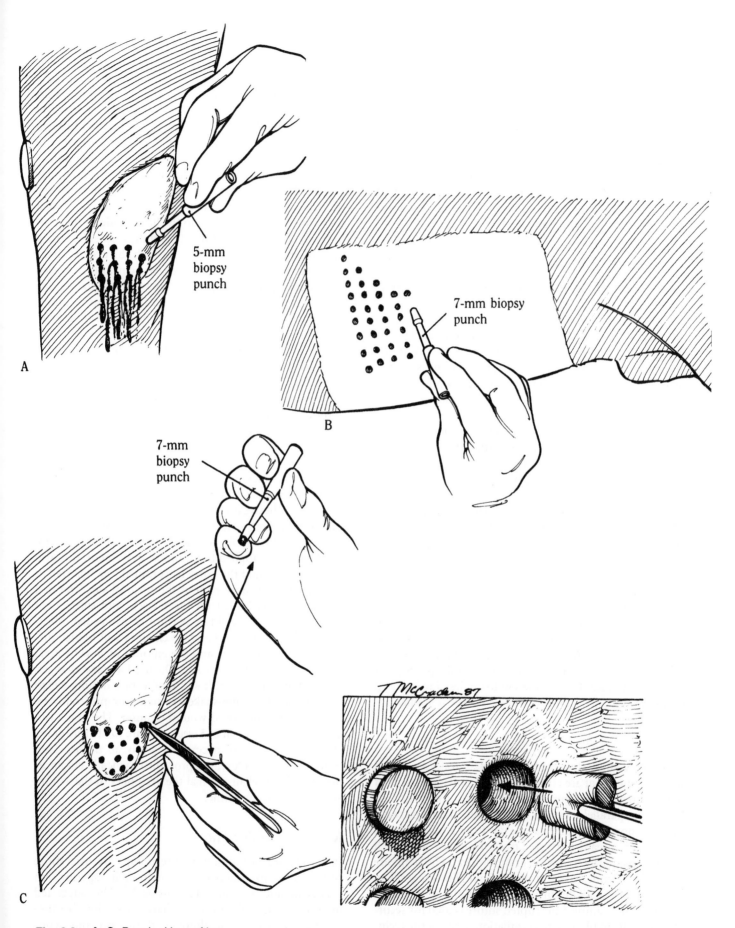

5-mm biopsy punch

7-mm biopsy punch

7-mm biopsy punch

A

B

C

Fig. 8.8. A–C. Punch-skin grafting.

Fig. 8.9. Tunnel grafting.

postoperatively, higher collagen content and fibroblast infiltration, and a decreased infiltration of polymorphonuclear leukocytes.[6,14]

References

1. Bailey, J.V. Repair of large skin defects on the limbs of horses. *Wien. Tierarztl. Mschr.*, 78:277–278, 280–282, 1991.

2. Beard, W.L., and Wilkie, D.A. Partial orbital rim resection, mesh skin expansion, and second intention healing combined with enucleation or exenteration for extensive periocular tumors in horses. *Vet. Ophthalmol.*, 5:23–28, 2002.

3. Bailey, J.V., and Jacobs, K.A.: The mesh expansion method of suturing wounds on the legs of horses. *Vet. Surg.*, 12:78, 1983.

4. Rose, V., Overstall, S., Moloney, D.M., and Powell, B.W. The H-flap: A useful flap for forehead reconstruction. *Br. J. Plast. Surg.*, 54:705–707, 2001.

5. Aasi, S.Z. Z-plasty made simple. 2011. Retrieved from *Dermatol. Res. Pract.* at http://www.ncbi.nlm.nih.gov/pmc/articles/PMC3123994/(accessedon3/6/2013.doi:10.1155/2010/982623

6. Bristol, D.G. Skin grafts and skin flaps in the horse. *Vet. Clin. Eq.*, 21:125–144, 2005.

7. Theoret, C.: Tissue engineering in wound repair: The three "R"s—repair, replace, regenerate. *Vet. Surg.*, 38:905–913, 2009.

8. Toth, F., Schumacher, J., Castro, F., and Perkins, J. Full-thickness skin grafting to cover equine wounds caused by laceration or tumor resection. *Vet. Surg.*, 39:708–714, 2010.

9. Wilmink, M.M., van den Boom, R., van Weeren, P.R., and Barneveld, A. The modified Meek technique as a novel method for skin grafting in horses: Evaluation of acceptance, wound contraction and closure in chronic wounds. *Equine Vet. J.*, 38:324–329, 2006.

10. French, D.A., and Fretz, P.B. Treatment of equine leg wounds using skin grafts: Thirty-five cases, 1975–1988. *Can. Vet. J.*, 31:761–765, 1990.

11. Stashak, T.S. Skin grafting in horses. *Vet. Clin. North Am. (Large Anim. Pract.*, 6:215, 1984.

12. Carson-Dunkerley, S.A., and Hanson, R.R. Equine skin grafting: Principles and field applications. *The Compendium*, 19:872–882, 1997.

13. Bristol, D.G.: The effect of tension on perfusion of axial and random pattern flaps in foals. *Vet. Surg.*, 21:223–227, 1992.

14. Gelman, C.L., Barroso, E.G., Britton, C.T., Haklin, M.F., and Staren, E.D.: The effects of lasers, electrocautery and sharp dissection on cutaneous flaps. *Plast. Reconstr. Surg.*, 94:829–833, 1994.

Chapter 9

EQUINE ORTHOPEDIC SURGERY

Dean A. Hendrickson, DVM, MS, DACVS

Objective

1. Discuss the indications for, techniques for, and complications of commonly used equine orthopedic surgical procedures, including the following:
   - Medial patellar desmotomy
   - Cunean tenectomy
   - Lateral digital extensor tenotomy
   - Inferior check ligament desmotomy
   - Superior check ligament desmotomy (after Bramlage)
   - Superficial digital flexor tenotomy
   - Deep digital flexor tenotomy
   - Sectioning of the palmar annular ligament of the fetlock
   - Palmar digital neurectomy
   - Amputation of the small metacarpal and metatarsal bones
   - Arthrotomy of the midcarpal joint
   - Arthrotomy of the fetlock joint

Medial Patellar Desmotomy

Indications

Upward fixation of the patella occurs when the patellar fibrocartilage and medial patellar ligament fix over the medial trochlear ridge of the femur, inhibiting flexion of the hock and stifle. Some predisposing factors are known, such as poor muscle tone and condition, hind limb conformation, stifle trauma, and hereditary factors.[1] An increased incidence of upward fixation of the patella is also seen in young horses and ponies, particularly Shetland ponies, and horses with straight hind limb conformation.[1,2] Good quality radiographs of the stifle joint are necessary to rule out osteochondritis dissecans, especially in young horses. This condition can mimic the signs of intermittent upward fixation of the patella and may be associated with straight limb conformation and distention of the femoropatellar joint as well.

Medial patellar ligament desmotomy should be considered a "last-resort" treatment for recurrent upward fixation of the patella. Depending on the duration and severity of the condition, many cases will respond to more conservative therapy. This is especially true in young horses that will improve after appropriate conditioning and development of quadriceps muscle tone through training. Medial patellar desmotomy induces thickening over the entire length of the medial patellar ligament after it heals, which ideally should allow the ligament to disengage from the notch on the medial ridge of the femoral trochlea and prevent locking. Counterirritants injected in and around the medial patellar ligament have also been used to treat more persistent cases with clinical success.[3]

Anesthesia and Surgical Preparation

This surgical procedure is performed with the animal standing. Depending on the temperament of the animal, tranquilization may be indicated. The area of the middle and medial patellar ligaments is clipped and surgically prepared. The tail is wrapped to avoid contamination of the surgical site. Two milliliters of local anesthetic are injected subcutaneously over the medial border of the middle patellar ligament. A 20-gauge, 1-inch needle is then inserted through this bleb, and the subcutaneous

Turner and McIlwraith's Techniques in Large Animal Surgery, 4th Edition. Dean A. Hendrickson and A. N. (Nickie) Baird.
© 2013 John Wiley & Sons, Inc. Published 2013 by John Wiley & Sons, Inc.

area around the distal part of the medial patellar ligament is infiltrated with local anesthetic.

Instrumentation

1. General surgery pack
2. Blunt-ended bistoury (tenotomy) knife
3. Curved Kelly forceps

Surgical Technique

A 1-cm incision is made over the medial border of the middle patellar ligament close to the attachment of the ligament to the tibial tuberosity. (The site of the skin incision in relation to the patellar ligaments is illustrated in Figure 9.1A.) Curved Kelly forceps are then forced through the heavy fascia and are passed beneath the medial patellar ligament. This creates a channel for the insertion of a bistoury knife beneath the medial patellar ligament (Figure 9.1B). The bistoury knife is inserted so the side of the knife lies flat beneath the patellar ligament. When the knife is positioned, the cutting edge is then turned outward (Figure 9.1C). With the left index finger palpating the end of the knife through the skin to ascertain its correct position, the surgeon cuts the ligament with a sawing movement (Figure 9.1D). One must ensure that the blade of the bistoury knife completely encloses the medial patellar ligament before it is severed. Once the ligament has been severed, the tendon of the sartorius muscle feels like a tense band medially and may lead the inexperienced operator to believe that the medial patellar ligament has not been completely severed. One or two sutures of nonabsorbable material are placed in the skin incision.

An alternate procedure has been described that achieves the same thickening effect of the medial patellar ligament as desmotomy. Medial patellar ligament splitting involves percutaneous splitting of the medial patellar ligament with a no. 15 blade. The proximal third of the medial patellar ligament is fenestrated, but the parapatellar fibrocartilage is not split (Figure 9.1B). The procedure is performed under the guidance of ultrasound and with the patient under general anesthesia and in dorsal recumbency. Medial patellar ligament splitting is described in detail elsewhere.[1] Another approach has been described where a 16-gauge needle is used to fenestrate the medial patellar ligament.[3] Either of these two approaches is more desirable than cutting the medial patellar ligament.

Postoperative Management

Antibiotics are not used routinely. Hand-walking is useful to control local swelling. The horse should be rested and hand-walked for a minimum of 2 weeks and preferably 4–6 weeks. Even with experienced operators, instances of severe swelling and lameness of varying duration are observed occasionally.

Complications and Prognosis

Complications that can arise during surgery include severing of the wrong ligament or inadvertent entrance into the femoropatellar joint with the bistoury. (This can potentially occur if the desmotomy is performed too proximad.) A complication that can be seen postoperatively is dehiscence of the skin incision and cellulitis (phlegmon) of the limb. These complications can be avoided by careful attention to aseptic technique during the procedure.

When used appropriately, medial patellar ligament desmotomy has a generally favorable prognosis, provided surgery is performed before any secondary gonitis develops. Unfortunately, the procedure is often performed on horses with undiagnosed lameness in which upward fixation of the patella is not the problem. In these cases, the results are less satisfactory.

A condition resembling chondromalacia patellae of man and associated with medial patellar desmotomy has been observed in our clinic.[4] On radiographs, spurring or fragmentation of the distal patella is noted. When viewed arthroscopically, cartilage lesions varying from softening and fibrillation to dissection and fragmentation of the articular cartilage have been seen. It is suggested that the lesions may be caused by maltracking of the patella within the trochlear groove, leading to more lateral positioning of the patella resulting from loss of the medial tensile pull of the medial patellar ligament. While it was originally thought that enforced rest for an extended period of time would reduce this problem, a recent study indicates that the patella will track abnormally for at least 120 days after transection of the medial patellar ligament.[5]

Lateral Digital Extensor Tenotomy

Relevant Anatomy

The lateral digital extensor muscle originates at the collateral ligament of the stifle, fibula, and lateral tibia; it proceeds distad, lateral to the tibia, and enters the tendon sheath just caudal to the lateral malleolus of the tibia. The tendon sheath is nonpalpable where it is covered by the fascia and extensor retinaculum of the hock. The tendon then continues distad and is palpable as it emerges from the tendon sheath at the level of the proximal third of the metatarsus (Figure 9.2A).

Indications

Lateral digital extensor tenotomy (myotomy) has been used for the treatment of equine stringhalt, a condition characterized by abnormal gait and involuntary hyperflexion of the hind limb.[6] Stringhalt has been defined as a distal axonapathy.[7] One proposed cause of the exaggerated hyperflexion of the hind limb is damage to the large,

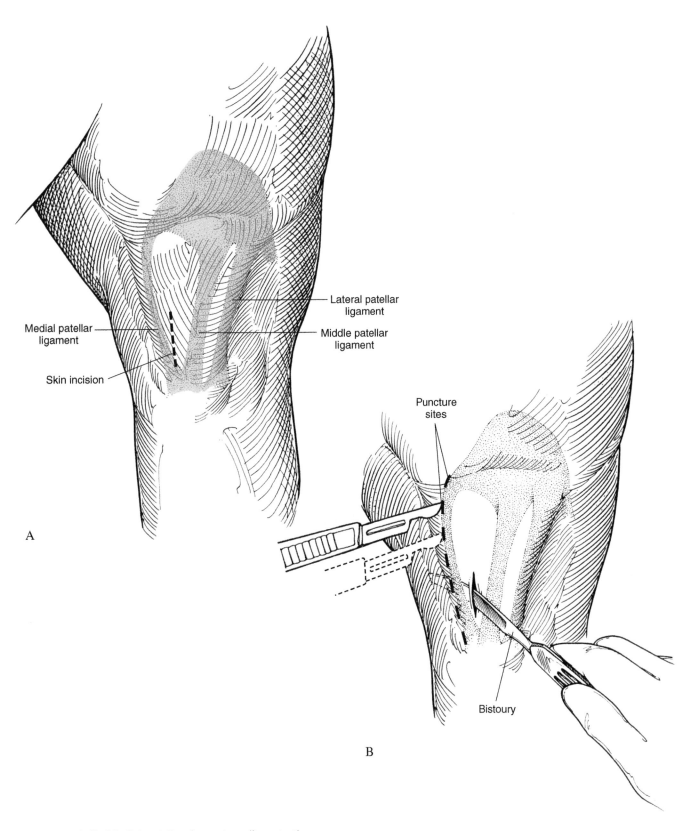

Medial patellar
ligament

Skin incision

Lateral patellar
ligament

Middle patellar
ligament

A

Puncture
sites

Bistoury

B

Fig. 9.1. **A–D.** Medial patellar desmotomy/fenestration.

115

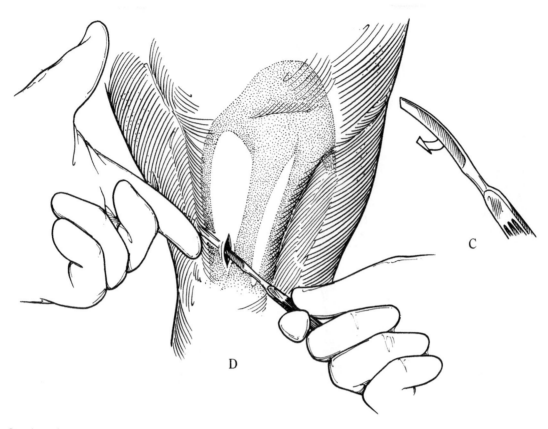

Fig. 9.1. *Continued.*

more vulnerable nerve fibers from the muscle spindles in the hind limb. The etiological agent of stringhalt is unknown; however, two general forms of the disease have been distinguished. Australian stringhalt is associated with ingestion of certain plant toxins, is distinguished by geographical and seasonal patterns of occurrence, and can occur bilaterally. Furthermore, it has been reported to spontaneously resolve itself and may be accompanied by forelimb and laryngeal abnormalties.[8,9] Conventional or "classic" stringhalt is not associated with the ingestion of plant toxin and occurs sporadically. This form of the disease has occurred subsequent to injury to the stifle or hock, particularly trauma that occurs to the dorsum of the metatarsus, upward fixation of the patella, painful foot diseases, and spinal cord disease.[8,10]

Although the exact cause of stringhalt is unknown, resection of the tendon and muscle belly (myotenectomy) has in some cases led to partial or even complete relief of the condition.[11] Benefits of this procedure are that it can be performed in the standing horse with local anesthesia and requires only two incision sites, approximately 2 and 6 cm long each.[12] The following technique involves resection of the tendon plus a large portion of the muscle belly of the lateral digital extensor tendon. This modified technique was designed to improve the surgical success rate.

Anesthesia and Surgical Preparation

It is preferable to perform this technique of lateral digital extensor tenotomy with the patient under general anesthesia because more attention can be paid to asepsis and hemostasis. If only a small amount of the muscle is removed, the surgery can be performed under local anesthesia with the animal standing. In this situation, the local anesthetic should be injected about 2 cm above the lateral malleolus of the tibia directly into the muscle belly of the lateral digital extensor. The second injection of local anesthetic should be made in the area below the hock and above the lateral digital extensor tendon, just before it joins the long digital extensor tendon.

The area over the surgical site is clipped and shaved. Two surgical sites are prepared: The first is a large area over the muscle belly, above the hock; and the second is a smaller area over the distal end of the tendon where it merges with the long digital extensor tendon (Figure 9.2A).

Instrumentation

1. General surgery pack
2. Blunt-ended bistoury (tenotomy) knife

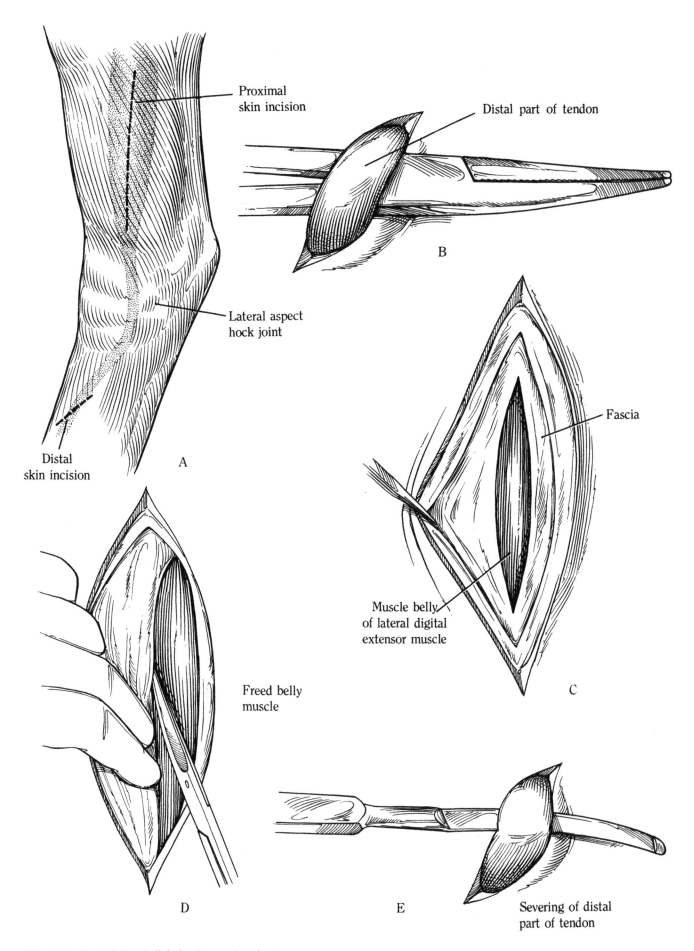

Fig. 9.2. **A–H.** Lateral digital extensor tenotomy.

The labels within the figure read:

- Proximal skin incision
- Distal part of tendon
- Lateral aspect hock joint
- Distal skin incision
- Fascia
- Muscle belly of lateral digital extensor muscle
- Freed belly muscle
- Severing of distal part of tendon
- A
- B
- C
- D
- E

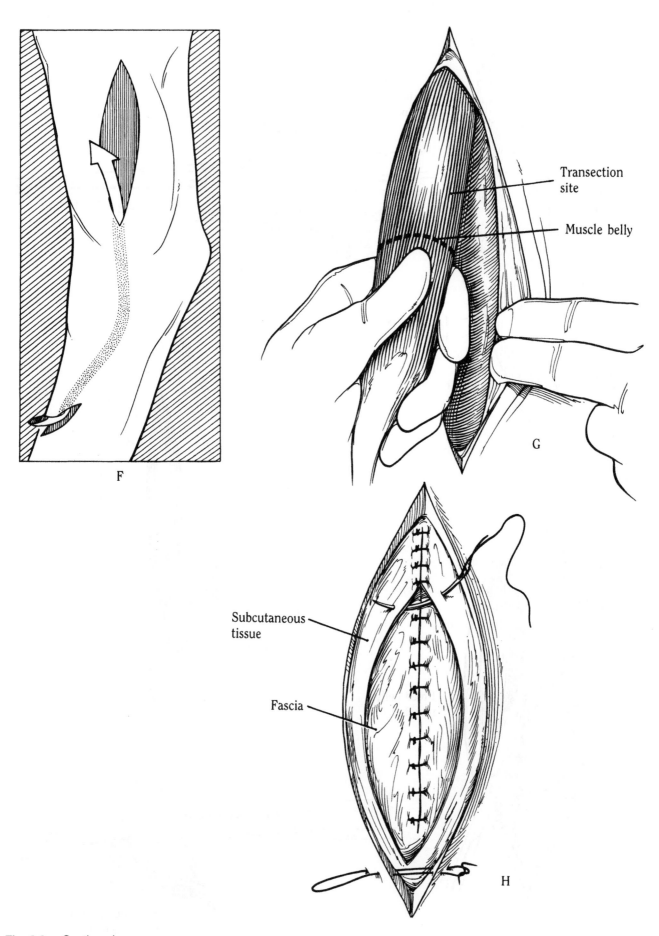

Transection site

Muscle belly

Subcutaneous tissue

Fascia

F

G

H

Fig. 9.2. *Continued.*

Surgical Technique

The distal incision is made over the lateral digital extensor tendon immediately proximal to its junction with the long digital extensor tendon. An incision is made directly over the tendon; the tendon is exposed and isolated by dissecting bluntly beneath the tendon and elevating it using either curved Kelly forceps or Ochsner forceps (Figure 9.2B). Pulling on the tendon at this stage reveals movement of the corresponding muscle belly of the lateral digital extensor tendon; this will assist the surgeon in locating the incision over the muscle belly.

The second incision is made over the muscle belly parallel to the direction of the muscle fibers. The incision should continue through the overlying fascia until the fleshy portion of the muscle belly is visible (Figure 9.2C). The fascia overlying the muscle belly is thick, and the fibers are directed diagonally. Once the muscle belly is freed (Figure 9.2D), the surgeon goes to the first incision over the distal aspect of the lateral digital extensor tendon and severs the tendon (Figure 9.2E). Prior to severing the tendon, one should make sure that the tendon in the distal incision corresponds to the muscle in the proximal incision. Then a pair of Ochsner forceps is placed under the musculotendinous junction; by exerting traction on it, the entire tendon is stripped from its sheath, which overlies the lateral aspect of the hock (Figure 9.2F). The muscle belly is then elevated from the incision and is severed at an oblique angle (Figure 9.2G).

The surgeon should attempt to oversew the muscle stump. This may be difficult because of excess tension, but we believe it reduces postoperative seroma formation. The stump of the muscle is oversewn by grasping the fascia surrounding the muscle belly on the one side and apposing it to the fascia on the opposite side of the muscle belly. Simple horizontal mattress sutures are placed using a synthetic absorbable material. The fascia is closed with simple interrupted or continuous sutures of an absorbable suture material, followed by closure of the subcutaneous tissues with a similar material in a simple interrupted or continuous pattern (Figure 9.2H). The skin is closed with a synthetic, monofilament, nonabsorbable suture material in a simple interrupted pattern. The distal incision is closed in one layer using a similar material in the skin. The wounds are covered with nonadherent dressings, and the entire limb is bandaged.

If the condition is bilateral, the horse is rolled over (if it is under general anesthesia), and the identical procedure is performed on the other pelvic limb.

With the original technique, in which only a small amount of muscle belly is severed, postoperative bandaging is less critical. With this modified muscle-belly severing technique, however, bandaging is essential to minimize seroma formation caused by hemorrhage from the muscle stump. A bandage for this purpose consists of soft cotton and extends from the proximal tibia distad to the pastern.

Postoperative Management

Bandaging is generally required for 2–3 weeks, and sutures are removed 2–3 weeks postoperatively. Box-stall rest is indicated until the surgical sites are healed. When the sites are healed, hand-walking is commenced for about 2 weeks. After this period of hand-walking, normal training is resumed.

Complications and Prognosis

Dehiscence of the skin sutures sometimes occurs because of the stringhalt nature of the gait, and although it has been suggested that the wounds be resutured,[11] it is preferable to allow healing by secondary intention. Other complications include persistence of clinical signs, seroma formation, and hemorrhage.

The results of this procedure in treating stringhalt have been inconsistent. Although many studies show that it is at least beneficial in alleviating some of the hind limb hyperflexion,[10] flexion of the tarsal cural joint involves other muscles, including the lateral digital extensor, long digital extensor, and cranial tibial muscle.[9] One recent study reported excellent long-term recovery in horses affected by acquired bilateral stringhalt (Australian stringhalt) that received lateral digital myotenectomies.[6] Other treatments for stringhalt vary from rest and removal from pasture to medical treatments including administration of phenytoin, mephenesin, or baclofen.[6] Clients are advised of these aspects when they present a horse to the clinician for surgery. If the client wants, the surgery is performed. Despite the uncertain pathogenesis, the operation offers the only real treatment possibility in horses that do not respond to conservative treatment.

Inferior (Distal) Check Ligament Desmotomy

Relevant Anatomy

The inferior (distal) check ligament, also known as the *deep digital flexor accessory ligament*, originates from the palmar carpal ligament and joins the deep digital flexor tendon in the metacarpal region. As described previously, the inferior check ligament functions as part of the stay apparatus in the horse to prevent overstretching of the flexor tendon and limit the amount of overextension possible in the metacarpophalangeal joint.

Indications

Inferior check ligament (deep digital flexor accessory ligament) desmotomy has been described as treatment for chronic desmitis of the deep digital flexor accessory ligament and chronic lameness associated with heel pain in horses.[13,14] More commonly, this procedure is indicated as treatment for cases of flexure deformity of the distal inter-phalangeal (coffin) joint or metacarpophalangeal joint (fetlock) that involve contracture of the deep digital flexor tendon (DDF). This includes conditions such as clubfoot and some caudal foot lameness.[14,15] Surgical treatment of flexural deformities is indicated only in cases that have not responded to conservative methods of therapy, which are described in detail in other texts. If after 1–2 months of conservative treatment methods are not successful, inferior check ligament desmotomy may be indicated.[16]

Flexure deformities may be congenital or acquired at any age in horses. Suggested causative factors for acquired flexure deformities included nutrition, genetics, and pain.[16] Some authors have suggested that excessive feeding in some rapidly growing breeds may result in bone growth that exceeds the elongation rate of the associated tendons. Other potential causes of this disease are speculated to be pain and altered weight bearing associated with orthope-dic disease, especially physeal dysplasia.[16]

In terms of function and cosmetics, inferior check des-motomy is a better technique than deep flexor tenotomy for the treatment of distal interphalangeal flexure defor-mities, except when the dorsal surface of the hoof is beyond vertical.[17]

An ultrasound-guided technique for inferior check desmotomy has been described as well.[15] Suggested advan-tages to this procedure include selection of the incision site, a smaller incision, no subcutaneous suturing, and decreased tissue swelling after surgery.[15]

Anesthesia and Surgical Preparation

Surgery is performed with the patient under general anes-thesia and in lateral recumbency. A lateral or medial approach may be used, but the lateral approach avoids the medial palmar (common digital) artery on the medial side; it is the easiest approach and is recommended for the inexperienced surgeon. A medial approach has one advantage, however, in that, if a blemish develops, it will be on the medial side of the limb and may not be as obvious. If only one leg is affected, the animal is posi-tioned so that the side of the leg to be operated on is uppermost. If both legs are affected, the horse is placed in dorsal recumbency and the legs are suspended from the ceiling. Then the carpometacarpal area is clipped and is surgically prepared.

Instrumentation

1. General surgery pack

Surgical Technique

A 3–4-cm incision is made over the cranial border of the DDF tendon centered at the junction of the proximal one-third and distal two-thirds of the cannon bone. The position of the incision is illustrated in Figure 9.3A, and

the relevant anatomy is illustrated in Figure 9.3B. Follow-ing the skin incision, the loose connective tissue over the flexor tendons is dissected bluntly and the paratenon is incised (Figure 9.3C). The superficial and deep flexor tendons must be identified, but they need not be dissected from each other. Blunt dissection is directed craniad to expose the inferior check ligament, and a cleavage plane is identified between the proximal part of the DDF tendon and the inferior check ligament. This cleavage plane is used to separate the check ligament from the DDF tendon (Figure 9.3D). Forceps are inserted between the check ligament and the DDF tendon to separate the structures; then the check ligament is lifted from the incision and is incised with a scalpel (Figure 9.3E). The author[16] prefers to remove a 1-cm segment of the check ligament. This surgical manipulation sometimes disrupts the synovial sheath of the carpal canal, the distal extremity of which extends most of the way down inside the cleavage plane. This event seems to be of little consequence, however. The foot of the patient is then extended manually. The ends of the check ligament become separated, and com-plete severance of all parts of the check ligament can be ascertained.

The paratenon and superficial fascia are closed in a single layer with simple continuous sutures of synthetic, absorbable material. The skin is closed with nonabsorb-able sutures in a suture pattern of the surgeon's choice.

Postoperative Management

A sterile dressing is placed over the incision, and the limb is bandaged from the proximal metacarpus to the coro-nary band. To apply more pressure over the surgical site (in an attempt to minimize swelling and reduce the potential blemish) a 4-inch roll of gauze bandage is placed over the incision and is held in position with pressure from an overlying bandage. The hoof is trimmed to normal conformation. Phenylbutazone (1–2 g) is admin-istered intravenously to reduce postoperative pain and to facilitate lowering of the heel. Antibiotics are not admin-istered routinely. Toe extensions may be indicated in more severe cases. Sutures are removed at 12–14 days, and ban-daging may be discontinued 3–4 days later.

Complications and Prognosis

Scarring at the incision site is a common complication of inferior check ligament desmotomies. Proponents of the ultrasound-guided technique for this procedure have reported a reduction in scarring when this method is used.[18] Normal thickening of the check ligament occurs following desmotomy; however, this has not been shown to adversely affect tendon function after healing.[19] Biome-chanical studies show that following transection of the accessory ligament, the load is redistributed to the super-ficial flexor tendon and shifted to the deep digital flexor toward the end of the stance phase.[20] Transfer of the load

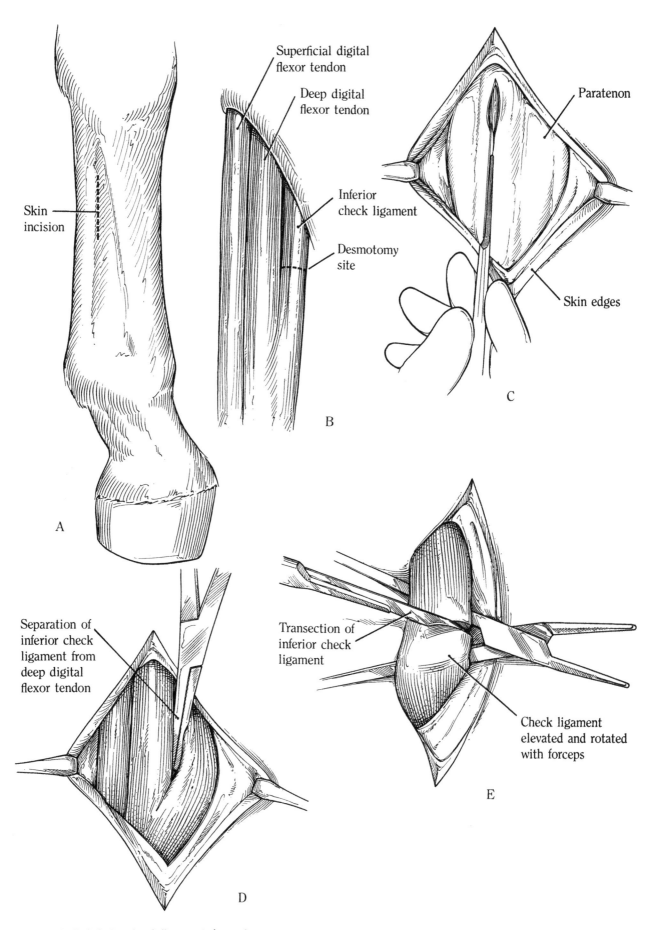

Skin incision

Superficial digital flexor tendon

Deep digital flexor tendon

Inferior check ligament

Desmotomy site

A

B

Paratenon

Skin edges

C

Separation of inferior check ligament from deep digital flexor tendon

D

Transection of inferior check ligament

Check ligament elevated and rotated with forceps

E

Fig. 9.3. **A–E.** Inferior check ligament desmotomy.

to the contralateral limb was not observed, and only minor hyperflexion of the metacarpophalangeal joint of the limb that received desmotomy occurred.[20] Overloading of the flexor tendon during locomotion was not considered a concern assuming high-load situations following surgery are avoided, such as jumping.

The results of athletic performance in horses afflicted with flexural deformities after surgery are favorable. A retrospective study of 40 horses treated for distal interphalangeal flexure deformities reported that 9 months to 4 years after surgery, 35 horses were not lame and were used as athletes.[20] Of the other 7 horses, 6 had complications related to the deformity, whereas 1 had complications resulting from surgery.[20] Another study reported that ultrasound-guided inferior check ligament desmotomy corrected 40 of 42 cases of clubfoot and both cases of fetlock deformities (2 horses). The prognosis for the horse returning to athletic function has been suggested to be correlated with the age of the horse receiving surgical treatment; Standardbred foals that received desmotomy at an older age had a decreased chance of racing and training soundly.[21]

Generally, the prognosis is poor for horses afflicted with desmitis of the deep digital flexor accessory ligament that is associated with adhesions or tendinitis of the superficial flexor tendon. Desmotomy of the accessory ligament has been shown to restore most of these horses to soundness and even use as a pleasure horse.[13]

Superior Check Ligament Desmotomy (After Bramlage)

Relevant Anatomy

The superficial digital flexor muscle belly is located between the larger deep digital flexor muscle belly and the flexor carpi ulnaris on the caudal aspect of the forelimb. The superior check ligament (the accessory ligament of the superficial digital flexor muscle), which inserts on the caudal surface of the radius, functions in the stay apparatus in the horse.[22] Together with the inferior check ligament (the accessory ligament of the deep digital flexor muscle), it prevents overextension of the fetlock during weight bearing. The cephalic vein runs superficially up the forearm and is used to locate the incision site in this procedure. Branches arising from this vein may require ligation. The brachial artery runs down the medial aspect of the humerus and gives rise to several branches. At the elbow, it becomes the median artery, which runs with the median nerve and courses under the flexor carpi radialis, giving rise to the common interosseous artery.[22] Just proximal to the carpus, the median artery divides into three branches: the palmar branch; the radial artery; and the main branch, which runs through the carpal canal with the flexor tendons and becomes the medial palmar artery. The median nerve also divides proximal to the radiocar-

pal joint and gives rise to the medial and lateral palmar nerves. There is a nutrient artery that runs near the proximal aspect of the superior check ligament that should, if possible, be avoided.

Indications

Superior check ligament desmotomy was initially described as a surgical treatment for metacarpophalangeal flexural deformities in young horses.[23] Reported results vary,[24,25] however, and it is now recognized that the (SDF) tendon is not necessarily the primary unit in metacarpophalangeal flexural deformities.[26] In cases where the SDF appears to be the most involved structure, superior check ligament desmotomy may be indicated.

Superior check ligament desmotomy has been reported as a treatment for superficial digital flexor tendinitis in racehorses.[27] The rationale for the surgery is that it interrupts the transfer of the weight-bearing load on the tendon to the distal radius, bringing the muscle and tendon proximal to the superior check ligament (and therefore enhanced elasticity to the functional unit) into use during weight-bearing.[28]

The technique described is a modification of that previously described.[29] The approach is more caudal, and the limits of the superior check ligament are more easily defined. In addition, the closure of the medial wall of the flexor carpi radialis sheath facilitates elimination of dead space and minimizes the potential for hematoma formation and adhesions.

Anesthesia and Surgical Preparation

Surgery is performed with the patient under general anesthesia and either in lateral recumbency with the affected leg down or in dorsal recumbency with the leg suspended. The latter position is preferable in terms of hemostasis. The leg is clipped from midradius to midmetacarpus. The medial side of the antebrachium is surgically prepared.

Instrumentation

1. General surgery pack

Surgical Technique

A 10-cm skin incision is made cranial to the cephalic vein, over the flexor carpi radialis tendon and extending from the level of the distal chestnut proximad. The incision is continued through the subcutaneous tissue and antebrachial fascia (Figure 9.4A). A transverse branch of the cephalic vein might require ligation (the incision can often be continued under it). The fascial sheath of the flexor carpi radialis is incised (Figure 9.4B), and Gelpi retractors are placed to expose the medial wall of the sheath, which adheres to the superior check ligament. A stab incision is made through the craniolateral wall of the

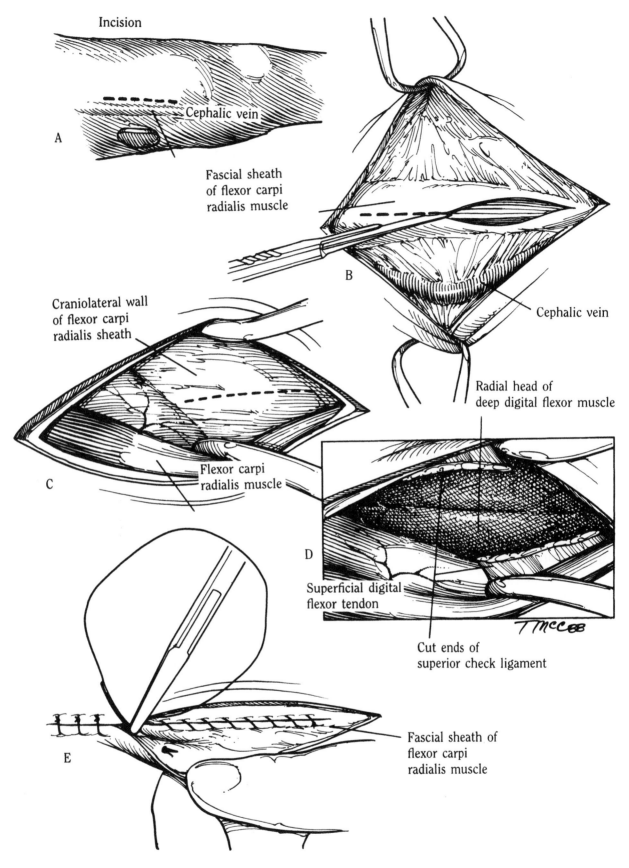

Incision

Cephalic vein

A

Fascial sheath
of flexor carpi
radialis muscle

B

Cephalic vein

Radial head of
deep digital flexor muscle

Craniolateral wall
of flexor carpi
radialis sheath

Flexor carpi
radialis muscle

C

D

Superficial digital
flexor tendon

Cut ends of
superior check ligament

E

Fascial sheath of
flexor carpi
radialis muscle

Fig. 9.4. Superior check ligament desmotomy.

123

sheath and superior check ligament (Figure 9.4C). The incision is continued proximad and distad to sever the ligament completely. Complete incision through the check ligament is evidenced by visualizing the muscular portion of the radial head of the deep digital flexor tendon beneath and separation of the superficial digital flexor muscle palmad (Figure 9.4D). An artery (nutrient artery for the superficial digital flexor tendon) may be present at the proximal border of the check ligament. After complete transection of the ligament, the membranous roof of the carpal synovial sheath is seen distally, and the muscle belly of the radial head of the deep digital flexor tendon is seen in central and proximal areas of the incision.

The incision in the flexor carpi radialis sheath is closed with a simple continuous pattern using 2-0 synthetic absorbable material. The antebrachial fascia and subcutaneous tissue is closed with a continuous suture of 2-0 synthetic nonabsorbable material (Figure 9.4E). The skin is closed with interrupted sutures of 2-0 nonabsorbable material.

Postoperative Management

A sterile dressing is placed over the incision, and a pressure bandage is applied. Phenylbutazone is administered postoperatively, but antibiotics are not used routinely. Sutures are removed at 12–14 days, and bandaging may be discontinued 3–4 days later.

Complications and Prognosis

Biomechanical studies have suggested that superior check desmotomy used to treat horses with superficial flexor tendinitis may predispose these horses to developing suspensory desmitis. The superior check ligament plays a vital role in maintaining proper metacarpophalangeal and fetlock joint angles in the horse. Following superior check ligament desmotomy, these angles are decreased, which subsequently increases strain on the superficial digital flexure tendon and suspensory ligament and might predispose the horse to other injuries.[30] In one study, Thoroughbred racehorses that received this procedure were shown to be 5.5 times more likely to develop suspensory desmitis than those that were treated nonsurgically.[26]

The efficacy of this procedure in returning racehorses inflicted with tendinitis to full athletic performance is controversial.[31] Most clinical studies of superior check desmotomy have been conducted in Thoroughbred and Standardbred racehorses, despite the fact that superficial flexor tendinitis is common in all sport horses, especially jumpers and 3-day event horses.[31] The prognosis in Standardbred racehorses appears to be slightly better for returning to athletic performance than that for Thoroughbreds, although the results are highly varied. One study showed that 50 of 61 Standardbred racehorses

(83%) returned to racing after treatment for tendinitis.[27] However, only 57% of the 61 horses went on to complete 20 or more starts. Similar results were found in another study, which reported that 35 of 38 (92%) horses returned to racing and 71% of horses started 5 or more races without recurring tendinitis.[31] The prognosis for Thoroughbred racehorses is generally lower in the literature. Reported percentages of horses that returned to racing and completed multiple starts range from 53% to 73%.[31,32] In some studies, these percentages have not substantially exceeded those calculated for Thoroughbred racehorses that are managed with minimal exercise and rehabilitation.[26,31] A minimally invasive technique has been described using an arthroscope and a lateral approach.[33] This technique provides a better cosmetic outcome and less postoperative care than the traditional open approach.

Superficial Digital Flexor Tenotomy

Relevant Anatomy

The tendons of the deep and superficial digital flexors share a tendon sheath as they pass through the carpal canal. The tendon of the superficial digital flexor remains superficial up until the fetlock, where it dives deep to insert on the distal tubercles of the first phalanx and the fibrocartilage of the second phalanx.[22] At the level of the first phalanx, the superficial digital flexor tendon forms a sleeve through which the tendon of the deep digital flexor passes to insert on the third phalanx. Local thickenings of deep fascia, the annular ligaments, hold the flexor tendons in place at the fetlock.[22]

The principal vessels and nerves of the distal limb exist on the palmar surface of the distal limb and run superficially between the borders of the suspensory ligament and the flexor tendons. The medial palmar artery, which passes through the carpal canal, is the main blood supply to the distal limb. Smaller metacarpal arteries arising from the median artery run with the suspensory ligament as well. The medial palmar artery branches into the medial and lateral digital arteries, which supply the digit, just proximal to the sesamoids. The medial and lateral nerves (branches of the median nerve) and the palmar and dorsal branches of the ulnar nerve innervate the distal limb. The medial and lateral palmar nerves run superficially in the groove between the suspensory ligament and flexor tendons until midway down the metacarpus, where the medial branch forms an anastomosis with the lateral palmar nerve.[22] Like the arteries, these will continue to the digit as the medial and lateral digital nerves.

Indications

Superficial digital flexor tenotomy is indicated for the treatment of selected cases of flexure deformity of the metacarpophalangeal (fetlock) joint. This condition has been described previously as SDF tendon contracture, but it has become evident that in most cases, more than the SDF tendon is involved.[34] The deep digital flexor tendon is commonly involved, and in a chronic case, the suspensory ligament may be involved as well. In an appropriate patient, however, tenotomy of the superficial flexor tendon may return the fetlock to normal alignment.

The technique of superior check (accessory ligament of the SDF) desmotomy has been advocated as an alternate treatment for flexure deformity of the metacarpophalangeal joint.[35] Effective division of the superior check ligament is more difficult than inferior desmotomy, however, and the value of the operation in treating flexure deformities of the metacarpophalangeal joint is controversial.[25,35]

Anesthesia and Surgical Preparation

This technique may be performed with the appropriate patient under local analgesia or in lateral or dorsal recumbency under general anesthesia. The midmetacarpal area is prepared surgically.

Instrumentation

1. General surgery pack
2. Blunt-ended tenotomy knife

Surgical Technique

Tenotomy may be performed blindly through a stab incision using a tenotomy knife or under direct visualization through a larger skin incision. The latter technique is illustrated here.

A 2-cm skin incision is made over the junction of the superficial and deep digital flexor tendons at the level of the midmetacarpus (Figure 9.5A). The paratenon is incised, and forceps are used to separate the SDF tendon from the deep digital flexor tendon. A cleavage plane is

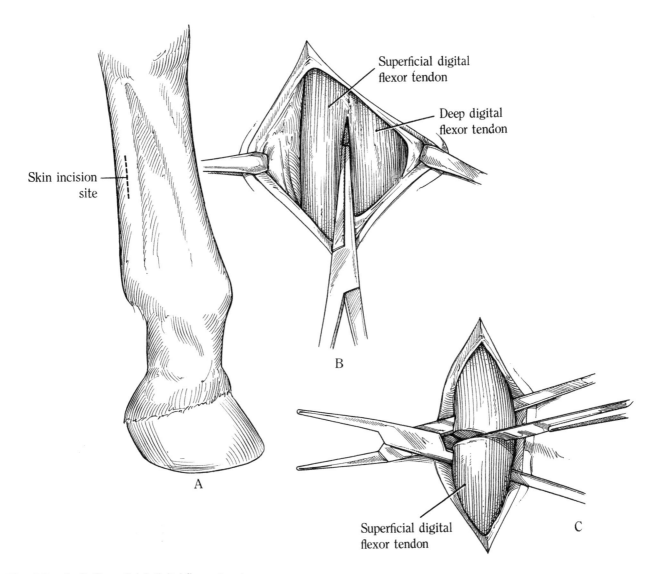

Skin incision site

Superficial digital flexor tendon

Deep digital flexor tendon

B

Superficial digital flexor tendon

A

C

Fig. 9.5. A–C. Superficial digital flexor tenotomy.

obvious (Figure 9.5*B*). When the SDF tendon is separated, it is incised with a scalpel (Figure 9.5*C*). Following tenotomy, the skin is sutured with nonabsorbable material.

When the surgeon has become familiar with the technique under direct visualization, it is simple to perform the surgery blindly by inserting a tenotomy knife blade through a small skin incision, manipulating it between the superficial and deep digital flexor tendons, rotating it 90°, and then severing the tendon. The stab incision is closed with a single suture.

Postoperative Management

A sterile dressing is placed over the incision, and the leg is bandaged from the proximal metacarpus distad. Phenylbutazone, 1–2 g, is administered to facilitate return to function, and the animal is placed on an exercise regimen immediately. The sutures are removed 10–12 days after the operation, at which point bandaging is discontinued. If this technique fails to correct the deformity, additional procedures, such as inferior check desmotomy, may need to be performed. In addition, in some cases, inferior check ligament desmotomy is the initial treatment of choice in patients with flexure deformities of the metacarpophalangeal joint.[34,36]

Complications and Prognosis

This procedure is generally recommended for unresponsive cases of metacarpophalangeal joint deformity in an effort to salvage the horse as a pasture pet or for breeding purposes.[34] The prognosis is generally guarded, healing is uncosmetic, and the procedure overall is painful. Arthrodesis of the metacarpophalangeal joint can be performed for nonresponsive, severe cases of flexure deformities as well.

Deep Digital Flexor Tenotomy

Relevant Anatomy

Refer to the previous section on superficial digital flexor tenotomy for a description of structures relevant to this procedure.

Indications

DDF tenotomy is indicated for the treatment of severe cases of flexural deformity of the distal interphalangeal joint and also as an aid in the management of chronic refractory laminitis.[36,37] If a distal interphalangeal joint flexural deformity has progressed to the extent that the dorsal surface of the distal phalanx has passed beyond vertical, secondary contraction of the joint capsule and peritendinous attachments of the distal segment of the deep flexor tendon may lock the digit in its fixed position.

In such cases, a good response to inferior check ligament desmotomy cannot be anticipated, but the patient may respond to a DDF tenotomy.

The most common explanation for pedal bone rotation in horses with severe laminitis is separation of the interdigitating sensitive and insensitive laminae at the dorsal aspect of the hoof wall and the continued pull of the DDF tendon on the solar surface of the distal phalanx. The rationale for DDF tenotomy in cases of severe laminitis is to reduce the dynamic forces favoring rotation and to reduce the pressure of the distal phalanx on the corium of the sole.[38] Results of a retrospective study support the technique's effectiveness as a salvage procedure in horses with chronic refractory laminitis.[38]

Tenotomy of the DDF tendon can be performed at either the midmetacarpal/metatarsal level or the midpastern region but the currently favored location is at the mid-metacarpal/metatarsal region.[36,37]

Anesthesia and Surgical Preparation

The surgery at the midmetacarpal/metatarsal level can be performed in either the standing animal or under general anesthesia and in lateral recumbency. A pneumatic tourniquet and Esmarch's bandage are advantageous to provide hemostasis in either position. The leg is clipped from above the carpus/tarsus to below the fetlock, and the area is surgically prepared.

Instrumentation

1. General surgery pack
2. Blunt-ended tenotomy knife

Surgical Technique

The preferred surgical approach at the midmetacarpal region is performed as described for the midmetacarpal superficial digital flexor tenotomy, transecting the deep digital flexor instead. It can easily be performed in the standing horse with the use of sedation and a local block. Both closure and resection of the synovial sheath have been recommended by different authors.[37,38] We recommend closure of the synovial sheath, based on the finding in one study that closure did not apparently impair tendon healing.[38]

Postoperative Management

A sterile dressing is placed over the incision, and the limb is bandaged from the hoof to the carpus. Phenylbutazone is administered as necessary. In cases of flexural deformity, the hoof is trimmed by shortening the heels as much as possible. This may be done gradually. Hand-walking is performed. Corrective shoeing may also be necessary. If postoperative dorsiflexion develops, shoes with caudally extended branches should be applied.

In horses with laminitis, shoeing is an important adjunctive therapy. Reversed, extended heel shoes have been recommended initially, with later substitution with flat shoes and pads.[38]

Complications and Prognosis

Results of a retrospective study support the technique's effectiveness as a salvage procedure in horses with chronic refractory laminitis.[38] Transection of the deep digital flexor tendon will also decrease the pain associated with the acute refractory stage of laminitis, but it does not reverse the pathological changes within the digital lamina.[39] Of horses that received deep digital flexor tenotomies for treatment of chronic laminitis, 77% survived greater than 6 months and 59% survived greater than 2 years.[40]

Sectioning of the Palmar (or Plantar) Annular Ligament of the Fetlock

Relevant Anatomy

There are three annular ligaments of the fetlock: the palmar, proximal digital, and distal digital. The palmar annular ligament of the fetlock runs from the abaxial surface of the proximal sesamoid bones and transverses the palmer aspect of the fetlock joint. With the intersesamoidean ligament, it creates a canal through which the superficial and deep digital flexor tendons pass. (Figure 9.6A).

Indications

This surgical procedure is indicated for the treatment of constriction of or by the palmar or plantar annular ligament, tendinitis in the digital sheath, or posttraumatic adhesions of the digital sheath.[41–44] The problem is associated with injury or infection, and the condition may develop in several ways. Direct injury to the annular ligament with subsequent inflammation may cause fibrosis, scarring, and a primary constriction of the ligament. The constricted ligament, in turn, exerts pressure on the superficial and/or deep flexor tendon. A primary injury to the superficial and/or deep flexor tendon with subsequent tendinitis ("bowed tendon") can have the same result because it is associated with swelling of the SDF tendon against the inelastic annular ligament. In some situations, both types of injuries may be involved.

The restriction of free tendon movement and tenosynovitis result in pain and persistent lameness. Prolonged permanent damage to the tendon may result. The syndrome can also arise as a primary chronic digital sheath synovitis of unknown cause, with excess production of synovial fluid and fibrous tissue deposition at the proximal reflection of the synovial sheath onto the flexor tendons.[42] Some authors have considered this pathogenesis to be the most common (the cause of the synovitis remains obscure).[42] Fluid distention of the digital flexor tendon sheath above and below the constricted annular ligament causes the characteristic "notched" appearance on the palmar (or plantar) aspect of the fetlock.[41]

Anesthesia and Surgical Preparation

The patient is placed under general anesthesia with the affected leg uppermost. The use of an Esmarch's bandage and a pneumatic tourniquet facilitates the surgery. A routine preparation for aseptic surgery is performed from the proximal metacarpus distad.

Instrumentation

1. General surgery pack
2. Blunt-ended tenotomy knife

Surgical Technique

There are many described techniques for performing an annular ligament desmotomy. The open approach has been generally dropped in favor of the other approaches, including the closed approach with scissors, the closed approach with a tenotomy knife, and the tenoscopic guided approach. Only the closed approach will be described here.

This simplified version of the surgery can be performed with the patient under anesthesia (preferred) or standing. Although it does not allow complete visualization of the tendon sheath contents, it does obviate potential problems of wound dehiscence and synovial fistulation that have been experienced with the open technique.

A 2-cm skin incision is made over the proximal outpouching of the digital flexor sheath; and, using Mayo scissors, a subcutaneous tunnel is created distad to the distal extremity of the annular ligament (Figure 9.6B). Mayo scissors are then positioned so that one arm is in the subcutaneous tunnel and one within the sheath; and, with appropriate care to avoid the palmar or plantar vessels and nerve, the annular ligament is incised (Figure 9.6C). Attention is also paid not to sever tendinous tissue within the sheath, and one must know the limits of the annular ligament. Conversely, the digital sheath can be distended with saline, and a stab incision can be made through the skin and into the sheath. A blunt tenotomy knife can be inserted into the sheath and turned at a 90° angle to the annular ligament to facilitate transection (Figure 9.6A). The skin alone is closed using 2-0 synthetic nonabsorbable suture material.

Postoperative Management

A sterile dressing is placed over the incision, and a pressure bandage is applied. Antibiotics are not used routinely.

Fig. 9.6. **A.** Drawing showing location of palmar/plantar annular ligament transection with blunt tenotomy knife. **B** and **C.** Closed technique with scissors.

Hand-walking is begun in 3 days and is maintained on an increasing plane to preclude the formation of adhesions. The sutures are removed at 14 days, and bandaging is maintained for 3 weeks. With uneventful healing, the main criterion for returning the horse to work is the time necessary for healing of the tendinitis in the superficial flexor tendon.

Complications and Prognosis

Dehiscence of the incision and the development of synovial fistulation are rare complications of the open technique. Such patients are placed on antibiotics, and careful wound management and bandaging are performed. The use of the closed technique virtually obviates this complication.

If extensive changes have not occurred in the superficial or deep flexor tendons, the prognosis is good, but the presence of adhesions or gross pathologic changes decreases the probability for success. Intrasynovial injections of high molecular weight sodium hyaluronate may be helpful in reducing adhesion formation. Aggressive physical therapy is helpful in reducing pathologic adhesions. In a recent study evaluating palmar/plantar annular ligament injury, the method of treatment, the thickness of the PAL, or the presence of subcutaneous fibrosis did not significantly affect the prognosis. Less than 50% of horses were able to return to athletic function with PAL desmopathy alone to having the best outcome. Bilateral thickening of the PAL or concurrent forelimb and hind limb injuries had a negative effect on prognosis, as did the simultaneous presence of subcutaneous fibrosis and lesions within the DFTS.[44] Tenoscopic evaluation and treatment has the possible benefit of more effectively treating complex cases involving adhesions and synovial masses.[5]

Palmar Digital Neurectomy

Relevant Anatomy

The lateral and medial palmar digital nerves are continuations of the lateral and medial palmar nerves. The palmar digital nerve is identified just palmar to the digital artery approximately 0.5 cm below the skin surface and deep to the ligament of the ergot. At the fetlock, the medial and lateral palmar nerves each give rise to dorsal branches.

Indications

Palmar, or posterior, digital neurectomy is used to relieve chronic heel pain. The most common indication is navicular disease that is not responsive to corrective shoeing and medical therapy, but it is also used in horses with fracture of the navicular bone, selected lateral-wing fractures of the distal phalanx, and calcification of the collateral cartilages of the distal phalanx.[45] This surgical procedure is not benign, and it is not a panacea. A number of potential complications should be explained to the owner prior to surgery. In the hands of a good operator, however, palmar digital neurectomy is a form of long-term relief from the pain of those conditions just listed.

Anesthesia and Surgical Preparation

Neurectomy may be performed under local analgesia with the animal standing or under general anesthesia. If the surgery is performed with the animal standing, it is preferable to inject the local analgesic agent over the palmar nerves at the level of the abaxial surface of the sesamoid bones. The nerves can be palpated in this area, and the infiltration of this area avoids additional trauma and irritation at the surgery site. If neurectomy is performed in a field situation immediately following the use of a diagnostic block of the palmar digital nerve, however, this same block may be used for the surgical procedure. However, the author generally recommends waiting for 10 days after performing a palmar digital nerve block before performing a neurectomy in order to reduce inflammation in the region. General anesthesia is convenient to use, and for the more involved technique of epineural capping, it is certainly indicated.

The area of the surgical incision is clipped, shaved, and prepared for surgery in a routine manner. Plastic adhesive drapes are useful to exclude the hoof as a source of contamination.

Instrumentation

1. General surgery pack
2. Iris spatula (epineural capping technique)
3. CO_2 laser

Surgical Technique

In both the simple guillotine method and the technique of epineural capping, the approach to the nerve is the same. In the simple guillotine technique, an incision 2 cm long is made over the dorsal border of the flexor tendons (Figure 9.7A). If epineural capping is to be performed, the incision is generally 3–4 cm long and is continued through the subcutaneous tissue. It is important that the tissues be subjected to minimal trauma. An incision over the dorsal border of the flexor tendons generally brings the operator close to the palmar digital nerve. Variation exists, but the relationship of vein, artery, nerve, and the ligament of the ergot assists the surgeon's orientation (Figure 9.7B). At this stage of the dissection, the surgeon should look for accessory branches of the palmar digital nerve. These branches are commonly found near the ligament of the

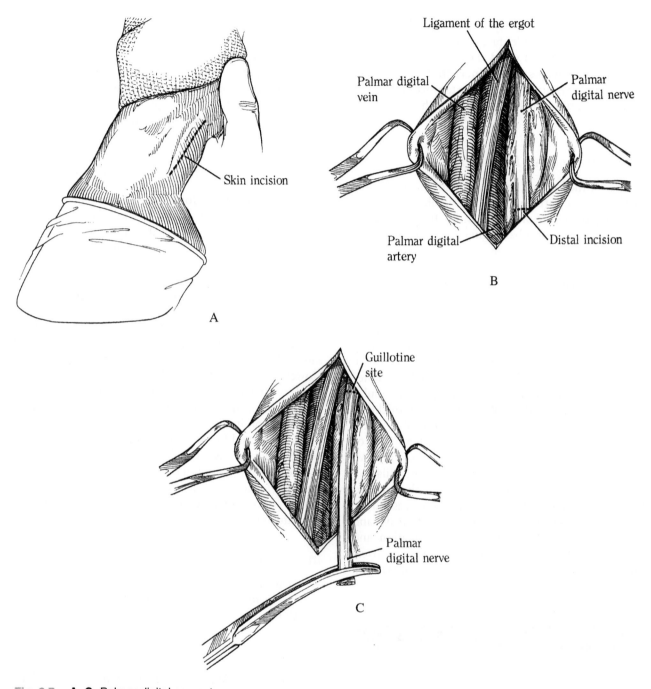

Fig. 9.7. A–C. Palmar digital neurectomy.

ergot. If an accessory branch is found, a 2-cm portion is removed using a scalpel.

Guillotine Technique

The nerve is identified and is dissected free of the subcutaneous tissue. The structure can be identified as nerve if it puckers after it is stretched, if scraping its surface reveals the longitudinal strands of the axons, or if a small incision into the nerve body reveals cut transverse sections of bundles of nerve fibers. The nerve is severed at the distal extremity of the incision. Then a hemostat is placed on the nerve, which is stretched while being cut with a scalpel or CO_2 laser at the proximal limit of the incision (Figure 9.7C). This sharp incision is made in such a fashion that the proximal portion of the nerve springs up into the tissue planes and out of sight. It is believed that the severance of untraumatized nerve and its retraction up into the tissue planes helps reduce the problems of painful neuromas. The concept behind using the CO_2 laser is that it seals the nerve ending, even further reducing the possibility of a painful neuroma.

The skin is closed with interrupted sutures of nonabsorbable material.

Pull-Through Technique

The pull-through technique is an extension of the Guillotine technique. The first part of the procedure is performed as previously described. The main difference is that, instead of transecting the nerve at the proximal site of the incision as in the guillotine technique, traction is placed on the distal nerve, and a second incision of 1 cm is made over the nerve at the base of the proximal sesamoid bone. The digital nerve is then pulled through the proximal incision and a guillotine technique is used to transect the nerve.[46]

Postoperative Management

Antibiotics are not used routinely. A sterile dressing is placed on the incision, and a pressure bandage is maintained on the leg for at least 21 days. To minimize postoperative inflammation, 2 g of phenylbutazone are administered daily following surgery for 5–7 days. Sutures are removed 10 days after the operation, and the horse is rested for 60 days.

Complications and Prognosis

Complications of neurectomy include painful neuroma formation, rupture of the deep digital flexor tendon, reinnervation, persistence of sensation because of failure to identify and sever accessory branches of the nerve, and loss of the hoof wall. Neuromas are the most common complications and can arise when the axons in the proximal stump regenerate axon sprouts, which cause pain and hypersensitivity.[47] One retrospective study of 50 horses that received palmar digital neurectomies, the majority by transection and electrocoagulation, reported that 17 horses (34%) had complications, with recurrence of heel pain being the most common.[48] Only 3 of the 17 horses developed neuromas, although this number may have been higher due to undetectable painful neuromas that could not be palpated. In 2 years, 63% of all the horses that received neurectomies were still sound. More recently, a study of 24 horses that received neurectomies using the guillotine technique reported no postoperative complications. The majority of these horses (22 of the 24) were treated for lameness associated with abnormal radiographic findings of the navicular bone and associated structures; the collateral cartilages of the hoof, or in one case, pedal osteitis.[49] Twenty-two of these horses returned to full athletic performance, including jumping, dressage, camp drafting, cutting, and endurance competition. When using the pull-through technique, 88% of the horses were sound at one year post surgery.[46]

Amputation of the Splint (II and IV Metacarpal and Metatarsal) Bones

Relevant Anatomy

The second and fourth metacarpal bones, or splint bones, are attached to the abaxial surface of the medial and lateral proximal sesamoids by fibrous bands.[49] Thus, frequent hyperextension of the fetlock that results in stretching of these bands may be a predisposing factor for fracture of the splint bones.[49] Fracture generally occurs at the most distal third of the splint bone.

Indications

Amputation of the small metacarpal or metatarsal (splint) bones is indicated when these bones are fractured. Horses that race over fences and Standardbreds appear to be most susceptible to this type of injury.[49] Splint bone fractures in Standardbred horses are often associated with suspensory desmitis as well.

The lameness caused by fractures of the splint bone is generally mild and may be an incidental finding in a radiographic examination. If the skin has been broken, osteitis or osteomyelitis at the fracture site may result. These cases are accompanied by more soft-tissue swelling and lameness than are closed fractures of the splint bone.[50]

Occasionally, undisplaced fractures of the splint bone heal following suitable rest, but constant movement at the fracture site generally results in nonunion with an attending callus.[50] The decision to remove the fractured distal end of a splint bone is often controversial. Dealing with the suspensory desmitis alone may be sufficient, and removal of the distal splint bone may be unnecessary.[51]

If infection and accompanying osteomyelitis are present, surgical debridement-curettage, or sequestrectomy may be necessary to resolve the infectious process, regardless of the health of the suspensory ligament.[52]

Anesthesia and Surgical Preparation

General anesthesia is recommended for this operation. The horse is placed in either lateral recumbency with the affected splint bone uppermost or dorsal recumbency with the injured leg suspended. The latter method has advantages when more than one splint is to be operated on, and it achieves natural hemostasis during the surgical procedure.

A tourniquet facilitates the surgery if the animal is in lateral recumbency. The surgical site is shaved and prepared for aseptic surgery.

Instrumentation

1. General surgery pack
2. Curved osteotome

3. Chisel
4. Mallet
5. Periosteal elevator

Surgical Technique

A variable-length incision is made directly over the splint bone, extending from approximately 1 cm distal to the distal extremity of the splint bone to approximately 2 cm proximal to the proposed site of amputation (Figure 9.8A). The subcutaneous fascia is incised along the same line as the incision, through the periosteum. The periosteum is elevated off the affected part of the splint bone. The distal end of the splint bone is undermined with the aid of sharp dissection and is freed from surrounding fascia (Figure 9.8B). Then the end is grasped firmly with forceps, such as Ochsner forceps. With further sharp dissection, the splint bone is separated from its attachments to the third metacarpal or metatarsal bone. Some of the attachments to the third metacarpal or metatarsal bone may need to be severed with the aid of a chisel (Figure 9.8C). A curved osteotome can also be used to sever these attachments.

The splint bone should be amputated above the fracture site or the area of infection with the aid of a chisel or osteotome. The splint bone should be removed (a large curette is sometimes necessary to remove diseased bone adequately).[53] The proximal end of the splint bone should

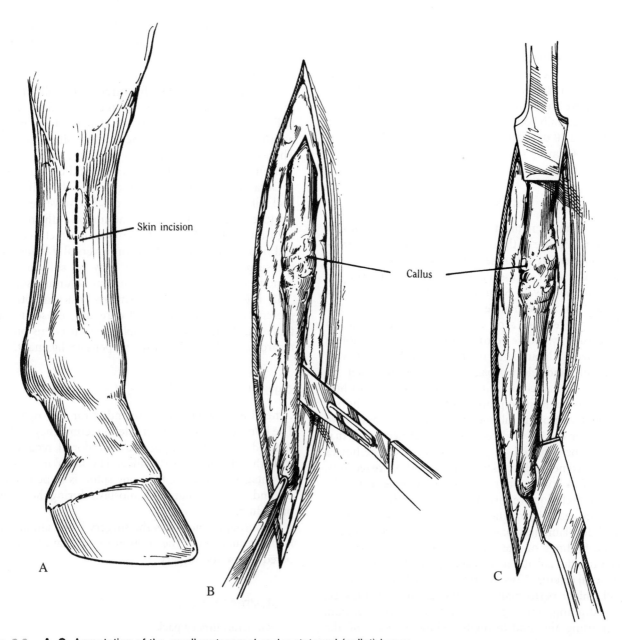

Fig. 9.8.   A–C. Amputation of the small metacarpal and metatarsal (splint) bones.

D   E

Fig. 9.8. **D** and **E.** Bone plate fixation of proximal splint bone fractures.

be tapered to avoid leaving a sharp edge (Figure 9.8C), and any loose fragments removed or flushed out of the surgical site. The periosteum should be sharply excised to reduce the chances of periosteal proliferation. If infection is present, unhealthy scar tissue must be excised with sharp dissection, and all sequestra removed. Any bleeding should be controlled at this time. When infection is present, generally the region is vascular because of acute and chronic inflammation.

If the fracture is not infected and is very proximal, the fracture should be repaired by use of a small bone plate with screws only placed into the splint bone (Figure 9.8D). If the fracture is infected and proximal, the distal end should be removed and the proximal segment anchored using a contoured bone plate fixed to the splint bone and cannon bone (Figure 9.8E).[11,53,54] Bone screws alone may be more likely to cycle and break. If this is not performed, the proximal fragment may become displaced because of the inadequate amount of interosseous ligament holding it in place.

When amputating a lateral splint bone in the pelvic limb, one must be careful to avoid incising the large, dorsal metatarsal artery III (great metatarsal artery), which lies above and between the third and fourth metatarsal bones in the interosseous space.[55] If large amounts of fibrous tissue are present because of an infectious process, the artery may be difficult to dissect from the soft tissue component. If the artery is inadvertently severed, it can be ligated without causing problems associated with loss of blood supply to the distal limb.

Following removal of the splint bone, the subcutaneous tissue should be closed with a synthetic absorbable suture. Considerable dead space may result from removal of the bone, especially if much bony and fibrous tissue reaction was present. Some patients with a severe infectious process or significant dead space may require a Penrose drain for a few days (see Chapter 7, "Principles of Wound Management and the Use of Drains"). However, a good pressure bandage is often adequate to reduce dead space. Only in rare instances is an ingress-egress system of flushing indicated. The skin should be closed with a monofilament nonabsorbable suture using a simple interrupted pattern. The incision is covered with an antimicrobial dressing and is placed under a pressure bandage.

Postoperative Management

Tetanus prophylaxis is administered. Antibiotics are used in cases of acute (active) osteitis or osteomyelitis, although with appropriate preoperative wound management and thorough wound debridement, the infection usually resolves without the need for preoperative antimicrobial therapy.[53] The limb should be kept under a pressure bandage for 3–4 weeks. Despite careful hemostasis, the surgical procedure is generally accompanied by some hemorrhage. It is therefore wise to change the bandage in the first 1–2 days postoperatively. After that time, pressure bandages are changed every 5–7 days, or sooner if needed. If drains are in place, they should generally be removed the second or third postoperative day. Skin sutures should be removed 10–14 days after surgery.

Complications and Prognosis

In Standardbred horses, suspensory desmitis rather than the fractured splint bone may limit the prognosis for return to athletic soundness.[51,56]

Arthrotomy of the Fetlock Joint and Removal of an Apical Sesamoid Chip Fracture

Relevant Anatomy

The suspensory apparatus in the horse—which includes the proximal sesamoid bones, distal sesamoidean ligaments, and the suspensory ligament—has two important functions: to prevent hyperextension of the fetlock joint and to store and redistribute some of the weight-bearing force from the joint to the limb. Injury to the suspensory apparatus is common in horses, particularly in performance breeds such as Thoroughbreds and Standardbreds.

Often, it manifests as a fracture in the proximal sesamoid bones, of which apical fractures are usually the most common.[57]

Indications

The removal of apical sesamoid fracture fragments can be performed via arthroscopy or arthrotomy. If left unoperated, the result will be either a fibrous union or displacement of the fragment proximad, which, in turn, can lead to exostosis formation and joint-surface irregularity.[58]

Anesthesia and Surgical Preparation

This surgical procedure is performed with the horse under general anesthesia and, depending on the surgeon's preference, the horse may be placed in lateral or dorsal recumbency. With dorsal recumbency and the leg suspended, natural hemostasis is achieved. If surgery is performed in lateral recumbency, Esmarch's bandage and a tourniquet are generally used. Prior to anesthetic induction, the patient's leg is clipped from proximal cannon to coronary band all the way around the leg. Following anesthetic induction, the area of the surgical incision is shaved, and routine surgical preparation is performed. Draping may include the use of a plastic adhesive drape.

Instrumentation

1. General surgery pack
2. Weitlaner retractor
3. Bone curette
4. Rongeurs
5. Periosteal elevator

Surgical Technique

The limb is maintained in an extended position while surgical entry into the joint is made. With the leg in this position, it is easier to identify the branch of the suspensory ligament. An incision approximately 5 cm long is made over the palmar or plantar recess (volar pouch) of the metacarpo- (metatarso-) phalangeal joint immediately dorsal and parallel to the branch of the suspensory ligament and palmar or plantar to the distal aspect of the metacarpus or metatarsus (Figure 9.9A). The incision extends from approximately 1 cm below the distal extremity of the splint bone to the proximal border of the collateral sesamoidean ligament. The incision is continued through the thin subcutaneous areolar connective tissue in the same line, and Weitlaner retractors are placed to facilitate exposure of the joint capsule. It may be easier to identify the joint capsule if the joint has been distended with saline prior to making the incision. A 3-cm incision is made through the joint capsule (fibrous joint capsule plus synovial membrane) to enter the joint (Figure 9.9B). Care is taken to avoid the collateral sesamoidean ligament

A—Skin incision
B—Third metacarpal bone
C—Proximal phalanx
D—Proximal sesamoid bone

Weitlaner retractors

Incision through joint capsule

Suspensory ligament

Apical fragment

Closure of joint capsule

Fig. 9.9. **A–E.** Arthrotomy of fetlock joint for removal of apical sesamoid fracture.

distally and the vascular plexus on the palmar (plantar) aspect of the distal metacarpus or metatarsus proximally. Following entry into the joint, the fetlock is flexed, and the edges of the joint capsule are retracted to expose the palmar articular surface of the third metacarpus and the articular surface of the proximal sesamoid bone.

The apical fragment to be removed is identified, and it is incised from the suspensory ligament using a no. 15 scalpel blade or periosteal elevator (Figure 9.9C). Trauma to the suspensory ligament is minimized by careful, sharp dissection. As the soft tissue attachments are severed, the chip is removed using Ochsner forceps or small rongeurs (Figure 9.9D). The fracture site is curetted smooth, and the joint is vigorously flushed with sterile Ringer's solution. Intraoperative radiographs should be taken to confirm complete removal. The hypertrophic synovial membrane is also removed.

The fibrous joint capsule is closed with a layer of simple interrupted or continuous sutures of synthetic absorbable suture material. The sutures in the fibrous joint capsule should not penetrate the synovial membrane. Preplacement of the sutures in the joint capsule facilitates accurate apposition and a tight seal, but is not necessary when using a simple continuous pattern. Following closure of the joint capsule, 8–10 ml of Ringer's solution (to which 1 million U of potassium penicillin may be added) are flushed into the joint using a 20-gauge needle (Figure 9.9E). The subcutaneous fascia is closed with a simple continuous pattern using synthetic absorbable material, and the skin is closed with simple interrupted or near-far-far-near sutures of monofilament nonabsorbable material. The tourniquet is removed, a sterile dressing is placed over the incision, and a firm bandage is placed on the leg.

Postoperative Management

The use of antibiotics is optional. The skin sutures are removed in 10–12 days, and the bandage is maintained on the leg for another 10 days. Convalescent time after removal of an apical sesamoid chip should be at least 4 months, but it varies, depending on the degree of concurrent injury in the suspensory ligament and other soft tissues.

Complications and Prognosis

The prognosis depends largely on the size of the fracture fragment and the presence and degree of suspensory desmitis.[59] Sport horses with large apical fragments accompanied by suspensory branch injury may require 6–12 months of recovery and have a poor prognosis. Nonsport horses without preexisting injury generally have a very favorable prognosis. Surgical removal carries the best prognosis for horses with proven speed when they are operated on within 30 days of injury and have no evidence of suspensory desmitis or osteoarthritis. The prognosis for return to racing was 65% for those horses that had raced previous to injury.[58] In Standardbreds, conservative therapy dramatically reduced the racing performance when preinjury values were compared to postinjury values.[58]

References

1. Tnibar, M.A. Medial patellar ligament splitting for the treatment of upward fixation of the patella in 7 equids. *Vet. Surg.*, *31*:462–467, 2002.
2. Dugdale, D. Intermittent upward fixation of the patella and disorders of the patellar ligaments. *In* Current Therapy in Equine Medicine. Edited by N.E. Robinson. Philadelphia, W.B. Saunders, 2006.
3. Reiners, S.R., May, K., DiGrassie, W., and Moore, T. How to perform a standing medial patellar ligament splitting. *In* 51 Annual Convention of the American Association of Equine Practitioners, AAEP, 2005, Seattle, WA, USA. Ithaca: International Veterinary Information Service (www.ivis.org), 2006; Document No. P2684.1205.
4. McIlwraith, C.W. Osteochondral fragmentation of the distal aspect of the patella in horses. *Equine Vet. J.*, *22*:157, 1990.
5. Baccarin, R.Y., Martins, E.A., Hagen, S.C., and Silva, L.C. Patellar instability following experimental medial patellar desmotomy in horses. *Vet. Comp. Orthop. Traumatol.*, *22*:27–31, 2009.
6. Torre, F. Clinical diagnosis and results of surgical treatment of 13 cases of acquired bilateral stringhalt (1991–2003). *Equine Vet. J.*, *37*:181–183, 2005.
7. Cahill, J.I., Goulden, B.E., and Jolly, R.D. Stringhalt in horses: A distal axonopathy. *Neuropathol. Appl. Neurobiol.*, *12*:459, 1986.
8. Crabill, M.R., Honnas, C.H., Taylor, D.S., Schumacher, J., Watkins, J.P., and Snyder, J.R. Stringhalt secondary to the dorsoproximal region of the metatarsus in horses: 10 cases (1986–1991). *J. Am. Vet. Med. Assoc.*, *205*:867–869, 1994.
9. Slocombe, R.F., Huntington, P.J., Friend, S.C.E., Jeffcott, L.B., Luff, A.R., and Finkelstein, D.K. Pathological aspects of Australian stringhalt. *Equine Vet. J.*, *24*:174–183, 1992.
10. Cahill, J., and Goulden, B.E. Stringhalt—Current thoughts on aetiology and pathogenesis. *Equine Vet. J.*, *24*:161–162, 1992.
11. Stashak, T.S. ed. Adams' Lameness in Horses. 4th Ed. Philadelphia, Lea & Febiger, 1987, p. 723.
12. Adams, S.P., and Fessler, J.F. eds. Atlas of Equine Surgery. Philadelphia, W.B. Saunders, 2000, pp. 381–383.
13. Todhunter, P.G., Schumacher, J., and Finn-Bodner, S.T. Desmotomy for treatment of chronic desmitis of the accessory ligament of the deep digital flexor tendon in a horse. *Can. Vet. J.*, *38*:637–639, 1997.
14. Turner, T.A., and Rosenstein, D.S. Inferior check desmotomy as a treatment for caudal hoof lameness. *In* Proceedings of the 88th Annual Meeting of the American Association of Equine Practitioners, 1992, pp. 157–163.
15. Wagner, D.C., Grant, B.D., Kaneps, A.J., and Watrous, B.J. Long-term results of desmotomy of the accessory ligament of the deep digital flexor tendon (distal check ligament) in horses. *J. Am. Vet. Med. Assoc.*, *187*:1351, 1985.
16. Hunt, R.J. Flexural limb deformities. *In* Current Techniques in Equine Lameness and Surgery. 2nd Ed. Edited by N.A. White, J.N. Moore. Philadelphia, W.B. Saunders, 1998, pp. 326–328.

17. McIlwraith, C.W., and Fessler, J.F. Evaluation of inferior check ligament desmotomy for treatment of acquired flexor tension contracture. *J. Am. Vet. Med. Assoc., 172*:293, 1978.

18. White, N. Ultrasound-guided transection of the accessory ligament of the deep digital flexor muscle (distal check ligament desmotomy) in horses. *Vet. Surg., 24*:373–378, 1995.

19. Wagner, P.C. Flexure deformity of the metacarpophalangeal joint (contracture of the superficial digital flexure tendon). *In* Current Practice of Equine Surgery. Edited by N.A. White, J.N. Moore. Philadelphia, J.B. Lippincott, 1990, pp. 476–480.

20. Buchner, H.H.F., Savelberg, H.H.C.M., and Becker, C.K. Load redistribution after desmotomy of the accessory ligament of the deep digital flexor tendon in adult horses. *Vet. Q., 18*(Suppl.):70–74, 1996.

21. Stick, J.A., Nickels, F.A., and Williams, A. Long-term effects of desmotomy of the accessory ligament of the deep digital flexor muscle in Standardbreds: 23 cases (1979–1989). *J. Am. Vet. Med. Assoc., 8*:1131–1132, 1992.

22. Dyce, K.M., Sack, W.O., and Wensing, C.J.G. Textbook of Veterinary Anatomy. 2nd Ed. Philadelphia, W.B. Saunders, 1996, p. 585.

23. Bramlage, L.R. Personal communication, 1987.

24. Fackelman, G.E. Flexure deformity of the metacarpophalangeal joints in growing horses. *Compend. Contin. Educ., 9*:51, 1979.

25. Wagner, P.C., Shires, G.M., Watrous, B.J., Kaneps, A.J., Schmotzer, W.B., and Riebold, T.W. Management of acquired flexural deformity of the metacarpophalangeal joint in Equidae. *J. Am. Vet. Med. Assoc., 187*:915, 1985.

26. Gibson, K.T., Burbidge, H.M., and Pfeiffer, D.U. Superficial digital flexor tendonitis in Thoroughbred racehorses: Outcome following non-surgical treatment and superior check desmotomy. *Aust. Vet. J., 75*:631–635, 1997.

27. Hogan, P.M., and Bramlage, L.R. Transection of the accessory ligament of the superficial digital flexor tendon for treatment of tendinitis: Long term results in 61 Standardbred racehorses (1985–1992). *Equine Vet. J., 27*:221–226, 1995.

28. Bramlage, L.R. Superior check ligament desmotomy as a treatment for superficial digital flexor tendonitis: initial report. *In* Proceedings of the 32nd Annual Convention of the American Association of Equine Practitioners in 1986, 1987, pp. 365.

29. Jann, H.W., Beroza, G.A., and Fackelman, G.E. Surgical anatomy for desmotomy of the accessory ligament of the superficial flexor tendon (proximal check ligament) in horses. *Vet. Surg., 15*:378, 1986.

30. Alexander, G.R., Gibson, K.T., Day, R.E., and Robertson, I.D. Effects of superior check desmotomy on flexor tendon and suspensory ligament strain in equine cadaver limbs. *Vet. Surg., 30*:522–527, 2001.

31. Ross, M.W. Surgical management of superficial flexor tendonitis. *In* Diagnosis and Management of Lameness in the Horse. Edited by M.W. Ross, S.J. Dyson. Philadelphia, W.B. Saunders, 2003, pp. 714–721.

32. Ordidge, R.M. Comparison of three methods of treating superficial digital flexor tendinitis in the racing Thoroughbred by transection of its accessory ligament alone (proximal check ligament desmotomy) or in combination with either intra-lesional injections of hyaluronidase or tendon splitting. *Proc. Am. Assoc. Equine Pract., 42*:164, 1996.

33. Southwood, L.L., Stashak, T.S., Kainer, R.A., and Wrigley, R.H. Desmotomy of the accessory ligament of the superficial digital flexor tendon in the horse with use of a tenoscopic approach to the carpal sheath. *Vet. Surg., 28*:99–105, 1999.

34. McIlwraith, C.W. Tendon disorders of young horses. *In* Equine Medicine and Surgery. 3rd Ed. Edited by R.A. Mansmann, E.S. McAllister. Santa Barbara, CA, American Veterinary Publications, 1982.

35. Fackelman, G.E. Flexure deformity of the metacarpophalangeal joints in growing horses. *Compend. Contin. Educ., 1*:S1, 1979.

36. McIlwraith, C.W. Diseases of joints, tendons, ligaments, and related structures. *In* Adams' Lameness in Horses. 4th Ed. Edited by T.S. Stashak. Philadelphia, Lea & Febiger, 1987, p. 339.

37. Fackleman, G.E., Auer, J.A., Orsini, J., and von Salis, B. Surgical treatment of severe flexural deformity of the distal interphalangeal joint in young horses. *J. Am. Vet. Med. Assoc., 182*:949, 1983.

38. Allen, D., Jr., White, N.A., 2nd, Foerner, J.F., and Gordon, B.J. Surgical management of chronic laminitis in horses: 13 cases (1983–1985). *J. Am. Vet. Med. Assoc., 189*:1605, 1986.

39. Hunt, R.J., Allen, D., Baxter, G.M., Jackman, B.R., and Parks, A.H. Mid-metacarpal deep digital flexor tenotomy in the management of refractory laminitis in horses. *Vet. Surg., 20*:15–20, 1991.

40. Eastman, T.G., Honnas, C.M., Hague, B.A., Moyer, W., and von der Rosen, H.D. Deep digital flexor tenotomy as a treatment for chronic laminitis in horses: 35 cases (1998–1997). *J. Am. Vet. Med. Assoc., 214*:517–519, 1999.

41. Fortier, L.A., Nison, A.J., Ducharme, N.G., Nohammed, H.O., and Yeager, A. Tenoscopic examination and proximal annular ligament desmotomy for treatment of equine "complex" digital sheath tenosynovitis. *Vet. Surg., 28*:429–435, 1999.

42. Gerring, E.L., and Webbon, P.M. Fetlock annular ligament desmotomy: A report of 24 cases. *Equine Vet. J., 16*:113, 1984.

43. McGhee, J.D., White, N.A., and Goodrich, L.R. Primary desmitis of the palmar and plantar annular ligaments in horses: 25 cases (1990–2003). *J. Am. Vet. Med. Assoc., 226*:83–86, 2005.

44. Owen, K.R., Dyson, S.J., Parkin, T.D., Singer, E.R., Kristoffersen, M., and Mair, T.S. Retrospective study of palmar/planar annular ligament injury in 71 horses: 2001–2006. *Equine Vet. J., 40*:237–244, 2008.

45. Mathews, S., Dart, A.J., and Dowling, B.A. Palmar digital neurectomy in 24 horses using the guillotine technique. *Aust. Vet. J., 81*:402–405, 2003.

46. Maher, O., Davis, D.M., Drake, C., Myhre, G.D., Labbe, K.M., Han, J.H., and Lejeune, S.S. Pull-through technique for palmar digital neurectomy: Forty-one horses (1998–2004). *Vet. Surg., 37*:87–93, 2008.

47. Cummings, J.F., Fubini, S.L., and Todhunter, R.J. Attempts to prevent equine post neurectomy neuroma formation through retrograde transport of two neurotoxins, doxorubicin and ricin. *Equine Vet. J., 20*:451–456, 1988.

48. Jackman, B.R., Baxter, G.M., Doran, R.E., Allen, D., and Parks, A.H. Palmar digital neurectomy in horses: 57 cases (1984–1990). *Vet. Surg., 22*:285–288, 1993.

49. Dyson, S.J. The metacarpal region. *In* Diagnosis and Management of Lameness in the Horse. Edited by M.W. Ross, S.J. Dyson. Philadelphia, W.B. Saunders, 2003, pp. 362–375.

50. Haynes, P.F. Diseases of the metacarpophalangeal joint and the metacarpus. *In* Symposium on Equine Lameness. *Vet. Clin. North Am. Large Anim. Pract., 2*:33, 1980.

51. Verschooten, F., Gasthuys, F., and De Moor, A. Distal splint bone fractures in the horse: An experimental and clinical study. *Equine Vet. J., 16*:532, 1984.

52. Harrison, L.J., May, S.A., and Edwards, G.B. Surgical treatment of open splint bone fractures in 26 horses. *Vet. Rec., 128*:606–610, 1991.

53. Allen, D., and White, N.A. Management of fractures and exostosis of the metacarpals II and IV in 25 horses. *Equine Vet. J., 19*:326, 1987.

54. Peterson, P.R., Pascoe, J.R., and Wheat, J.D. Surgical management of proximal splint bone fractures in the horse. *Vet. Surg., 16*:367–372, 1987.

55. Milne, D.W., and Turner, A.S. An Atlas of Surgical Approaches to the Bones of the Horse. Philadelphia, W.B. Saunders, 1979.

56. Bowman, K.F., Evans, L.H., and Herring, M.E. Evaluation of surgical removal of fractured distal splint bones in the horse. *Vet. Surg., 11*:116, 1982.

57. Ruggles, A.J., and Gabel, A.A. Injuries of the proximal sesamoid bones. *In* Current Techniques in Equine Surgery and Lameness. Edited by N.A. White, J.N. Moore. Philadelphia, W.B. Saunders, 1998, pp. 403–408.

58. Spurlock, G.H., and Gabel, A.A. Apical fractures of the proximal sesamoid bones in 109 Standardbred horses. *J. Am. Vet. Med. Assoc., 183*:76, 1983.

59. Richardson, D.W. The metacarpophalangeal joint. *In* Diagnosis and Management of Lameness in the Horse. Edited by M.W. Ross, S.J. Dyson. Philadelphia, W.B. Saunders, 2003, pp. 348–362.

Chapter 10

EQUINE UROGENITAL SURGERY

Dean A. Hendrickson, DVM, MS, DACVS

Objectives

1. Describe a technique for routine castration and discuss potential serious complications.
2. Discuss several approaches for performing a cryptorchidectomy.
3. Describe common urogenital surgical techniques in the mare, including Caslick's operation for pneumovagina, urethroplasty, cesarean section, and repair of third-degree perineal lacerations.
4. Describe techniques for performing circumcision and penile amputation in the male.

Castration

Relevant Anatomy

In the male horse, the scrotum is located high between the hind limbs on the ventral portion of the caudal abdomen. The left testicle in the horse is commonly larger and more caudad than the right.[1] Externally, the median or scrotal raphe divides the scrotum into roughly equal left and right halves.

The scrotum contains the testicles, the distal components of the spermatic cord, the cremaster muscles, and the epididymis. There are four primary layers of the scrotum: the outermost skin and associated connective tissue, the smooth muscle fibers of the tunica dartos, the loose connective tissue of the scrotal fascia, and the innermost parietal vaginal tunic.[1] The testes are comprised of parenchyma encapsulated by a fibrous layer, the tunica albuginea. Most of the parenchyma consists of seminiferous tubules.[1] The remaining interstitial tissues are comprised of Leydig cells, blood vessels, lymphatic vessels, and immune cells.[1] The head of the epididymis is attached to the dorsolateral surface of the testicle and terminates in a coiled tail at the posterior end. The ductus deferens continues from the epididymis with the spermatic cord, which runs from the testicles to the vaginal rings. The spermatic cords contain the ductus deferens, testicular artery, pampiniform plexus, lymph vessels, nerves, and smooth muscle, which are all enclosed by the parietal layer of the vaginal tunic.

Indications

Castration is usually performed to facilitate the management of a particular animal when it is in the company of females or other males. Castration can be performed at any time; however, the colt is often left intact for 12–18 months to allow for development of certain desirable physical characteristics. Other animals may be castrated at a later age when it is no longer desirable to maintain them as stallions. Prior to castration, it should be ascertained that the animal is healthy and that both testes are descended. If a horse is anesthetized and only one testis is descended, the surgery should be aborted unless the surgeon is comfortable with cryptorchid castration.

Many methods of castration are available. This section describes a two-phase emasculation preceded by separate dissection of the common tunic because the authors believe it is the optimal technique for the prevention of untoward sequelae. In the technique of "closed" castration, the common vaginal tunic is dissected, but not opened; and emasculation of the entire cord within the tunic is performed as a single procedure. Because several structures are enclosed within the jaws of the emasculator, there is a greater chance that a vessel will be emasculated inadequately. This technique should be restricted to

---

Turner and McIlwraith's Techniques in Large Animal Surgery, 4th Edition. Dean A. Hendrickson and A. N. (Nickie) Baird.
© 2013 John Wiley & Sons, Inc. Published 2013 by John Wiley & Sons, Inc.

patients with small testes. In a modified-closed technique, the vaginal tunic is sharply incised over the spermatic cord, the vascular structures exteriorized and emasculated, followed by emasculation of the entire cord.

In the "open" technique, the common tunic is opened with the initial skin incision, and prior dissection of the tunic from the subcutaneous tissue is not performed. This method is commonly used without any problems, but the chances of inadequate tunic removal with consequent hydrocele are increased.

A technique of primary closure in multiple layers with ablation of the scrotum has been described.[2] In this technique, the ventral scrotum is ablated. The testicles are removed by emasculation combined with transfixation ligatures. Additional skin may have to be removed, so the scrotum is completely ablated when the skin edges are apposed. Closure of the subcutaneous and subcuticular tissues is performed in three or four layers. This method is certainly more time consuming than other procedures, but postoperative scrotal swelling is usually eliminated.[2]

Anesthesia and Surgical Preparation

Castration may be performed on the standing animal under local analgesia or with the animal in recumbency under general anesthesia. The technique depends on the temperament of the animal, the experience of the surgeon, and in some situations, the tradition and environment in which the horse is castrated.

For castration of the standing animal, a tranquilizer or sedative may be administered to the horse, and local infiltration analgesia is performed. A combination of detomidine hydrochloride (20–40 µg/kg) or xylazine hydrochloride (0.3–0.5 mg/kg) and butorphanol tartate (0.01–0.05 mg/kg) is commonly used and provides reliable sedation.[3,4] Following surgical preparation of the area, the skin is infiltrated on a line 1 cm from the median raphe with 10 ml of local analgesic solution; this infiltration is continued into the subcutaneous tissue. Local analgesia can be injected directly into the testis. It is also important to infiltrate the spermatic cord in the region of emasculation with a long 18- to 20-gauge needle.

For castration of the recumbent animal, several anesthetic regimens are available and suitable. Anesthesia may be induced by intravenous administration of a xylazine (1.0 mg/kg) and ketamine hydrochloride (2.2 mg/kg) mixture.[5] If the procedure is prolonged, a second dose may be given intravenously according to the desired time of anesthesia. Alternatively, guaifenesin in combination with thiamylal sodium may be used; or if rapid induction is desired, thiamylal sodium or thiopental sodium alone is suitable.

For a right-handed operator, the horse is cast with the left side down. The upper hind leg is tied craniad, and the surgical site is prepared. Clipping or shaving is not necessary. It can be easier to position the horse in dorsal recumbency using bales to hold the horse in place.

Instrumentation

1. General surgery pack
2. Emasculators
3. LDS stapler (US Surgical)

Surgical Technique

This castration technique is illustrated here in the recumbent animal. Prior to making the first incision, it is helpful to inject local anesthetic into the testis and spermatic cord. This will reduce the movements during the procedure and lengthen the effective time of the general anesthetics. Castration is performed through separate incisions for each testis, with incisions located approximately 1 cm from the median raphe (Figure 10.1A). The lower testis is grasped between the thumb and forefingers, and the first skin incision is made for the length of the testis (Figure 10.1B). The incision is continued through the tunica dartos and scrotal fascia, leaving the common tunic (tunica vaginalis parietalis) intact. At the same time, pressure exerted by the thumb and forefingers causes the testis, which is still contained within the common tunic, to be extruded (Figure 10.1C). The testis is then grasped in the left hand (for a right-handed operator), and the subcutaneous tissue is stripped from the common vaginal tunic as far proximally as possible (Figure 10.1D). The use of a gauze sponge can facilitate the stripping of the subcutaneous tissue from the common tunic. At this point, a closed, a modified closed, or an open technique can be performed. For the open technique, the surgeon incises the common tunic over the cranial pole of the testis (Figure 10.1E) and, hooking a finger within the tunic to maintain tension, continues the incision proximad (Figure 10.1F).

The testis is now released from within the common tunic. The mesorchium is penetrated digitally to separate the vascular spermatic cord from the ductus deferens, common tunic, and external cremaster muscle (Figure 10.1G). The latter structures are severed, with attention to removing as much of the common tunic as possible (Figure 10.1G). The severance of this musculofibrous portion of the spermatic cord may be performed conveniently with emasculators, and the crush need only be applied for a short period of time. The testis is then grasped, and the spermatic vessels are emasculated (Figure 10.1H).

Care must always be taken to apply the emasculator correctly without incorporating skin between its jaws and to prevent stretch on the spermatic cord at the time of emasculation. An optional preliminary to emasculation is to place forceps proximally on the cord as a safeguard against loss if a failure occurs during emasculation. The emasculator remains in position for 1–2 minutes, depending on the size of the cord, and is then released.

Another technique that can minimize the amount of hemorrhage following castration is to use an LDS stapling

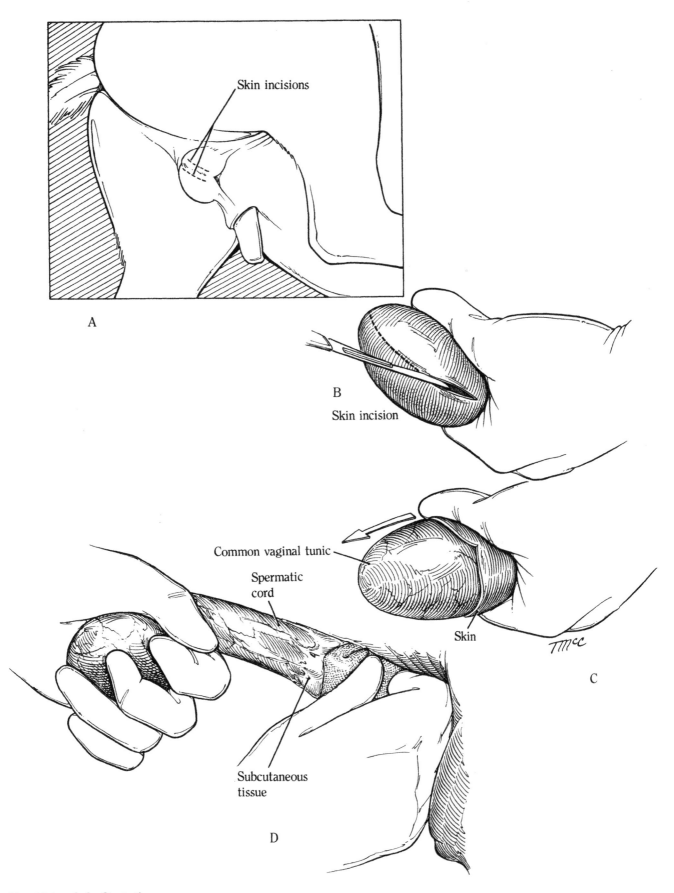

Skin incisions

A

B
Skin incision

Common vaginal tunic

Spermatic cord

Skin

Subcutaneous tissue

C

D

Fig. 10.1. **A–L.** Castration.

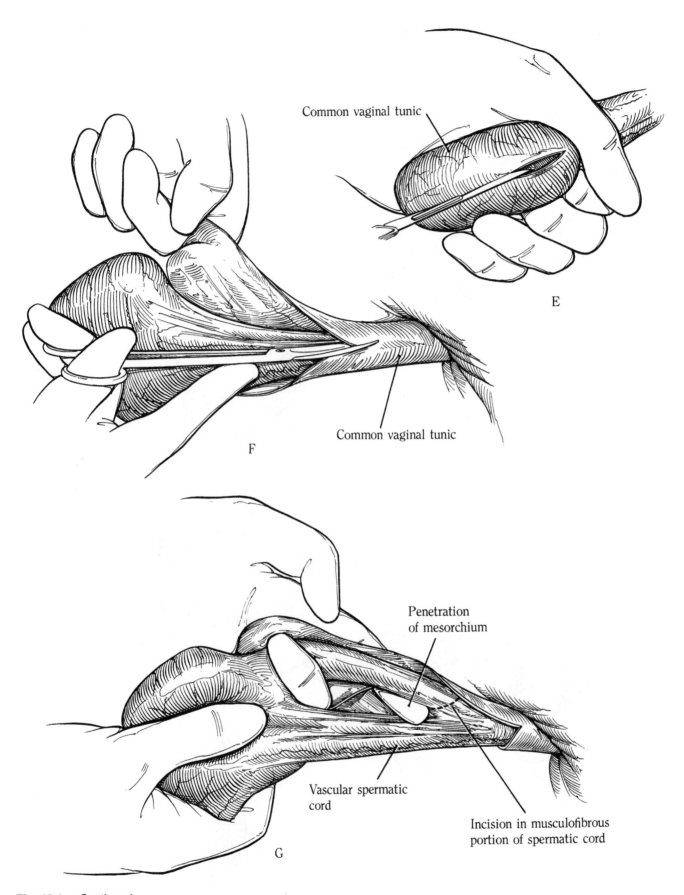

Common vaginal tunic

Common vaginal tunic

E

F

Penetration
of mesorchium

Vascular spermatic
cord

Incision in musculofibrous
portion of spermatic cord

G

Fig. 10.1. *Continued.*

H

I

Fig. 10.1. *Continued.*

J

K

L

Fig. 10.1. *Continued.*

device to ligate the spermatic vasculature. The testis is approached as previously described, up to the point just following stripping of the subcutaneous fascia (Figure 10.1A–D). At this point a small incision is made into the vaginal tunic over the spermatic cord (Figure 10.1I). The vascular portion of the spermatic cord is exteriorized. An LDS stapling device (Covidien, Mansfield, MA) with the dividing blade removed is used to place two ligating staples around the vasculature (Figure 10.1J). The vasculature is transected distal to the staples (Figure 10.1K), and the emasculator is placed over the tunic and the testis removed (Figure 10.1L).

The skin incisions are enlarged by pulling them apart with the fingers until a 10-cm opening is obtained. The median raphe may also be removed to further facilitate drainage. However, this may cause more hemorrhage. Any redundant adipose tissue or fascia is also removed.

Postoperative Management

Tetanus immunization is administered, and antibiotics usually are not indicated. The horse should be kept under close observation for several hours after castration to make sure that it is not hemorrhaging, and under general observation for the first 24 hours for other complications and periodically during the first week following surgery. During the first 24 hours, the horse should be confined with limited exercise. Uneventful healing is the usual result with good drainage and satisfactory exercise. The animal should be forcibly exercised twice daily from the day following surgery until healing is complete. The new gelding should be separated from mares for at least a week to ensure that no pregnancies will occur.[6] It has been suggested that a gelding can impregnate a mare up to 60 days after castration.

Complications and Prognosis

Complications of equine castration are uncommon, but they can be life threatening to the horse and of great concern to the surgeon. To minimize postoperative complications, good communication with the client is required.

A number of possible complications may arise following castration, such as

1. Severe hemorrhage is usually associated with inadequate emasculation of the testicular artery of the spermatic cord, but considerable hemorrhage can occur from one of the branches of the external pudendal vein in the scrotal wall or septum, if accidentally ruptured,[7] or in the transected external cremaster muscle.
2. Excessive swelling of the surgical site can arise because of inadequate drainage or inadequate exercise, or a hydrocele may form because of collection of fluid in a common tunic that has been inadequately resected.

3. Evisceration may occur through an inguinal hernia.
4. Acute wound infection and septicemia may occur; scirrhous cord formation is due to chronic infection and generally can be related to poor technique and inadequate exercise or drainage.
5. Persistent masculine behavior can occur following removal of two normal testes.
6. Penile paralysis.

Hemorrhage

Minor hemorrhage may occur for several hours, but significant hemorrhage beyond approximately 12 hours may require surgical intervention. If the source of hemorrhage is the testicular artery, ligation using a synthetic absorbable suture material may be required. This procedure may warrant general anesthesia if the horse is difficult to manage. Curved forceps, such as Mixter curved hemostatic forceps, are helpful. Standing laparoscopy can be used to look for intraabdominal bleeding.

Edema

Edema of the scrotum and prepuce, a more common complication of castration, usually begins on the third or fourth postoperative day and is often associated with inadequate exercise. Simply turning the gelding out to pasture without forced exercise is often inadequate because of postoperative pain. Horses with excessive edema of the scrotum and prepuce should be checked for a temperature rise because it may indicate impending infection. To help reestablish drainage, a sterile surgical glove is donned, and the scrotal incision is opened cautiously. Parenteral antibiotics, such as procaine penicillin G, may be indicated, as well as a conscientious program of forced exercise. Phenylbutazone may be indicated to reduce soreness and to encourage pain-free movement. Long-standing chronic infections with abscess formation in the inguinal canal may need surgical exploration and abscess drainage.

Visceral Prolapse

Visceral prolapse through the inguinal canal and open scrotum is the most serious potential complication of castration. Eventration of the intestine or omentum may occur within the first few hours after castration before swelling has closed the inguinal canal, but it has been observed up to 6 days after surgery.[8] The incidence of herniation following routine castration is fairly low; one study reported evisceration of the small intestine in 4.8% of the 568 colts that were castrated.[5] Furthermore, there was no association found between open and closed techniques of castration and the incidence of herniation or evisceration in these horses.[5] Some authors believe a half-closed castration technique, which involves opening of the vaginal cavity and ligation of both the parietal vaginal tunic and spermatic cord, minimizes the risk of herniation and evisceration.[9] It has been suggested that breeds such as draft horses, Standardbred horses, warmbloods, and some mustangs have a higher incidence of eventration and should have a ligature placed around the spermatic cord when being castrated.

The postoperative complication rate is high for repair of intestinal prolapse, and the condition requires immediate attention.[5] If management of the eventration is beyond the capabilities of the surgeon, the offending viscera, unless it is extensive, can be replaced in the scrotum; the scrotum can be packed with sterile gauzes and temporarily closed with several simple interrupted sutures; and, following the appropriate fluid therapy and parenteral antibiotics, the animal can be referred to an equine surgical facility.

If the eventration is to be managed where the horse was gelded because referral is out of the question, preoperative planning is essential. The appropriate instruments, drapes, and isotonic solutions for lavage must be obtained, and preoperative broad-spectrum antibiotic therapy should commence. Plans for balanced, movement-free general anesthesia must also be made.

With the animal under general anesthesia and in dorsal recumbency, the offending viscera is cleaned by lavage of balanced electrolyte solutions. The incision and scrotal area are prepared for aseptic surgery as thoroughly as possible. Debris, such as straw or blood clots, may have to be manually removed from the bowel in the earlier stages of preparation for surgery. Small segments of bowel, if viable and relatively uncontaminated, can be replaced in the abdomen. Some enlargement of the inguinal ring may be required if the bowel has become congested and edematous. Greater lengths of intestine may be sufficiently contaminated or devitalized causing resection and anastomosis to be required. The internal ring may have to be enlarged, a portion of normal bowel exteriorized, and then anastomosis performed. If a portion of omentum is the only abdominal content involved, it can be excised, and remaining healthy omentum can be replaced in the abdomen.

Closure of the internal ring is usually impossible, but closure of the external ring using preplaced simple interrupted synthetic absorbable suture material is necessary, as described in the next section of this chapter on cryptorchidectomy.

Packing of the external canal, as shown in Figure 10.2J, is then performed. Fluid therapy should be instituted, as well as other adjunctive therapy for shock, such as flunixin meglumine. The prognosis following eventration is always guarded. A long-term complication may be adhesion of bowel to the inguinal ring (discussed later in this section).[10]

Persistent Masculine Behavior

Many practitioners and horsemen believe that if a stallion is "cut-proud" (a small quantity of epididymis was not removed during surgery), he will continue to show stal-lionlike behavior. That removal of identifiable epididymal tissue or another piece of a long spermatic cord has resolved the problem in some instances and lends some support to this idea.[7] Testicular or adrenal tissue has not been demonstrated in these removed segments, however, and the problem has been proposed to be psychological.[11] If one suspects that testicular tissue is still present in a gelding, we suggest measuring testosterone levels 30–100 minutes after injecting 6000–12,000 IU of human chorionic gonadotropin (HCG).[12]

Wound Infection

Wound infection may be either acute or chronic. Acute infection can be treated by enlarging the scrotal incisions to allow drainage and by increasing exercise. Antibiotics may be useful. Chronic infection, or scirrhous cord formation, generally requires a second surgery to remove the abnormal tissue. This procedure generally requires more surgical time, and plans should be made accordingly.

Penile Paralysis

Penile paralysis (paraphimosis), a rare complication, is usually seen when phenothiazine tranquilizers have been used. If the penis is flaccid and does not retract in 4 to 8 hours, mechanical support of the penis is indicated. *Priapism* is an abnormally prolonged erection of the penis, not associated with sexual desire.[13] It also has been associated with the use of phenothiazine tranquilizers; but fortunately, it is an even rarer complication of castration. Priapism has been treated medically using an anticholinergic agent, benztropine mesylate.[14] The condition has also been treated by drainage and irrigation of the corpus cavernosum penis, along with creation of a vascular shunt between that structure and the corpus spongiosum penis.[11] Description of this procedure is beyond the scope of this book, and the references should be consulted for further details.[13]

Adhesions

Other long-term complications of castration are uncommon, but they are serious and require surgical management. Adhesions of small intestine may occur following ascending infection.[15] We have seen this condition cause a chronic low-grade colic because of incomplete obstruction of the lumen of the small intestine. Muscular hypertrophy, fibrosis, and thickening of the bowel wall aboral to the adhesion usually result. A ventral midline celiotomy, in combination with an inguinal approach, may be required to treat an adhesion in this region. Following identification of the offending bowel and the extent of the adhesion, the adhesion is broken down by carefully separating the bowel from the inguinal region. If the adhesion is of long duration, blind transection of the adhesion with scissors may be required. Standing laparoscopy may be

Fig. 10.2. **A–S.** Cryptorchidectomy.

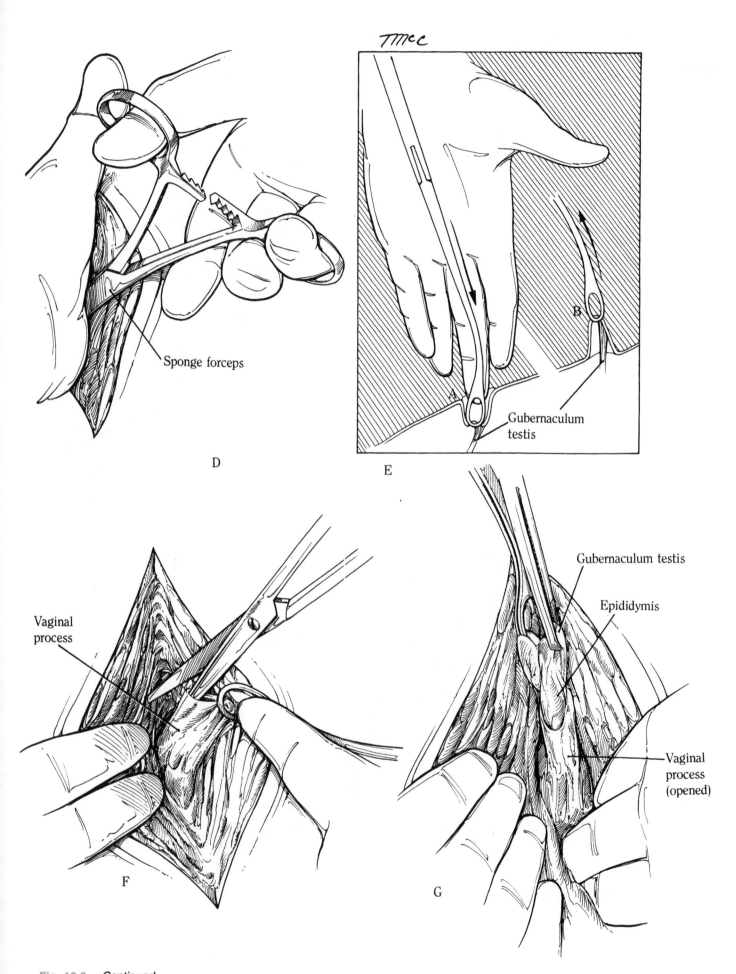

TMcC

Sponge forceps

Gubernaculum testis

D

E

Vaginal process

Gubernaculum testis

Epididymis

Vaginal process (opened)

F

G

Fig. 10.2. *Continued.*

H

I

J

Testis

Sterile
Gauze

Fig. 10.2. *Continued.*

K

L

M

Fig. 10.2. *Continued.*

Testis

N

O

P

Fig. 10.2. *Continued.*

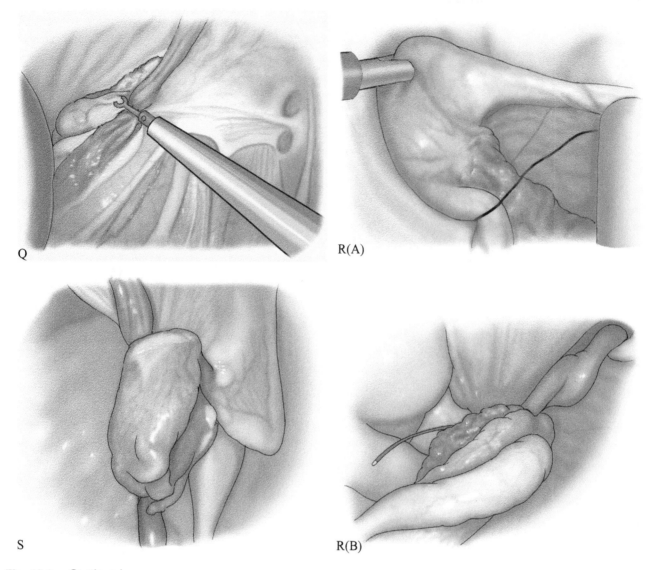

Q

R(A)

S

R(B)

Fig. 10.2. *Continued.*

helpful in diagnosing and treating adhesions. With either method, the risk of tearing the intestinal wall and contaminating the abdominal cavity with intestinal contents is real and may be fatal. Peeling the bowel off the adhesion has been successful, but it leaves a raw, bleeding edge that itself is prone to future adhesion formation. Daily rectal examinations, if the horse's size and temperament permit, allow the surgeon to "wipe away" carefully any potentially adhering bowel from these raw surfaces.

Cryptorchidectomy by the Inguinal, Parainguinal, and Flank Approach

Relevant Anatomy

In the fetal colt, the testes descend from the abdominal cavity through the inguinal canal to the scrotum just prior to birth or within 2 weeks after.[16] The entrance of the canal from the abdominal cavity, the deep inguinal ring, is located at the caudal border of the internal abdominal oblique muscle. The canal terminates externally at an opening in the aponeurosis of the external abdominal oblique muscle, called the *superficial inguinal ring*. If one or both testes fails to reach the scrotum, it may remain within the abdomen or the canal itself resulting in cryptorchidism. If the testis has traversed the vaginal ring but has not reached the scrotum, the horse is considered an inguinal cryptorchid ("high flanker"). If the testis has not traversed the vaginal ring and has not descended into the inguinal canal, the horse is considered an abdominal cryptorchid. In this case, the vaginal process with the attached gubernaculum will usually be developed and it may be inverted into the abdominal cavity or descended into the canal.[16] Cryptorchidism may be unilateral or bilateral and, in cases of inguinal cryptorchids, may spontaneously resolve itself after a year or more following birth. Horses with abdominal testis(es) will not spontaneously resolve. If the condition does not resolve, then surgical removal of the retained testis(es) is necessary. In a retrospective study of 16 unilaterally castrated horses and 44 cryptorchid horses, there was not statistical difference in the left- versus right-sided retained testes.[17] In another report, the left testis was found in the abdomen in 75% of cryptorchid horses compared to 42% of right testes.[4] This is more in line with the author's experience.

The previous section contains additional pertinent anatomy for this technique. For both the inguinal and paraguinal approaches, a thorough understanding of the orientation of the gonadal structures is crucial to successfully locating the testis. In particular, the surgeon relies on the attachment between the tail of the epididymis and the vaginal process to do so.

Indications

There are multiple techniques used for cryptorchidectomy. They can be used to remove both abdominally retained and inguinally retained testis. The most commonly used techniques are the inguinal, paraguinal, and standing laparoscopic techniques. Each will be described.

A rectal examination performed on a cryptorchid patient may enable one to ascertain whether the cryptorchid testis(es) is abdominal or inguinal. Inguinal testes may be nonpalpable on external examination of the inguinal canal. The rectal palpation of the ductus deferens through the vaginal ring indicates that the testis is in the inguinal canal. If the ductus deferens cannot be palpated passing through the vaginal ring, the testis is considered to be within the abdomen. We do not routinely perform a rectal examination prior to cryptorchidectomy. Because of altered behavior frequently seen in these cases, the horses are usually fractious and are therefore at an increased risk for rectal perforation. Unlike the broodmare, these animals have not usually been subjected to routine rectal palpation, and this further increases the risk. Arabians, because of a smaller anus and rectum, may be particularly predisposed to this problem. Transrectal ultrasound can be used to diagnose an intraabdominal testis; however, it is not always possible to find the testis. In one report, the use of transabdominal ultrasonography successfully identifies the location of the testis in 93% of horses.[18]

Anesthesia and Surgical Preparation

The horse is placed under general anesthesia for the inguinal and paraguinal approach and positioned in dorsal recumbency. General anesthesia can be induced with xylazine and ketamine and maintained using "triple drip" (see Chapter 2, "Anesthesia and Fluid Therapy"). The inguinal area is prepared for aseptic surgery in a routine manner and draped.

Instrumentation

1. General surgery pack
2. Sponge forceps
3. Emasculator
4. Spay hook (parainguinal approach)

Surgical Technique

Inguinal Approach

The horse is anesthetized and placed into dorsal recumbency. A 12- to 15-cm skin incision is made over the external inguinal ring and is continued through the superficial fascia. (The site of the incision is illustrated in Figure 10.2A.) Sharp dissection is then abandoned in favor of blunt dissection with fingertips to separate the subcutaneous inguinal fascia and to expose the external inguinal ring. Large branches of the external pudendal vein are in this region, and trauma to these vessels should be avoided. Dissection is continued beyond the external inguinal ring and through the inguinal canal until the vaginal ring is located with the finger (Figure 10.2B). With an inguinal cryptorchid, the testis contained within the common vaginal tunic would be located in the canal at this time (Figure 10.2C). The common tunic is isolated, and the testis is removed as previously described for normal castration. A closed castration technique is generally used.

With an abdominal cryptorchid, however, the testis will not be obvious. In this situation, the vaginal ring is located, and curved sponge forceps are carefully introduced through the inguinal canal so that the jaws are placed through the vaginal ring into the vaginal process (Figure 10.2D). The partially opened jaws of the forceps are pressed against the vaginal process and are closed (Figure 10.2E). The forceps grasp the vaginal process and associated gubernaculum testis, and the forceps are then withdrawn (Figure 10.2E). This is the critical part of the technique and the most difficult part for the inexperienced surgeon, because excessive force ruptures the vaginal process. The cordlike gubernaculum may then be palpated within the everted vaginal process by rolling it between the thumb and forefinger. When the gubernaculum is identified, the vaginal process is opened with Metzenbaum scissors (Figure 10.2F), and the gubernaculum is grasped with Ochsner forceps. Traction on the gubernaculum causes the tail of the epididymis to be presented (Figure 10.2G). Generally, gentle traction on the epididymis pulls the testis through the vaginal ring. Pushing around the vaginal ring with the fingers at the same time usually is sufficient to deliver the testis, but manual dilation of the vaginal ring is necessary in some cases.

At this point, the testis is positively identified (Figure 10.2H) and is emasculated (Figure 10.2I). In some instances, the testis cannot be retracted sufficiently to enable emasculation, so the cord is ligated and the testis sharply amputated. If the opening made in the vaginal process to deliver the testicle is considerable and if intestinal herniation is a possibility, the external inguinal ring is closed using a large-diameter synthetic absorbable suture material in either a preplaced interrupted pattern or a simple continuous pattern. The strong aponeurosis of the external abdominal oblique muscle is opposed to the fascia on the opposite side of the ring. The dead space is then closed using a no. 2-0 synthetic absorbable suture material. Conversely, a sterile gauze bandage may be packed over the external inguinal ring (Figure 10.2J); this protects against herniation while normal swelling obliterates the inguinal canal. Finally, the skin is sutured with a synthetic absorbable suture, either in a continuous pattern or with simple interrupted sutures with long ends (Figure 10.2J). If the opening in the vaginal process is small (barely enough to squeeze the testicle through), packing will usually be unnecessary. Surgical judgment and some experience will decide whether to pack the external ring or not.

The foregoing technique cannot be used in certain instances, such as when accidental rupture of the vaginal process, vaginal ring, or medial wall of the inguinal canal results in the loss of vital landmarks or when the horse has been subjected to a previous, unsuccessful attempt at surgery. In these situations, the first alternative is digital exploration of the boundaries of the vaginal ring to locate the gubernaculum and the ductus deferens or epididymis. Occasionally, the testes are encountered during the digital exploration. If these methods fail to locate the testis, manual exploration of the abdomen with the entire hand may be necessary. The hand may be admitted through a dilated (ruptured) vaginal ring or through the internal abdominal oblique muscle. The internal abdominal oblique muscle forms the medial wall of the inguinal canal and is thin and easily penetrated in this location. If the testis or ductus deferens is not found immediately, the ampullae should be located at the dorsal aspect of the bladder and traced craniad to the ductus deferens and testis. Termination of the ductus deferens with no epididymis or testis suggests the absence of a testis.

Parainguinal Approach

To perform the parainguinal approach, the horse is anesthetized and placed in dorsal recumbency as described for the inguinal approach. The ventral abdomen is aseptically prepared and draped to allow access to the inguinal areas. A 10-cm incision is made to allow access to the inguinal areas. A 10-cm incision is made through the skin parallel to and 4 cm axial to the inguinal canal (Figure 10.2K). The inguinal canal is explored as for the inguinal approach (Figure 10.2B) to assess the presence of an inguinal testis. If there is an inguinal testis, it is removed as previously described. If no inguinal testis is present, an incision of similar length is made into the external rectus sheath using a scalpel blade. It is important to not make the inci-

sion any deeper than the sheath. The rectus abdominus muscle is bluntly divided, and the internal rectus sheath is bluntly penetrated along with the peritoneum. A spay hook is placed through the incision into the peritoneal space. The tip of the spay hook is swept through the region of the vaginal ring to pick up the gubernaculum (Figure 10.2L,M). The gubernaculum is removed from the abdomen and traction is placed until the testis is removed from the abdomen. The testis is emasculated (Figure 10.2N). The external rectus sheath is closed in a simple continuous pattern using no. 1 polyglyconate (Figure 10.2O). The subcutaneous tissue and skin are closed respectively using a no. 2-0 synthetic absorbable suture material using a simple continuous pattern.

Standing Flank Approach

To perform the flank approach, the horse is sedated and placed into standing stocks. It is important to determine on which side of the abdomen the retained testis is located, as it is not possible to remove the contralateral testis from the flank. The flank of the appropriate side is clipped and aseptically prepared for surgery. The skin and flank musculature is anesthetized with local anesthetic in either an inverted L pattern or as a line block. A 15-cm skin incision is made in the midportion of the paralumbar fossa through the skin and external abdominal oblique muscles, centered at the level of the most distal portal shown for the laparoscopic approach. (Figure 10.2P) The internal abdominal oblique and transverse abdominus are penetrated along their fibers in a grid fashion. The testis is identified and exteriorized from the incision and emasculated. The external abdominal oblique fascia is closed with an absorbable suture material in a continuous pattern. The skin is closed with a nonabsorbable suture material in a continuous pattern.

Postoperative Management

Tetanus immunization is administered. If gauze packing is placed, it is removed at 24 hours postoperatively. Sutures and gauze pack are removed, the horse is discharged, and the owner is given instructions for routine post castration management. If suture closure of the inguinal canal is performed, we prefer to hospitalize the horse for 72 hours. Horses can begin exercise in 2 weeks.

Complications and Prognosis

The potential postoperative complications following cryptorchid surgery are the same as described previously for routine castration. Management of the complications is the same for both procedures, and the reader is referred to "Complications and Prognosis" in the section earlier in this chapter titled "Castration." The noninvasive approaches described here are considered superior to the invasive technique. Complications of the invasive technique may be severe, whereas the most common reported complication of the noninvasive technique is failure to identify the vaginal process or ring. Nonetheless, there are inherent risks associated with the noninvasive approach, such as trauma to abdominal structures or inadvertently clamping bowel instead of the vaginal process. Severe swelling may occur, but it can be resolved with hydrotherapy. The prognosis is very favorable with either technique. The author prefers the parainguinal approach because it is easier to close the external rectus sheath than the external inguinal ring. Scrotal ablation and primary closure techniques have been described with apparently fewer complications, better cosmetic results (less postoperative swelling), and less postoperative discomfort. Further details of these methods are available.[2]

Laparoscopic Cryptorchidectomy

Relevant Anatomy

The anatomical structures relevant to this procedure are the same as discussed in the previous sections. The perspective is different, however, due to the flank approach. The testis will hang from the dorsal body wall at the mesorchial attachment and is very easy to locate and identify even if previous surgical attempts have been made.

Indications

This technique is an effective, less-invasive, method for removal of cryptorchid testes than a flank or inguinal approach. The benefits of laparoscopy in horses include a shorter convalescence time, better visualization, and more complete exploration of the abdominal cavity. This technique describes the use of hand-tied or pretied ligatures to facilitate intraabdominal amputation of cryptorchid testes in the standing horse.

Anesthesia and Surgical Preparation

For standing laparoscopic procedures in the horse, fasting should begin prior to surgery to prevent intestinal contents from interfering with visualization in the abdomen. The surgery is performed in stocks, generally, with the tail wrapped and secured either to the horse or stocks. The appropriate flank or flanks are aseptically prepared for surgery depending on the location of the abdominally retained testes. Both flanks should always be prepared on bilateral cryptorchids or where the castration history is unclear. Sedation is achieved intravenously with xylazine (0.5 mg/kg) combined with butorphanol (0.05 mg/kg). Further sedation is achieved with either continuous IV infusion of detomidine (20 mg detomidine in 1 L polyionic replacement fluids) through a jugular catheter or with detomidine injected into the epidural space (40 g/kg detomidine brought to a total volume of 10–12 ml with

sterile saline). The skin and musculature of the left flank is desensitized with local portals site blocks (Figure 10.2P) or with an inverted L block using local anesthetic, such as 2% Lidocaine or 2% Mepivacaine (see Chapter 2).

Instrumentation

1. General surgery pack
2. 3–4 surgical drapes
3. Additional towel clamps
4. Telescope (see Chapter 3, "Surgical Instruments")
5. Light source with attached light cord
6. Mare urinary catheter
7. Veress needle, teat cannula, or trochar catheter
8. Sharp and blunt trochars
9. 3–6 cannulas, 10 mm in diameter and 15–20 cm long
10. 10-mm serrated laparoscopic scissors
11. 1–2 10-mm acute claw graspers
12. Laparoscopic injection needle
13. Knot pusher
14. Endoscopic suture materials
15. Laparoscopic video camera (optional)

Surgical Technique

After draping, a 1-cm incision is made in the appropriate flank (left for left-sided of bilateral cryptorchids, right for right-sided cryptorchids) at the base of the tuber coxae, midway between the tuber coxae and the last rib. The incision should include the skin and the fascia of the external abdominal oblique muscle. A mare urinary catheter or a 10-mm diameter, 20-cm long cannula with a blunt trochar is placed through the incision, directed upward toward the opposite stifle, and inserted through the body wall in one continuous motion.[19] Presence in the peritoneal space is confirmed by listening for air being drawn into the abdomen. Insufflation tubing is attached to the cannula and insufflation with CO_2 begun. If a laparoscopic cannula is used, the laparoscope can be inserted to confirm presence in the peritoneal space. The abdomen is insufflated to a pressure of 12–15 mmHG.[20] Second and third portals are placed 10 cm dorsal and slightly rostral and 10 cm ventral, respectively, to the first portal (Figure 10.2P). The laparoscope is placed in the dorsalmost portal, and the abdomen explored. Instruments can be placed in the middle or ventral portals to lift the small colon to observe the opposite inguinal area and determine the location of the testes. The ipsilateral testis is identified (Figure 10.2Q) and grasped, and the mesorchium is infiltrated with 2% lidocaine using a laparoscopic injection needle. A laparoscopic slipknot (4–5 modified Modified Roeder using no. 1 polyglyconate) in a knot pusher is placed into a 5-mm reducing cannula and inserted in the middle cannula.[21,22] The loop is advanced into the abdomen, and an acute claw grasper is placed into the ventral cannula, through the loop; and the testis is grasped. The loop is placed over the testis onto the mesorchium and tightened (Figure 10.2*R*). The long end of the suture is cut and the mesorchium transected distal to the knot. The pedicle is assessed for bleeding (Figure 10.2*S*).

A single ligature is generally sufficient; however, a second one can be placed if necessary. In cases of bilateral cryptorchids, the right testis can generally be removed from the left side after placing a 4th cannula in the left flank and lifting the small colon.[19] After the testis has been amputated, the ventralmost incision is enlarged and the testis removed. The external abdominal oblique fascia is closed in the enlarged incision using no. 0 polyglyconate in a simple continuous pattern. The skin is closed with a synthetic, nonabsorbable suture material.

Postoperative Management

Generally, the convalescence time for laparoscopic procedures is shorter than other approaches. The horse should be kept in confinement for 3 days and then can return to full exercise. If only one testis was abdominal and the other was removed through standard castration, the horse should begin hand-walking at 24 hours postsurgery.

Complications and Prognosis

The complications that have been encountered in this procedure include peritonitis, wound infection, intestinal perforation, and hemorrhage. In the hands of a skilled surgeon, the prognosis for laparoscopic cryptorchidectomy is very good because this technique is generally considered less invasive than other approaches. The recovery time and contamination is reduced with this technique, and abdominal testes may be viewed and extracted more easily.

Caslick's Operation for Pneumovagina in the Mare

Relevant Anatomy

The external genitalia of the mare is comprised of the perineum and the vulva. The perineum describes the area extending from the base of the tail to the ventral commissure of the vulva.[16] Between the anus and vulva is the perineal body, formed by muscle fibers of the external anal sphincter and constrictor vulvae muscles.[16] The vulva consists of two labia, which meet at the ventral and dorsal commissures, and the clitoris. The labia are normally held together at the vulvar cleft by paired constrictor vulvae muscles. In most mares, the majority of the vulva is located ventral to the pelvic floor. Some mares, Thoroughbreds in particular, will have a slightly more dorsally orientated vulva, which can interfere with closure at the vulvar cleft and result in aspiration of air, endometritis, and sterility.

The vestibule is the termination of the internal genital tract and connects the vulva to the vagina. Normally, the vestibule slopes dorsally in the cranial direction and extends up to the transverse fold, which is the remnant of the hymen at the vaginovestibular junction.[23] The transverse fold of mucosa is identified approximately 5–10 cm cranial to the brim of the pelvis on the floor of the vagina. The urethral orifice opens just caudal to and underneath the transverse fold. Cranial to the transverse fold, the vagina continues to the fornix at the cervix. Most of the vagina is retroperitoneal, with the exception of the cranial portion that is covered with peritoneum.

Indications

The operation for pneumovagina in the mare is to prevent the involuntary aspiration of air into the vagina. Pneumovagina is caused by faulty closure of the lips of the vulva as a result of poor conformation or injury. Mares in which the lips of the vulva are tilted toward the anus are prone to vaginitis, cervicitis, metritis, and infertility due to contamination from material aspirated through the vulva. Old, thin, debilitated mares with sunken ani usually are more prone to pneumovagina. At least 80% of the vulval labia should be located ventral to the pelvic floor, and the vulval seal should be at least 2.5 cm deep and resistant to parting. In addition, the labia should be at an angle of at least 80° or nearly perpendicular to the horizontal.[23] Breeding or foaling injuries may also result in pneumovagina because the skin and mucosa of the labia become misshapen, resulting in a faulty seal. Some mares, especially in racing, may aspirate air even though they have good vulvar conformation, whereas others may have overlapping vulvar lips with relatively good conformation. These mares are also candidates for Caslick's operation. This operation is performed in combination with other surgery of the mare's perineum, such as repair of first-, second-, and third-degree perineal lacerations.[24]

Anesthesia and Surgical Preparation

Caslick's operation is performed with the animal under local anesthesia by direct infiltration of the vulvar labial margin. The surgery is best performed in a set of stocks, where dangers to the mare and operator are minimal; some mares require a twitch and, occasionally, tranquilization. Prior to the surgery, the feces should be manually removed from the rectum, and the tail should be bandaged and secured out of the surgical field. A thorough cleansing of the perineal region should be performed using a mild disinfectant solution, and all traces of the disinfectant solution should be removed by rinsing with water. Cotton or paper towels are recommended, rather than a scrub brush. Approximately 5 ml of local anesthetic are used for local infiltration into each side (Figure 10.3*A*,*B*).

Following desensitization of the required length of the mucocutaneous junction of the vulva and labia, a final preparation of the surgical site is performed using a

Fig. 10.3. A–I. Caslick's operation.

suitable, nonirritating antiseptic applied with cotton or gauze sponges.

Instrumentation

1. General surgery pack

Surgical Technique

Using tissue scissors, the surgeon removes a ribbon of mucosa approximately 3-mm wide from each vulvar labium (Figure 10.3C). To facilitate trimming the tissue, thumb forceps are used to grasp the ribbon of tissue and to apply downward pressure to stretch the area. A common mistake is to remove too much tissue. Consequently, many practitioners use a scalpel blade to incise into the local anesthetic bleb to create a fresh edge (Figure 10.3D). Most mares require that this operation be performed on successive years, and if excessive tissue is removed, subsequent repairs will be more difficult. The length of the vulva and labia to be sutured will vary, depending on the conformation of the individual mare. This length may vary from the upper half of the vulva to as much as 70% of its length. Once the ribbon of tissue is removed with scissors, or the scalpel incision made, the raw surface is generally much wider than one would anticipate because tissue edges under tension retract (Figure 10.3E). This tension is due to swelling caused by the local analgesic infiltration. Bleeding from the edges usually is minimal.

When the ribbon of tissue has been removed with either scissors or a scalpel blade, the raw edges are apposed using a simple continuous suture pattern (Figure 10.3F). A nonabsorbable, noncapillary suture material such as no. 2-0 nylon or no. 2-0 polypropylene is preferred. Vertical mattress, simple interrupted, and continuous interlocking patterns, and Michel clips, have also been used successfully. The suture pattern depends on individual preference, but the raw edges should be in good apposition no matter what pattern is used (Figure 10.3G).

To avoid excessive stress on the suture line at its ventral end during breeding or speculum examination, a "breeder's stitch" may be inserted ventral to Caslick's closure.

The area where the stitch is placed is desensitized and is infiltrated 2 cm in all directions from where the suture is to be placed (Figure 10.3G). Using sterile umbilical tape, the surgeon places a single interrupted suture at the most ventral part of Caslick's operation (Figure 10.3H). The stitch should not be so ventral that it interferes with breeding, nor should it be so loose that it may lacerate the stallion's penis (Figure 10.3I).

Postoperative Management

Generally, postoperative topical or systemic antibiotics are not indicated. The sutures can be removed 7–10 days postoperatively.

To prevent unnecessary damage at parturition, the vulvar labia should be surgically separated (episiotomy), and the Caslick's operation should be performed 1 or 2 days after foaling. It may also be necessary to separate the labia during natural mating or during manipulations of the reproductive tract for examination or therapy. If the labia become separated for any reason, the Caslick's surgery should be redone at the earliest opportunity to prevent pneumovagina.

Complications and Prognosis

Complications of this procedure include recurrence of pneumovagina and wound dehiscence. Certain mares may be candidates for other procedures, such as episioplasty and urine-pooling surgery, to achieve optimal fertility.[24] A mare that still has vaginal aerophagia following Caslick's operation should be considered a candidate for additional surgery. Animals in which the perineal region is sunken beneath both tuber ischii and in which the dorsal commissure of the vulva becomes horizontal, with rostral displacement of the anus, may not respond to Caslick's operation alone. Older, multiparous mares seem to be more prone to this condition, especially if they are unthrifty.

Urethroplasty by Caudal Relocation of the Transverse Fold

Relevant Anatomy

The urethral orifice opens just caudal to and underneath the transverse fold (the remnant of the hymen at the vaginovestibular junction). The transverse fold of mucosa is identified approximately 5–10 cm cranial to the brim of the pelvis on the floor of the vagina. Other relevant anatomy is discussed in previous sections of this chapter.

Indications

This reconstructive technique is indicated for treatment of urine pooling in the vagina, also known as *vesicovaginal reflux*. Urine pooling is more common in older, multiparous mares when sunken vaginas develop. The ventral floor of the vagina slopes cranioventrad, and uterine fluid and urine accumulate in the fornix of the vagina around the cervix. Vaginitis, cervicitis, endometritis, and temporary or permanent sterility may result. The aim of this operation is to promote caudal evacuation of urine and to prevent its pooling in the vagina.

Anesthesia and Surgical Preparation

The surgery is performed on the standing mare restrained in stocks. Tranquilization and epidural anesthesia are used. If the epidural anesthetic is ineffective, local infiltration of the surgical site can be performed. The tail is wrapped and is tied away from the surgical field. The vestibule and vagina are flushed with dilute povidone-iodine solution (not performed routinely by all surgeons), and the perineal area is prepared for aseptic surgery. The bladder should be emptied using a Foley catheter. The surgeon may elect to leave the catheter in place during surgery to help identify the incision and ensure that adequate tissue is available for closure.

Instrumentation

1. Long-handled surgical instruments
2. Self-retaining retractor (Glasser retractor)
3. Foley catheter

Surgical Technique

A self-retaining retractor (Glasser retractor) is placed in the vulva to expose the surgical area (Figure 10.4*A,B*). Long-handled instruments facilitate the performance of this procedure. The transverse fold is grasped at the center with a pair of thumb forceps and is retracted caudad approximately 5cm using moderate tension (Figure 10.4*C,D*). The dotted line in the figure indicates the line of mucosal resection. Using curved scissors or a scalpel, the surgeon removes the lateral edge or transects, respectively, the retracted transverse fold from the point of attachment of the thumb forceps to the junction of the fold with the vestibular wall (Figure 10.4*C,D*).[25] A scalpel blade is then used to carry the incision from the junction of the fold and the vestibular wall in a horizontal line to the vulvar lips. The incision must be dorsal enough so that the two lateral flaps can be sutured together without tension. A similar incision is made on the right side (Figure 10.4*E*). The suture line is started at the left lateral corner of the incision (Figure 10.4*F,G*). The mucosa is inverted to the midpoint of the urethral fold. A second suture line is started at the right lateral wall and closed similarly to the left. When the second suture line meets the first suture line, it is carried through to the end of the dissected folds to form a "Y"-shaped closure (Figure 10.4*H*).[25]

It is important to have minimal tension on the transverse fold when it is sutured into this new position; otherwise, the surgery will fail because of pressure necrosis at the sutures. In addition, the transverse fold should not be sutured more than 2cm from the floor of the vestibule, or the fold could be torn during copulation. It is also important that the new urethral aperture be of sufficient size so that normal urine flow is not restricted.

Postoperative Management

Tetanus prophylaxis is provided, and a course of systemic antibiotics is instituted. Caslick's operation is performed at the same time as the urethroplasty. The vagina is not interfered with for 2 weeks. After surgery, mares should not be sexually active for 30–60 days; during this time, any uterine infection should be treated. Artificial insemination should be used when possible.

Complications and Prognosis

Complications of this procedure include failure to resolve urine pooling secondary to suture line failure.

In a recent study good fertility was achieved following surgery and breeding during the same cycle as the repair.[26]

Cesarean Section in the Mare

Relevant Anatomy

The uterine body in the mare ranges from 18 to 20cm in length and occupies both retroperitoneal and peritoneal spaces.[27] The cervix, ranging from 5 to 8cm in length, is within the pelvic cavity dorsal to the bladder and urethra. The lumen of the cervical canal is lined by longitudinal mucosal folds that merge with the endometrial folds in the body.[27] The uterine horns are approximately 20–25cm in length and are suspended by the mesometrium, or broad ligament. The equine placenta has a diffuse attachment, and the cut edge of the uterus is felt to be prone to bleeding.

There are three primary layers to the uterine wall: the tunicae mucosa, muscularis, and serosa, referred to as the *endometrium, myometrium,* and *perimetrium,* respectively.[27] The innermost endometrium lines the lumen and consists mostly of epithelial and glandular tissue. The myometrium contains a highly vascularized layer and a thin, longitudinal layer of smooth muscle. The serosa is the outermost layer, which is composed of visceral peritoneum and two peritoneal sheets of the mesometrium.

The uterine artery, the uterine branch of the ovarian artery, and the uterine branch of the vaginal artery supply blood to the uterus and are contained within the broad ligament.

Indications

This operation is indicated for treatment of various types of dystocia in the mare. The most common indications are transverse presentation, some instances of uterine torsion, and instances of uterine rupture,[28] Although uterine torsion is best managed by a standing flank laparotomy and manual repositioning of the gravid uterus, a ventral midline celiotomy is indicated if the mare is intractable, if the uterus is ruptured, or if the torsion cannot be corrected with the animal in the standing position. In such cases, hysterotomy is performed first, making untwisting of the torsion easier.[29]

Vagina

Transverse fold

External urethral orifice

Vestibule

A

B (dorsal aspect)

C

TMᶜC

Fig. 10.4. **A–H.** Urethroplasty by caudal relocation of the transverse fold.

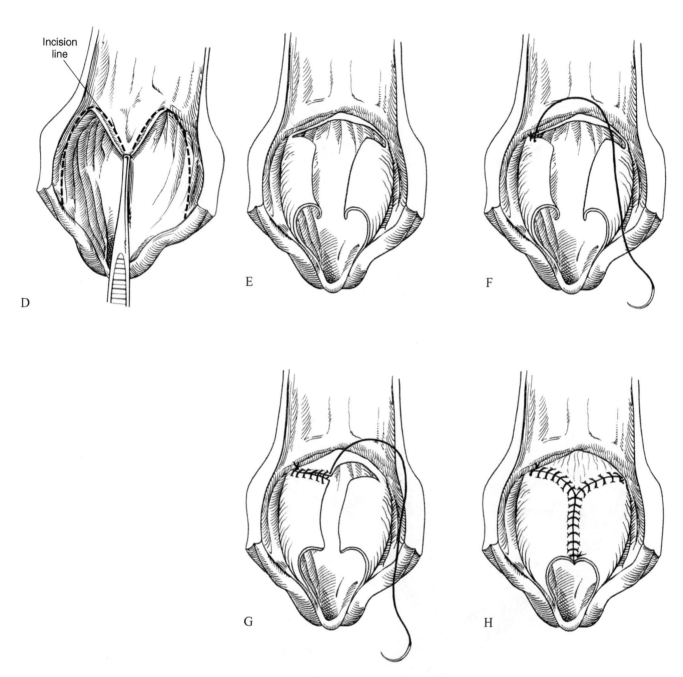

Fig. 10.4. *Continued.*

Fetal manipulation with the animal under general anesthesia or fetotomy, if the fetus is deemed nonviable, are also used in many instances of dystocia. The particular method used to handle a problem commonly depends on the experience and preference of the clinician. Repeated manipulations and attempts at fetotomy can damage the sensitive mucosal lining of the vagina and cervix, result in lacerations of the genital tract, and compromise the mare's future reproductive health.[30] If the surgeon lacks the equipment, is not familiar with the correct fetotomy technique, or lacks anesthetic assistance, a cesarean section may be the best option. Cesarean section should not be considered as a last resort in the mare.

Anesthesia and Surgical Preparation

Heavily pregnant mares present many challenges. However, newer anesthetic agents minimize the complications associated with cesarean section. The use of short-acting injectable agents along with inhalation agents such as isoflourane or sevoflourane, mechanical ventilation, and blood pressure support improve outcome for both the mare and the foal. See Chapter 2 for more in-depth coverage of anesthetic agents.

If the ventral midline approach is used, the mare is placed in dorsal recumbency and is clipped and prepared for aseptic surgery in a routine manner. According to the systemic status of the patient, appropriate fluid therapy and medication are administered.

Instrumentation

1. General surgery pack

Surgical Technique

The abdomen is entered through a ventral midline incision, which is used for the ventral midline laparotomy described in Chapter 12, "Equine Dental and Gastrointestinal Surgery." The uterus is located, and an incision site over a limb is chosen, just as in bovine cesarean section. This area is exteriorized as much as possible to minimize contamination of the peritoneal cavity. A more cranial limb should be chosen; otherwise, it may be difficult to close the hysterotomy incision because of caudal retraction of the uterus once the fetus is removed. The uterus is incised using a scalpel, and the foal is removed. Unless the allantochorion has already separated or will lift off easily, it should be left in the uterus.

Before closing the uterus when equine cesarean section is performed, any large bleeding vessels should be ligated. The allantochorion is separated for a distance of 2–5 cm from the margin of the uterine incision, and a continuous suture of rapidly absorbing synthetic suture material (Caprosyn) is placed around the entire margin of the uterine incision for hemostasis (Figure 10.5, inset).[31] The technique consists of a simple continuous pattern penetrating all layers of the uterus. It is necessary because the equine endometrium is only loosely attached to the myometrium, and there is little natural hemostasis for the large subendometrial veins. The uterus is closed with either an appositional pattern followed by an inverting pattern, or a double inverting layer of sutures using no. 1 polyglyconate (Maxon) or no. 2 lactomer 9-1 (Polysorb) (Figure 10.5). Although hemostatic sutures have been advocated in the past to reduce hemorrhage from hysterotomy sites, recent studies suggest that this practice does not decrease the incidence of anemia, and the time to place these sutures may outweigh any benefits.[32,33] Consequently, some surgeons prefer to simply perform a full thickness appositional suture to limit bleeding and speed in the closure of the uterus.

The abdomen is closed as for ventral laparotomy in the horse, which is described in Chapter 12. Great care should be exercised when separating the allantochorion at the margin of the uterine incision and avoiding its inclusion in the suture lines. If rupture has occurred, copious lavage of the abdomen with warm physiologic solutions during surgery is indicated because of the increased risk of contamination from uterine contents.

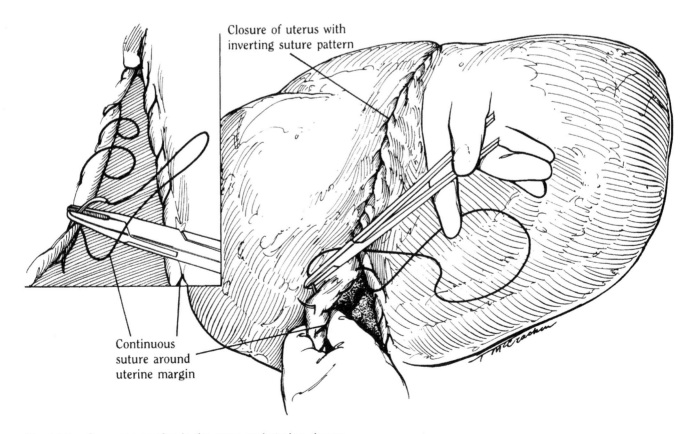

Closure of uterus with inverting suture pattern

Continuous suture around uterine margin

Fig. 10.5. Cesarean section in the mare and uterine closure.

Postoperative Management

Tetanus prophylaxis, antibiotics, and oxytocin are administered. Appropriate fluid therapy is continued or is instituted if the patient is compromised systemically.

As soon as the mare is standing and it is safe to milk her, colostrum should be obtained and given to the foal. The foal should be introduced to the mare as soon as the mare is stable enough on her feet not to be a danger to the foal. For the next 5–7 days, rectal or vaginal examination is indicated to assess uterine size.

Prolonged retention of the placenta is of significant concern in the horse, and the mare should be monitored and treated for retention of fetal membranes if necessary. Immediate forced traction of the placenta should be avoided in case the uterus is torn, especially in mares that have had uterine rupture. The placenta will usually pass on its own. If not, gentle manual removal with careful separation of the placenta from the uterine wall may eventually be indicated.

Complications and Prognosis

Anemia and bleeding from the hysterotomy site is a common and serious complication following cesarean sections. One study showed a 22% prevalence rate of this complication.[34] Although not as common, bleeding from uterine arteries can also occur and be fatal. Retained placenta, metritis, uterine tears, vaginal or cervical tears, colitis, peritonitis, decreased fertility, and incisional dehiscence are among some of the other reported complications that can occur following cesarean section.[33,35] Of these, retained placenta and decreased fertility are probably the most common.

The survival to discharge rate in one study was 84% for mares and 35% for foals. Mares that had dystocia for <90 minutes and were greater than 16 years of age had the fewest complications. Cumulative foaling rate before and after C-section was 77% compared to 52%.[28]

As discussed in the section of Chapter 12 on ventral midline laparotomy, fears regarding dehiscence or herniation following the use of this approach are unfounded.

Circumcision of the Penis (Reefing)

Relevant Anatomy

The penis of the horse is musculocavernous and can increase in size by up to three times during erection. There are two cavernous spaces of the shaft; the corpus cavernosum, formed by the union of the two crura, and the corpus spongiosum, which gives rise to the glans cranially. These erectile bodies are encapsulated in a thick, fibroelastic layer called the *tunica albuginea.*

The penis is attached caudally to the ischial arch of the pelvis through the paired crura. The urethral process is located at the fossa glandis, the ventral depression of the cranial aspect of the glans. The entrance to the inner sleeve of the prepuce, or sheath, is called the *preputial ring.* The preputial ring is the cranial border of the preputial fold.

Indications

This operation is indicated for the removal of neoplasms, granulomas (including those associated with repeated habronema infestation), and scar tissue or chronic thickening of the preputial membrane that prevents retraction of the penis.[7,36] Circumscribed lesions of the preputial ring may require only simple surgical removal and suturing of the skin edges. More extensive lesions cause deformity, and consequently, a complete ring of tissue is removed.

Anesthesia and Surgical Preparation

The horse is positioned in dorsal recumbency under general anesthesia. The penis is held in extension with towel clamps or a gauze loop around the neck of the glans, and the surgical area is prepared and draped for aseptic surgery. Catheterization of the urethra and the use of a tourniquet are optional.

Instrumentation

1. General surgery pack
2. Stallion catheter
3. Tourniquet

Surgical Technique

Figure 10.6*A* shows a lesion on the internal preputial membrane with the lines of excision demarcated. If the lesion involves the cranial rim of the inner prepuce, retraction of the inner lining will be essential before the incisions are made. The placement of a tourniquet proximally will improve visualization at the time of surgery. Two circumferential skin incisions are made cranial and caudal to the lesion (Figure 10.6*B*), and the preputial membrane is tensed by the use of towel forceps. A plane of dissection superficial to the deep fascia of the penis is found, and the tissue between the two circumferential incisions is removed. A third longitudinal incision connecting the two circumferential incisions facilitates the ease of dissection. One should be careful not to cut the large subcutaneous vessels around the penis during the blunt dissection. It is necessary to ligate one subcutaneous vein on each side of the penis. Once the tissue between the two circumferential incisions is removed, two healthy skin margins are left proximally and distally, ready for reapposition (Figure 10.6*C*). The edges are brought together and are closed with a layer of simple interrupted sutures of no. 2-0 glycomer 631 (Biosyn) (Figure 10.6*D*). If a subcutaneous layer is used, no attempt is made to secure this to the underlying tunica albuginea.

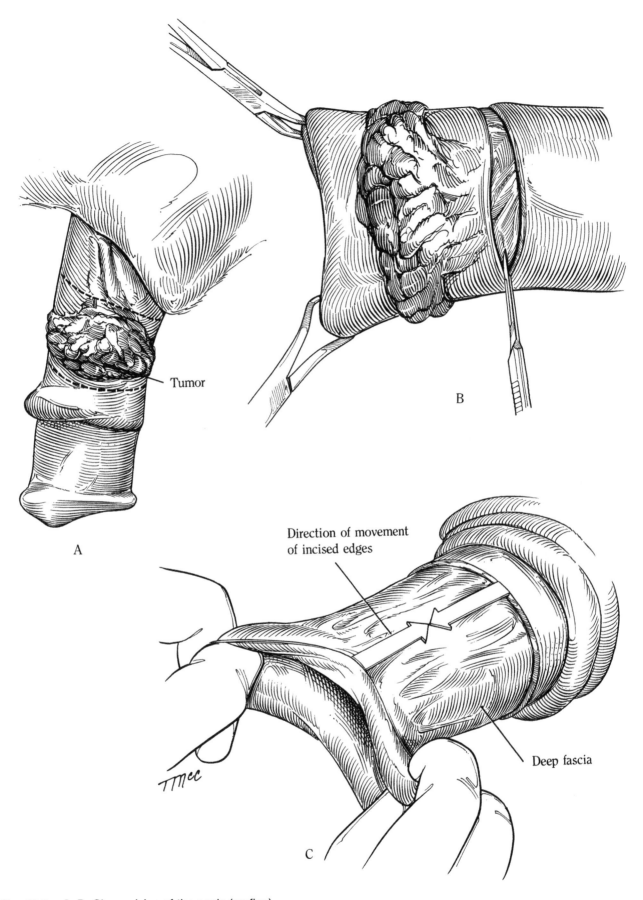

Tumor

Direction of movement
of incised edges

Deep fascia

A

B

C

Fig. 10.6.   **A–D.** Circumcision of the penis (reefing).

D

Fig. 10.6. *Continued.*

Postoperative Management

Tetanus prophylaxis is administered, and the use of post-operative antibiotics is recommended. The horse is hand-walked to help minimize preputial swelling, and sutures can be removed in 14 days. If this surgery is performed on a stallion, the animal should be isolated from mares for 3 to 4 weeks.[36]

Complications and Prognosis

The primary complication that may occur during this procedure is mild hemorrhage. This can generally be avoided by ligation of larger vessels and cautery of smaller vessels. Infection and suture dehiscence may occur if the stallion is not prohibited from sexual activity in the post-operative period. Overall, the prognosis for this procedure is good provided that the underlying tunics are not involved in the lesion.

Amputation of the Penis

Relevant Anatomy

Relevant anatomy for this procedure is described in the previous section.

Indications

The indications for penis amputation in the horse are invasive neoplastic lesions, granulomas associated with

habronemiasis, and intractable paralysis or priapism of the penis. The procedure is illustrated as it would be performed for a squamous cell carcinoma of the glans of the penis. In this situation, the penis is amputated at a point distal to that required for penile paralysis, and the operation is therefore easier. The proximal amputations are more difficult because of the greater diameter of the penis and the reflections of the prepuce. En bloc amputation, penile amputation with sheath ablation, and penile retroversion involve extensive resection and have been described for treatment of neoplasia that extends to subcutaneous tissues or regional lymph nodes.[37,38]

Anesthesia and Surgical Preparation

The horse is positioned in dorsal recumbency under general anesthesia. The penis is prepared for aseptic surgery in a routine manner, and a sterile catheter is passed to identify the urethra. A tourniquet of rubber tubing is applied proximal to the site of amputation (Figure 10.7A). The penis is also extended and stabilized using a gauze loop around the neck of the glans (not illustrated).

Instrumentation

1. General surgery pack

Surgical Technique

A triangular skin incision is made on the ventral aspect of the penis, and the incision is continued through the

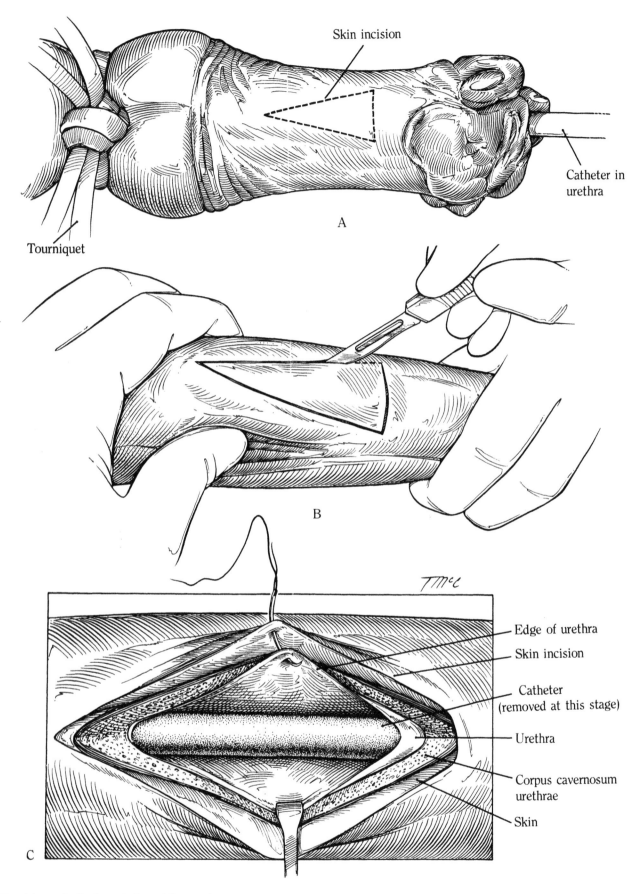

Skin incision

Catheter in
urethra

Tourniquet

A

B

Edge of urethra

Skin incision

Catheter
(removed at this stage)

Urethra

Corpus cavernosum
urethrae

Skin

C

Fig. 10.7. **A–G.** Amputation of the penis.

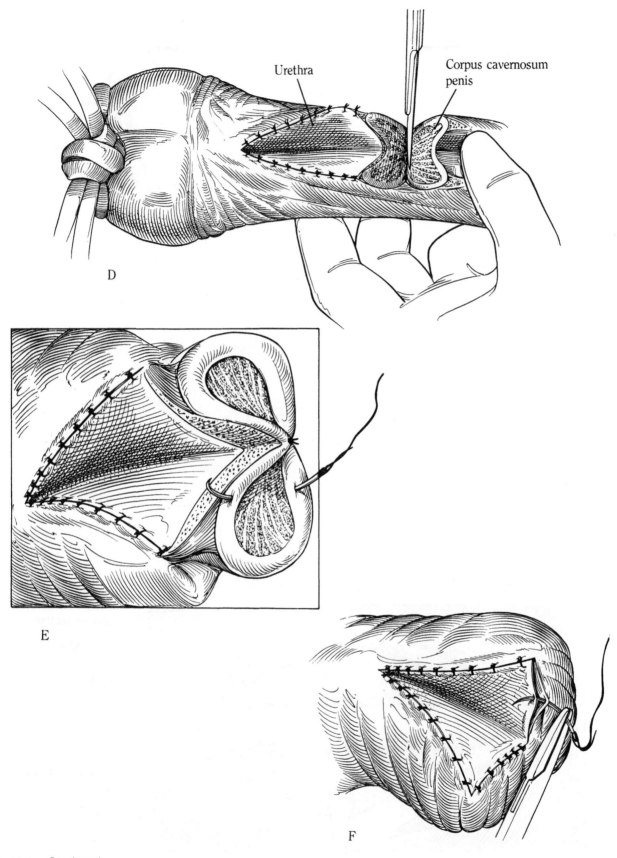

D

Urethra

Corpus cavernosum penis

E

F

Fig. 10.7. *Continued.*

Tourniquet

G

Fig. 10.7. *Continued.*

fascia and corpus spongiosum (Figure 10.7B). The apex of the triangle is located on the midline in a caudal direction. The triangle has a 3-cm base with sides approximately 4 cm in length. These incisions should extend down to the urethral mucosa, and the connective tissue within the triangle is removed and discarded. With the catheter as a guide, the urethral mucosa is split longitudinally on the midline from the base to the apex of the triangular defect. Then the catheter is removed.

The edges of the urethra are sutured to the skin edges along the sides of the triangular defect using simple interrupted sutures of no. 2-0 glycomer 631 (Caprosyn) (Figure 10.7C). The urethra and penis are then transected. The incision extends from the base of the triangle at a slightly oblique angle craniad toward the dorsal surface of the penis (Figure 10.7D). The principal blood vessels encountered are the branches of the dorsal arteries and veins of the penis that lie between the deep fascia and the tunica albuginea. Other vessels lying in the loose connective tissue beneath the superficial fascia may require ligation.

The tunica albuginea is closed over the transected corpus cavernosum penis using simple interrupted sutures of no. 0 polyglyconate (Maxon) (Figure 10.7E). The first suture is placed in the midline, and the next two sutures bisect these halves. Generally, seven sutures are used, and preplacement of the sutures to minimize excess tension on a single suture is preferable. The transected base of the urethral mucosa is then sutured to the skin using simple

interrupted sutures of no. 2-0 glycomer 631 (Caprosyn); these sutures should pass through the underlying stump (Figure 10.7F). Alternatively, the closure can be made in one layer using simple interrupted sutures, with four bites taken through urethral mucosa, ventral and dorsal tunica albuginea, and skin. At this point, the tourniquet is removed.

Another option that has been recently reported is the modified Vinsot technique that can be performed in the standing horse.[39] In this technique a linear urethrostomy is performed just proximal to the location of the amputation. A latex tourniquet is placed at the rostral aspect of the urethrostomy(Figure 10.7G). The distal end of the penis is allowed to necrose and fall off. This is a viable approach for horses that are unsuitable candidates for general anesthesia.

Postoperative Management

Tetanus prophylaxis is administered, and systemic antibiotics may be used for 4 to 5 days. Sutures should be removed in 14 days. A stallion should not be exposed to mares for 4 weeks.

Complications and Prognosis

Complications include edema of the prepuce, hemorrhage, dehiscence, granuloma formation, recurrence of neoplasia, and urethral stenosis.[37,38] Some hemorrhage will be observed following removal of the tourniquet, but excessive hemorrhage can cause a dissecting hematoma and wound breakdown. Minor dehiscence of the suture line, if it occurs, will not cause a significant problem; granulation and epithelialization will occur. Urethral stenosis should not be a problem if the triangulation technique is used. If wound dehiscence is extensive, however, stenosis secondary to fibrosis may result.

Horses treated with penile amputation for squamous cell carcinoma have a favorable prognosis. One study reported a 17% mortality rate due to recurrence,[38] while another indicated a 26% recurrence after partial phallectomy, compared to 18% with an en bloc resection.[40]

Aanes' Method of Repair of Third-Degree Perineal Laceration

Relevant Anatomy

The relevant anatomy for this procedure was discussed in previous sections of this chapter.

Indications

Perineal lacerations in the mare occur during parturition when the foal's limb(s) or head are forced caudad and dorsad.

The injury is seen predominantly in primiparous mares and is usually due to violent expulsive efforts by the mare in combination with some degree of malposition of the fetus, such as dorsopubic position or footnape posture. The injury is also seen following forced extraction of a large fetus or extraction before full dilation of the birth canal.[41]

First-degree lacerations occur when only the mucosa of the vagina and vulva are involved. Second-degree lacerations occur when the submucosa and muscularis of the vulva, anal sphincter, and the perineal body are involved, but there is no damage to the rectal mucosa. Third-degree perineal lacerations occur when there is tearing through the rectovaginal septum, musculature of the rectum and vagina, and the perineal body (Figure 10.8A).[42] Reconstruction of third-degree perineal lacerations is necessary to return the mare to breeding soundness. The communication between the rectum and vagina results in the constant presence of fecal material in the vagina. Reconstruction is performed occasionally in riding horses to eliminate the unpleasant sound made by air aspirated into the vagina.

Generally, surgery is not performed on an emergency basis. The torn tissues are edematous, necrotic, and grossly contaminated; and it is advisable to wait a minimum of 4 to 6 weeks before attempting repair. Repairs attempted earlier than this are usually unsuccessful. While waiting for repair, the mare should remain under close observation. The excessive straining caused by the injury can lead to prolapse of the viscera, including eversion of the urinary bladder.

The cervix should also be examined for lacerations prior to repair because lacerations of the cervix result in a poor prognosis for return to breeding soundness. Mares with lacerations of the cervix are more susceptible to endometritis and early abortion.[42] Upon discovery of the injury, tetanus immunization should be administered. Some cases may require a course of antibiotics. A preoperative diet of grass hay and alfalfa hay should be commenced to maintain proper fecal consistency. Diets consisting of a low-bulk, highly digestible complete feed, such as Buckeyer Maturity Senior, can reduce the bulk of the feces to minimize stress on the repair.

The following technique is performed in two stages: in the first operation, a shelf is constructed between the rectum and vagina; the second operation involves reconstruction of the perineal body. The aim of two-stage repair is reduction of the incidence of straining and subsequent tearing of sutures. Delaying reconstruction of the perineal body avoids reduction in the size of the rectal lumen, minimizes the accumulation of feces, and reduces the number of muscular contractions necessary to void feces. Moreover, suturing of rectal mucous membrane is avoided in this technique, which decreases straining because of suture irritation.[42] However, many surgeons will choose to complete the reconstruction in one stage,

using the same techniques. If the feces are appropriately soft, this can be very successful.

Anesthesia and Surgical Preparation

The mare is tranquilized and is placed in stocks; and an epidural anesthetic is administered (refer to Chapter 2 for details of epidural anesthesia in the horse). The tail is wrapped and tied in a cranial direction to avoid interference during surgery. Feces in the rectum and vagina are removed manually, and the perineal region is scrubbed with mild soap and water. The rectum and vagina are then cleansed with povidone-iodine solution (Betadine), and excess fluids are absorbed with moistened cotton.

During the first phase of the surgery, two temporary retaining sutures are placed on each side of the laceration, one at the level of the anal sphincter and one near the dorsal commissure of the vulva. These sutures are tied to the skin 8–10 cm lateral to the normal position of the anus and vulva. If assistants are available during surgery, they can use a pair of malleable retractors to enhance visualization of the surgical site (Figure 10.8B).

Instrumentation

1. General surgery pack
2. Malleable retractors
3. Long-handled needle holders, thumb forceps, and scalpel handles

Surgical Technique

Stage One

An incision is made along the scar tissue at the junction of the rectal and vaginal mucosa, commencing at the cranial end of the shelf and moving caudad toward the operator. The completed incision should extend from the shelf formed by the intact rectum and vagina, along the scar-tissue margin, to the level of the dorsal commissure of the vulva (Figure 10.8B).

The vaginal mucous membrane and submucosa are reflected ventrad from the line of the incision to form a flap of tissue approximately 2.5 cm wide. At the shelf, the rectum and vaginal mucosa are separated craniad for a distance of 2–3 cm. Hemorrhage from the incision is usually minimal and is not a problem.

At this point, the surgeon should determine whether further dissection is necessary by estimating the ease with which the vaginal mucosa can be brought into apposition. The mucosa should form the vaginal roof with minimal tension on the suture material.

Closure of the shelf is commenced by apposing the vaginal roof, using no. 0 polyglyconate, and tying on the midline of the vaginal roof just cranial to the defect. The knot becomes the cranial end of a continuous

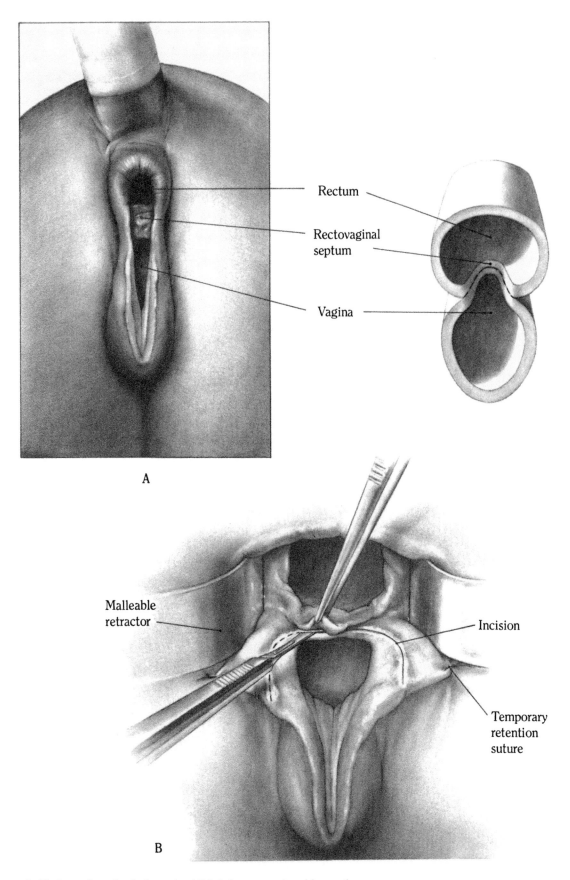

Labels in figure A: Rectum, Rectovaginal septum, Vagina

Labels in figure B: Malleable retractor, Incision, Temporary retention suture

A

B

Fig. 10.8. **A–H.** Aanes' method of repair of third-degree perineal laceration.

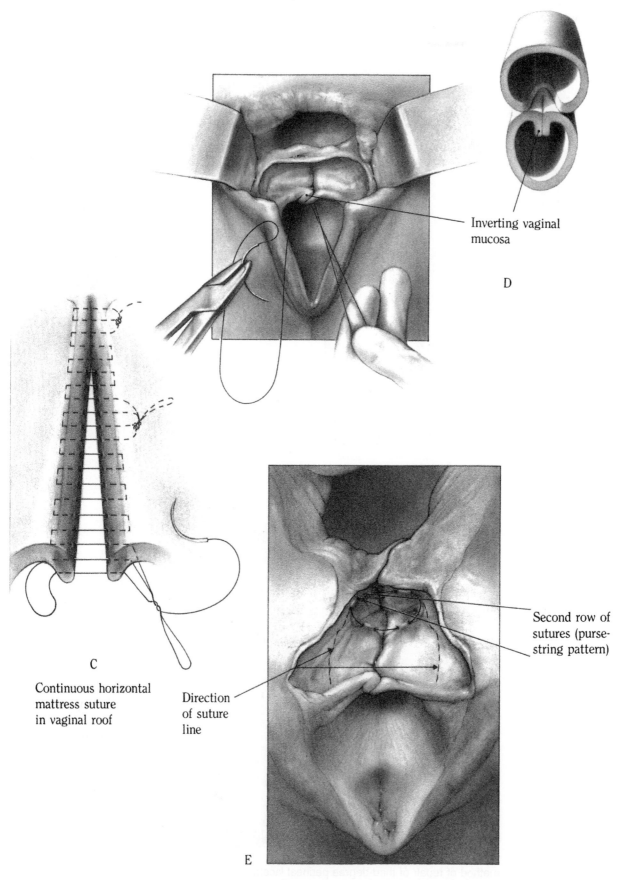

Inverting vaginal
mucosa

D

C

Continuous horizontal
mattress suture
in vaginal roof

Direction
of suture
line

Second row of
sutures (purse-
string pattern)

E

Fig. 10.8. *Continued.*

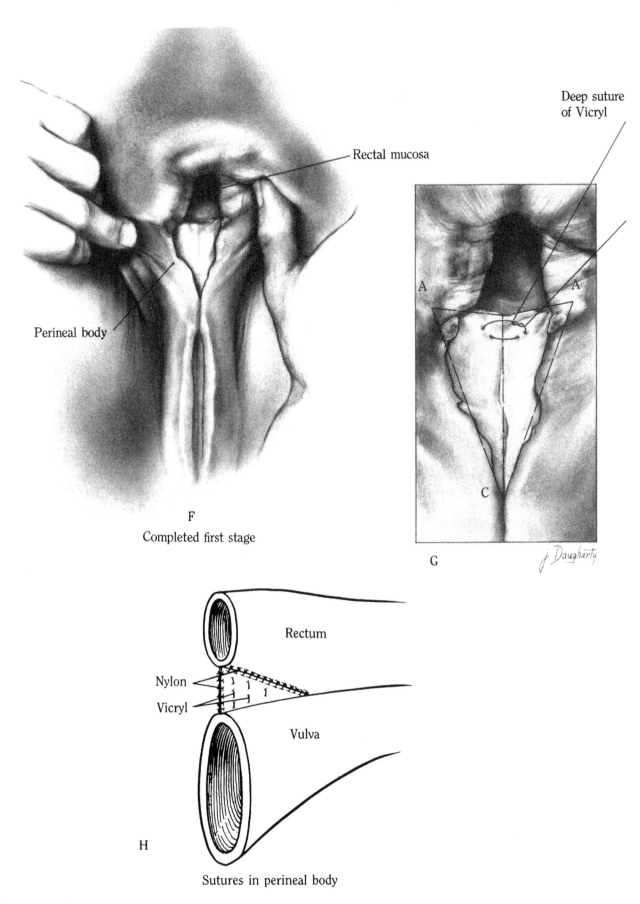

Rectal mucosa

Deep suture
of Vicryl

Perineal body

A   A

C

J. Daugherty

F

Completed first stage

G

Rectum

Nylon

Vicryl

Vulva

H

Sutures in perineal body

Fig. 10.8. *Continued.*

173

horizontal mattress suture pattern, inverting the vaginal mucosa and forming the first layer of the repaired roof of the vagina (Figure 10.8C,D).

The suture pattern should penetrate the edges of the vaginal mucous membrane and should be continued caudad for one-third to one-half of the laceration. The suture is tied and is tucked into the vagina until it is needed later in the repair (Figure 10.8C).

A second row of sutures of no. 0 or 1 polyglyconate (Maxon) is placed between the rectum and the vaginal wall. The suture is essentially a purse-string pattern, passing through the rectal submucosa, perivaginal tissue, and vaginal submucosa on both sides of the common vault. Each suture is tied immediately after it is placed (Figure 10.8E).

When the interrupted sutures are placed as far caudally as the newly sutured vaginal roof, the continuous horizontal mattress pattern of polyglyconate is resumed, and the vaginal mucosa is sutured in a caudal direction to the dorsal commissure of the vulva (Figure 10.8C). The interrupted sutures are continued caudad to the dorsal commissure of the vulva; one should keep the overall direction of this row horizontal. This method avoids narrowing of the rectal lumen. Sutures should not be placed in the rectal mucous membrane (Figure 10.8F).

Following the first stage of the operation, the mare should receive antibiotics for about 5 days. Approximately 2 weeks of healing should be allowed before proceeding with the second stage of the operation. Any exposed polyglactin 910 sutures should be removed a few days before the second operation. Conversely, the second stage can be performed immediately.[43] In one study, 14/17 mares were successfully repaired in a single procedure.[44] A single stage repair is preferred by the author.

Stage Two

Surgical preparation and anesthesia for the second stage of the procedure are similar to those for the first stage. The retrovestibular shelf is examined for healing, and if a small, granulating fistula remains, the second stage should be delayed until it is healed. When a large fistula remains, the shelf is converted to a third-degree perineal laceration, and the first stage is repeated. Local infiltration of lidocaine can be used, rather than epidural anesthesia.

To obtain fresh surfaces for reconstruction and healing of the perineal body, the newly formed epithelialized tissue must be removed. An incision that commences at the cranial margin of the perineal body is made. It extends peripherally along the scar tissue margin and ends at the dorsal commissure of the vulva, forming two sides of a triangle. An incision is made on the opposite side, and a superficial layer of epithelium is removed, creating two raw, triangular surfaces. The skin of the perineum is undermined and is reflected laterad to permit subsequent closure of the skin without undue tension (Figure 10.8G).

This step is not necessary if the reconstruction is performed in a single stage.

Closure of the deep layers of the perineal body should commence cranially with simple interrupted sutures of no. 0 or 1 polyglyconate (Maxon). This closure is completed with simple interrupted sutures of 2-0 polyglyconate placed within the epithelial edges of the rectum. The sutures are placed alternately until reconstruction of the perineal body is completed. No attempt is made to locate and to suture the ends of the anal sphincter muscle because they are usually surrounded by scar tissue. The dorsal portion of the vulvar lips is removed just as in Caslick's operation for pneumovagina. The skin of the perineum and lips of the vulva are closed with interrupted sutures of 2-0 nylon or polyglyconate (Figure 10.8H).

Postoperative Management

The mare is put back on a low bulk feed immediately after the operation. A stool softener, such as mineral oil, should be administered for at least a week. Antibiotics are administered for 5 days, and any nonabsorbable sutures in the perineum and lips of the vulva are removed 14 days after surgery.

Following healing, the mare should be examined for endometritis and treated accordingly. A uterine biopsy may be indicated. Natural service should be postponed for 6 months to allow the region to attain some strength. Some mares require artificial insemination because of a marked reduction in the size of the vulvar opening.

Complications and Prognosis

The complications of this surgery include dehiscence, abscessation and cellulitis, constipation, and fistula formation. Excessive straining after surgery can result from cystitis or fecal impaction of the rectum.[45] This should be treated with epidural analgesia or tranquilization. Urine pooling may occur due to excessive closure of the vulvar cleft or poor perineal conformation and may require one of the urethral extension operations described elsewhere in this chapter.

In most cases, the prognosis for future pregnancies following successful repair of a third-degree perineal laceration is excellent. A fertility rate of approximately 75% can be expected.[41] Recurrence of third-degree perineal lacerations at subsequent parturitions ranges from no injury to another third-degree perineal laceration. It is advisable to have an attendant present during future foalings to minimize the severity of damage in case dystocia occurs.[42]

References

1. Riegel, R.J., and Hakola, S.E. Illustrated Atlas of Equine Anatomy and Common Disorders of the Horse. Vol. II. Marysville, WA, Equistar Publications, 2000.

2. Barber, S.M. Castration of horses with primary closure and scrotal ablation. *Vet. Surg., 14*:2, 1985.

3. Schumacher, J. Testis. *In* Equine Surgery. Edited by J.A. Auer, J.A. Stick. St. Louis, MO, Saunders, 2006, pp. 775–810.

4. Searle, D., Dart, A.J., Dart, C.M., and Hodgson, D.R. Equine castration: Review of anatomy, approaches, techniques and complications in normal, cryptorchid and monorchid testes. *Aust. Vet. J., 77*:428–434, 1999.

5. Shoemaker, R., Bailey, J., Janzen, E., and Wilson, D.G. Routine castration in 568 draught colts: Incidence of evisceration and omental herniation. *Equine Vet. J., 36*:336–340, 2004.

6. Shideler, R.K., Squires, E.L., and Pickett, B.W. Disappearance of spermatozoa from the ejaculate of geldings. *J. Reprod. Fertil., 27*(Suppl.):25, 1979.

7. Walker, D.F., and Vaughan, J.T. Bovine and Equine Urogenital Surgery. Philadelphia, Lea & Febiger, 1980.

8. Boussauw, B., and Wilderjans, H. Inguinal herniation 12 days after a unilateral castration with primary wound closure. *Equine Vet. Educ., 8*:248–250, 1996.

9. Van Der Velden, M.A., and Rutgers, L.J.E. Visceral prolapse after castration in the horse: A review of 18 cases. *Equine Vet. J., 22*:9–12, 1990.

10. Thomas, H.L., Zaruby, J.F., Smith, C.L., and Livesey, M.A. Postcastration eventration in 18 horses: The prognostic indicators for long-term survival (1985–1995). *Can. Vet. J., 39*:764–768, 1998.

11. Pickett, B.W., Squires, E.L., Voss, J.L., and Wallach, S.J.R. Factors affecting sexual behavior of the equine male. *In* Proceedings of the 25th Annual Convention of the American Association of Equine Practitioners in 1979, 1980, p. 61.

12. Cox, J.E. Experiences with a diagnostic test for equine cryptorchidism. *Equine Vet. J., 7*:179, 1975.

13. Schumacher, J., and Hardin, D.K. Surgical treatment of priapism in a stallion. *Vet. Surg., 16*:193, 1987.

14. Sharrock, A.G. Reversal of drug induced priapism in a gelding by medication. *Aust. Vet. J., 58*:39, 1982.

15. Crouch, G.M., Snyder, J.R., and Harmon, B.G. Adhesion of the ileum to the inguinal ring in a gelding. *Equine Pract., 5*:32, 1983.

16. Dyce, K.M., Sack, W.O., and Wensing, C.J.G. Textbook of Veterinary Anatomy. 2nd Ed. Philadelphia, W.B. Saunders, 1996, p. 565.

17. Marshall, J.F., Moorman, V.J., and Moll, H.D. Comparison of the diagnosis and management of unilaterally castrated and cryptorchid horses at a referral hospital: 60 cases (2002–2006). *J. Am. Vet. Med. Assoc., 231*:931–934, 2007.

18. Schambourg, M.A., Farley, J.A., Marcoux, M., and Laverty, S. Use of transabdominal ultrasonography to determine the location of cryptorchid testes in the horse. *Equine Vet. J., 38*:242–245, 2006.

19. Trumble, T., and Hendrickson, D.A. Standing male equine urogenital endoscopic surgery. *Vet. Clin. North Am. Equine Pract., 16*:269–284, 2000.

20. Fischer, A.T. Equine Diagnostic & Surgical Laparoscopy. Philadelphia, W.B. Saunders, 2001.

21. Carpenter, E.M., Hendrickson, D.A., James, S., Franke, C., Frisbie, D., Trostle, S., and Wilson, D. A mechanical study of ligature security of commercially available pre-tied ligatures versus hand tied ligatures for use in equine laparoscopy. *Vet. Surg., 35*:55–59, 2006.

22. Shettko, D.L., Frisbie, D.D., and Henrickson, D.A. A comparison of knot security of commonly used hand-tied laparoscopic slipknots. *Vet. Surg., 33*:521–524, 2004.

23. Woodie, B. Vulva, vestibule, vagina, and cervix. *In* Equine Surgery. 3rd Ed. Edited by J.A. Auer, J.A. Stick. St. Louis, MO, Saunders, 2006, p. 835.

24. McIlwraith, C.W., and Turner, A.S. Equine Surgery: Advanced Techniques. 2nd Ed. Baltimore, MD, Williams & Wilkins, 1998.

25. McKinnon, A.O., and Beldon, J.O. A urethral extension technique to correct urine pooling (vesicovaginal reflux) in mares. *J. Am. Vet. Med. Assoc., 192*:647–650, 1988.

26. Jalim, S.L., and McKinnon, A.O. Surgical results and fertility following correction of vesicovaginal reflux in mares. *Aust. Vet. J., 88*:182–185, 2010.

27. Wenzel, J.G.W. Anatomy of the uterus, ovaries, and adnexa. *In* Large Animal Urogenital Surgery. 2nd Ed. Edited by D.F. Wolfe, D.H. Moll. Baltimore, MD, Williams & Wilkins, 1999, pp. 375–380.

28. Abernathy-Young, K.K., Leblanc, M.M., Embertson, R.M., Pierce, S.W., and Stromberg, A.J. Survival rates of mares and foals and postoperative complications and fertility of mares after cesarean section: 95 cases (1986–2000). *J. Am. Vet. Med. Assoc., 241*:927–934, 2012.

29. Pascoe, J.R., Meagher, D.M., and Wheat, J.D. Surgical management of uterine torsion in the mare: A review of 26 cases. *J. Am. Vet. Med. Assoc., 179*:351, 1981.

30. Frazor, G.S. Fetotomy technique in the mare. *Equine Vet. Educ., 13*:151–159, 2001.

31. Hopper, S.A. Equine cesarean section for acute dystocia. *In* Proceedings of the 11th Annual American College of Veterinary Surgeons in 2001, pp. 183–188.

32. Embertson, R.M. The indications and surgical techniques for cesarean section in the mare. *Equine Vet. Educ., 4*:31–39, 1992.

33. Freeman, D.E., Hungerford, L.L., Schaeffer, D., Lock, T.F., Sertich, P.L., Baker, G.J., Vaala, W.E., and Johnston, J.K. Caesarean section and other methods for assisted delivery: Comparison of effects on mare mortality and complications. *Equine Vet. J., 31*:203–207, 1999.

34. Freeman, D.E., Johnston, J.K., Baker, G.J., Hungerford, L.L., and Lock, T.F. An evaluation of the haemostatic suture in hysterotomy closure in the mare. *Equine Vet. J., 31*:208–211, 1999.

35. Watkins, J.P., Taylor, T.S., Day, W.C., and Varner, D.D. Elective cesarean section in mares: Eight cases (1980–1989). *J. Am. Vet. Med. Assoc., 197*:1639–1645, 1990.

36. Vaughan, J.T. Surgery of the male equine reproductive system. *In* The Practice of Large Animal Surgery. Edited by P. Jennings. Philadelphia, W.B. Saunders, 1984, p. 1088.

37. Doles, J., Williams, J.W., and Yarbrough, T.B. Penile amputation and sheath ablation in the horse. *Vet. Surg., 30*:327–331, 2001.

38. Mair, T.S., Walmsley, J.P., and Phillips, T.J. Surgical treatment of 45 horses affected by squamous cell carcinoma of the penis and prepuce. *Equine Vet. J., 32*:406–410, 2000.

39. Arnold, C.E., Brinsko, S.P., Love, C.C., and Varner, D.D. Use of a modified Vinsot techniques for partial phallectomy in 11 standing horses. *J. Am. Vet. Med. Assoc., 237*:82–86, 2010.

40. van den Top, J.G., de Heer, N., Klein, W.R., and Ensink, J.M. Penile and preputioal squamous cell carcinoma in the horse: A retrospective study of treatment of 77 affected horses. *Equine Vet. J., 40*:533–537, 2008.

41. Colbern, G.T., Aanes, W.A., and Stashak, T.S. Surgical management of perineal lacerations and rectovestibular fistulae in the mare: A retrospective study of 47 cases. *J. Am. Vet. Med. Assoc., 186*:265, 1985.

42. Aanes, W.A. Surgical management of foaling injuries. *Vet. Clin. North Am. Equine Pract., 4*:417–438, 1988.

43. Climent, F., Ribera, T., Arguelles, D., Nomen, C., and Prades, M. Modified technique for the repair of third-degree rectovaginal lacerations in mares. *Vet. Rec., 164*:393–396, 2009.

44. Belknap, J.K., and Nickels, F.A. A one-stage repair of third-degree perineal lacerations and rectovestibular fistulae in 17 mares. *Vet. Surg., 21*:378–381, 1992.

45. Schumacher, J. Perineal injuries of the horse. *In* Proceedings of the 6th Annual Convention of American College of Veterinary Surgeons in 1996, p. 205.

Chapter 11

SURGERY OF THE EQUINE UPPER RESPIRATORY TRACT

Dean A. Hendrickson, DVM, MS, DACVS

Objectives

1. Describe common upper respiratory surgical techniques, including tracheostomy, laryngotomy, two techniques for ventriculectomy and ventriculocordectomy, partial resection of the soft palate, and two surgical techniques for entry into the guttural pouches to facilitate drainage.
2. Discuss the indications and alternative treatments for each procedure.

Tracheostomy

Relevant Anatomy

The incision site for this procedure follows the ventral median of the proximal one-third of the neck, approximately 3 cm distad to the cricoid cartilage, or at the point where the sternocephalicus and omohyoideus muscle bellies diverge and converge, respectively. To visualize the trachea, the muscle bellies of the sternothyroideus and sternohyoideus, which lie on the ventral aspect of the trachea, will be separated. From this point, the tracheal rings will be visible. Dorsolateral to the proximal half of the trachea are the common carotid artery, the vagosympathetic trunk, and the recurrent laryngeal nerve, which are all enclosed in the carotid sheath.[1]

Indications

Tracheostomy may be performed on an emergency or elective basis. Emergency situations include obstructions of the upper airway, such as those caused by rattlesnake bite, regional lymph node abscessation due to *Streptococcus equi* infection, nasopharyngeal neoplasia, excessive guttural pouch distention with inspissated pus, or postsurgical edema. Elective tracheostomy may be performed following nasal surgery, such as nasal septum resection or laryngeal surgery, or whenever postoperative respiratory obstruction is anticipated. It is also indicated for retrograde pharyngoscopy and endotracheal intubation to permit arytenoidectomy or surgery in the oral cavity, as well as to provide oxygen insufflation into the trachea during any hypoxic crisis.[2] In elective situations, the tracheotomy may be temporary or permanent as well.

Anesthesia and Surgical Preparation

Elective tracheostomy is usually performed with the horse sedated in a standing position, preferably in the stocks so that the head may be supported with the neck extended. A 3-inch × 6-inch rectangle of hair is clipped over the middle third of the neck, and the area is scrubbed surgically. The surgical site is anesthetized by infusing local anesthetic in either a 10-cm line or an inverted "U" pattern beginning from about the 5th tracheal ring and extending dorsally over the 2nd tracheal ring (Figure 11.1A).[3]

Instrumentation

1. General surgery pack
2. Tracheostomy tube

Surgical Technique

The surgical site is variable, but it is generally at the junction of the middle and upper third of the neck (approximately the 2nd to 5th tracheal rings). With the operator standing on the right side of the horse (the reverse for a left-handed operator), a 10-cm incision is made through the skin and subcutaneous tissue; this is facilitated by

Turner and McIlwraith's Techniques in Large Animal Surgery, 4th Edition. Dean A. Hendrickson and A. N. (Nickie) Baird.
© 2013 John Wiley & Sons, Inc. Published 2013 by John Wiley & Sons, Inc.

Sternothyrohyoideus
muscles

C

Tracheal
rings

A

B

D

Fig. 11.1. **A–D.** Tracheostomy.

tensing the skin at the proximal end of the incision with the left hand and making the skin incision with the right hand (Figure 11.1*B*). Following incision of the skin and subcutaneous tissues, the bellies of the sternothyrohyoideus muscles are visible. These muscle bellies are bluntly divided in the midline with scissors or the tip of a hard-backed scalpel (Figure 11.1*C*). Then the tracheal rings are identified. The scalpel is inserted midway between two of the tracheal rings with a sharp thrust. This incision is made in a horizontal direction about 1 cm in either direction from the midline (no more than one-third the circumference of the trachea) (Figure 11.1*D*). When the incision is completed, the tracheostomy tube can be inserted. This method is used when a tracheostomy tube will be left in place for a short period of time. Generally, the incision is not closed and will heal well by secondary intention after the tracheostomy tube is removed.

Postoperative Management

The tracheostomy site should be cleaned daily with a sterile physiologic solution, such as saline solution. The area can be dressed with a suitable, nonirritating, triple antibiotic ointment at the same time. When the tracheostomy tube is in place, it should be removed and cleaned once or twice daily, depending on the amount of accumulated secretions. The site will usually heal uneventfully by secondary intention.

Complications and Prognosis

In an emergency situation, such as when the animal is in danger of suffocation, the surgeon may need to forego a complete aseptic preparation, which may predispose the animal to infection. Occasionally, subcutaneous emphysema develops where air is trapped between the wound edges and dissects along fascial planes. This condition is usually self-limiting, and its chances of occurrence are minimized by handling tissues gently and not dissecting around either side of the trachea. Tracheal stenosis is a potential complication of this surgery, and its likelihood depends on the length of time the tracheostomy tube is left in place and the width of the incision between the tracheal rings.

Laryngotomy, Laryngeal Ventriculectomy, and Ventriculocordectomy

Relevant Anatomy

The larynx is comprised of the unpaired cricoid, thyroid, and epiglottic cartilages and the paired arytenoid cartilages. The arytenoid cartilages articulate with the lateral surfaces of the cricoid cartilage, thus facilitating the dorsolateral and axial rotation of the arytenoids during adduction and abduction. This allows the glottis to completely close during swallowing and open maximally during exercise. If this movement is impaired, upper airway function during exercise may be compromised, resulting in respiratory noise (roaring), poor performance, and exercise intolerance. The arytenoid cartilages are particularly susceptible to inflammation and injury, which may result in exercise-induced respiratory noise, known as *roaring*, or paralysis in a condition known as *laryngeal hemiplegia*.

Indications

Laryngeal ventriculectomy is indicated for the treatment of laryngeal hemiplegia. It may be performed alone in some cases, or, in conjunction with laryngoplasty, which is described in *Equine Surgery: Advanced Techniques*.[4] Other surgical treatments for laryngeal hemiplegia include ventriculocordectomy, partial or full arytenoidectomy, and laryngeal reinnervation.[5] The degree of surgical treatment and the most appropriate technique necessary to produce the desired results in the patient are largely dependent on the use of the horse, the horse's level of performance, and the grade of laryngeal movements.[5] For the purpose of this text, ventriculectomy and ventriculocordectomy will be described.

Ventriculectomy, or sacculectomy, consists of the removal of the mucous membrane lining the laryngeal ventricle. This technique is accomplished by performing a laryngotomy through the cricoid membrane. Ventriculocordectomy is essentially a sacculectomy with the additional removal of a small wedge of tissue from the leading edge of the vocal fold.[6] Ventriculocordectomy is indicated for horses affected by vocal fold collapse and some show and draft horses with laryngeal hemiplegia. The technique of laryngotomy described here is also used for partial resection of the soft palate, arytenoidectomy, and the surgical treatment of epiglottic entrapment, pharyngeal cysts, or lymphoid hyperplasia.

Ventriculectomy and ventriculocordectomy are not indicated alone for treatment of laryngeal hemiplegia in sport horses or racehorses, because they will not produce abduction of the arytenoid cartilages and alleviate airway obstruction in these horses.[5] These procedures are, however, appropriate in animals in which the arytenoid cartilage is not adducted beyond the normal resting position, so the larynx appears symmetric at rest. For some show horses, these treatments will provide satisfactory reduction of respiratory noise by reducing soft tissue collapse during exercise.[5] Laryngoplasty is used when endoscopic examination shows that the arytenoid cartilage is displaced medially from the resting position. In these cases, ventriculectomy alone will not provide sufficient abduction of the vocal cord. Ventriculcordectomy can be used as the sole treatment for laryngeal paresis in cases with low grade recurrent laryngeal neuropathy.[7]

Laser-assisted ventriculectomy and ventriculocordectomy, either alone or in conjunction with laryngoplasty, are indicated for treatment of specific cases of laryngeal hemiplegia, as previously described. Although laser-assisted surgical techniques are considered advanced, they will be discussed here because they are important alternatives to many of the traditionally performed upper respiratory surgical techniques. This technique is usually performed using a neodymium:yttrium garnet or diode laser transendoscopically through an oral approach or by performing a laryngotomy. The transendoscopic laser-guided technique does not require a laryngotomy, and therefore it reduces anesthesia and convalescence time. Laser vocal cordectomy has been described as a potential treatment for laryngeal hemiplegia, but it has not been shown to reduce respiratory noise as effectively as ventriculocordectomy.[8]

Anesthesia and Surgical Preparation

Laryngotomy and ventriculectomy may be performed with the horse under general anesthesia and in dorsal recumbency or with the standing animal sedated and injected with local analgesic at the surgical site. Prior to surgery (ideally, 4 hours prior), the patient is given 2 g of phenylbutazone intravenously to minimize postoperative laryngeal edema. The surgical area at the caudal aspect of the mandible is clipped and prepared aseptically (Figure 11.2A).

To perform the endoscopically guided ventriculectomy, the horse is placed in standing stocks and sedated with 0.3 mg xylazine HCl. A jugular catheter is placed and a continuous infusion of 20 mg detomidine in 1 L polyionic fluids is used to maintain sedation. A flexible endoscope is passed nasally, and 20 ml of 2% carbocaine is used to bathe the surgery area.

Instrumentation

1. General surgery pack
2. Self-retaining retractor (Gelpi, Weitlaner, or Hobday's roaring retractor)
3. Laryngeal bur
4. Tracheostomy tube
5. Laser with fiber (980-nm diode laser with 3 m/600-m fiber preferred)
6. Protective eyewear

Surgical Technique

Ventriculectomy and Ventriculocordectomy

A skin incision centered at the caudal aspect of the mandible, approximately 10 cm long, is made from the surface of the cricoid cartilage to beyond the junction of the thyroid cartilages (Figure 11.2A). In some instances, the triangular depression between the thyroid cartilages and cricoid cartilage can be felt before the skin incision is made. When this is not possible, the central area of the skin incision is located by placing a horizontal line across the area where the rami of the mandible merge with the neck. The skin incision exposes the midline between the sternothyrohyoideus muscles, which are separated with scissors to expose the cricothyroid membrane. After initial separation with scissors, the muscles may be retracted digitally for the length of the skin incision. The cricothyroid membrane is cleared of adipose tissue, and at this stage, it may be necessary to ligate a small vein that commonly is present in the surgical site. The cricothyroid membrane is then incised, commencing with a stab incision, to penetrate the laryngeal mucosa (Figure 11.2B). The incision is then extended longitudinally from the cricoid cartilage caudad to the junction of the thyroid cartilages cranially. The wings of the thyroid cartilages are retracted with a self-retaining retractor (Gelpi, Weitlaner, or Hobday's roaring retractor).

If a small-diameter, cuffed endotracheal tube is used, ventriculectomy may be performed with the endotracheal tube in place; otherwise, removal of the tube will be necessary for identification of the laryngeal saccule and ventriculectomy. The laryngeal ventricle is identified by sliding the index finger craniad off the edge of the vocal cord and turning the finger laterad and downward toward the base of the ear to enter the ventricle. The laryngeal bur is passed into the ventricle as deeply as possible and twisted to grasp the mucosa (Figure 11.2C). A sagittal section of the larynx showing the location of the laryngeal ventricle is illustrated in Figure 11.2D. When the operator believes that the mucosa is engaged in the bur, the bur is carefully withdrawn from the ventricle by everting the ventricular mucosa (Figure 11.2E). At this stage, it is advisable to place a pair of forceps on the everted mucosa to avoid tearing or slippage as the mucosa is fully retracted. The forceps are attached to the mucosa, the bur is untwisted and removed, and the ventricular saccule is completely everted using traction. With retraction maintained by Ochsner forceps or a similar instrument placed across the saccule, the everted mucous membrane is resected with scissors as close to the base as possible without damaging associated cartilage (Figure 11.2F). It is common to perform the ventriculectomy bilaterally, but the clinical problem is usually associated with the left side. Following excision of the ventricle, any tags of remaining mucous membrane are removed. To perform a ventriculocordectomy, an additional 2-cm long and 2-mm wide crescent-shaped wedge is excised from the leading edge of the adjacent vocal fold after performing ventriculectomy.[6] The abaxial edge of the vocal fold and the axial border of the ventricle may be opposed and sutured using 2-0 PDS. This serves to limit hemorrhage and lessen cicatrix formation and redundant tissue folds.[6] Many surgeons do not close the mucosa.

The cricothyroid membrane is closed using 3-0 polyglytone 6211 (Caprosyn). The rest of the laryngotomy

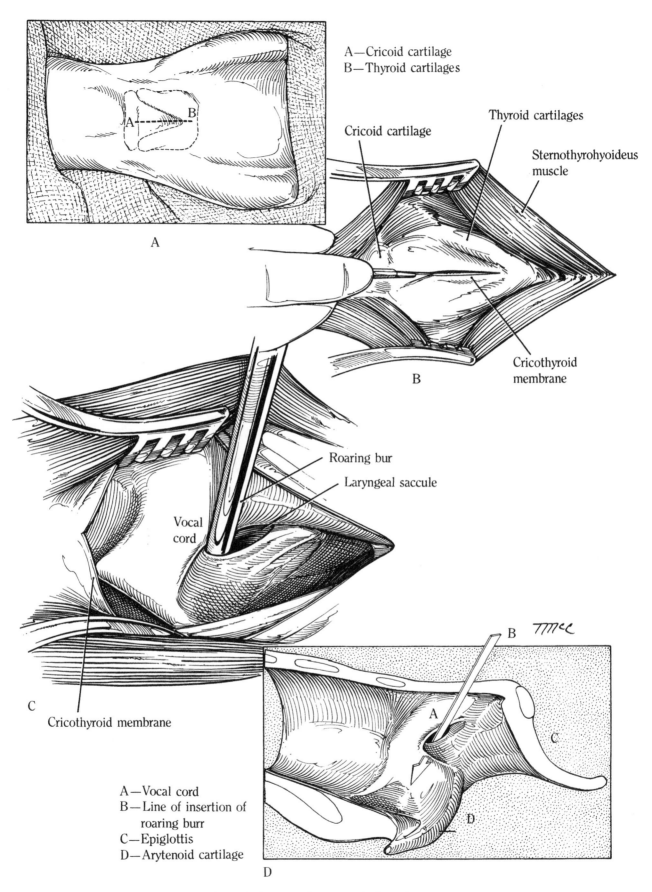

A—Cricoid cartilage
B—Thyroid cartilages

A

Cricoid cartilage

Thyroid cartilages

Sternothyrohyoideus muscle

Cricothyroid membrane

B

Roaring bur

Laryngeal saccule

Vocal cord

C

Cricothyroid membrane

A—Vocal cord
B—Line of insertion of roaring burr
C—Epiglottis
D—Arytenoid cartilage

B

A

C

D

D

Fig. 11.2. **A–H.** Laryngotomy, laryngeal ventriculectomy, laser ventriculocordectomy.

181

A—Vocal cord
B—Eversion of laryngeal saccule
C—Cricothyroid membrane
D—Roaring bur

A—Vocal cord
B—Everted laryngeal saccule
C—Cricothyroid membrane
D—Sternothyrohyoideus muscle

Fig. 11.2. *Continued.*

H

Fig. 11.2. *Continued.*

incision is not sutured, but is left open, because the respiratory tract mucosa cannot be aseptically prepared and contamination of the incision can occur with subsequent infection and abscessation as potential problems. The laryngotomy wounds heal satisfactorily by secondary intention; therefore, suturing this wound is not considered justifiable. Conversely, a tracheostomy tube can remain in the laryngotomy site while the horse recovers from anesthesia.

Laser Ventriculectomy/Ventriculocordectomy

The laser fiber is placed through the biopsy channel of the flexible endoscope and the endoscope placed into the nasal passage of the horse (Figure 11.2G). The laser is set at 15 watts, and the laser fiber extended through the end of the scope. The laser should never be fired if the fiber tip is not easily seen on the monitor. Because the fiber lasers create significant collateral damage, only the surface mucosa need be ablated (Figure 11.2H). In many instances, both ventricles are ablated along with the vocal cords to minimize noise after surgery. Care should be taken to avoid lasering the most ventral commissure of the vocal folds to reduce the chance of cicatrix formation. There is no laryngotomy incision to care for using this approach.

Postoperative Management

Antibiotics are not administered routinely. The laryngotomy wound is cleaned twice daily. The animal is confined for the 2–3 weeks it takes for the wound to heal.

After this period, the horse is hand-walked. The horse may be put back to work 8 weeks following surgery.

The tracheostomy tube is usually left in the laryngotomy opening until the patient recovers from anesthesia. If there is undue trauma during surgery—more likely with some of the more involved procedures performed by a laryngotomy approach—it may be advisable to leave the tracheostomy tube in place in case laryngeal edema develops. We do not perform a separate tracheostomy without a specific, critical indication.

Complications and Prognosis

Ventriculectomy or ventriculocordectomy performed alone has less risk of complications than these procedures performed in conjunction with laryngoplasty, described in *Advanced Techniques of Equine Surgery.*[4] A study in draft horses showed that ventriculectomy alone significantly improved athletic performance to a level deemed satisfactory by owners in 87% of these horses.[9] In one report, 86% of owners considered the surgery worthwhile, 3% did not consider it worthwhile, and 11% were unsure.[7] Postoperative complications are rare and generally minor.[10] The most commonly reported complication of laryngoplasty is coughing, which may be performance limiting in some horses.[11]

Complications associated with laser ventriculectomy and ventriculocordectomy are generally few; and in general, horses will ingest food and water without apparent discomfort in 6 hours postoperatively.[12] Thermal damage to surrounding tissue, inadequate removal of ventricular mucosa due to poor visualization, excessive tissue sloughing, mucocele formation, laser burns to the contralateral vocal cord, and arytenoid cartilage necrosis have been documented following laser ventriculocordectomy, however.[12] Complete healing of the surgical site was affirmed by endoscopic evaluation at 47 days postoperatively.[12] A histologic study showed that there was no collateral damage to the laryngeal cartilage when using a diode laser in contact fashion at 20 watts.[13]

Partial Resection of the Soft Palate

Relevant Anatomy

The soft palate forms the floor of the nasopharynx and extends from the caudal border of the hard palate to the base of the larynx. The soft palate itself is comprised of oral and nasopharyngeal mucous membranes, the palatine gland and associated ductile openings, the palatine aponeurosis, and the palatinus and palatopharyngeus muscles.[14] At its most caudal-free margin, the soft palate continues dorsally to form two lateral pillars that join to form the palatopharyngeal arch, named for the palatinus muscle of which the pillars are composed.[14] The position of the soft palate is largely controlled by the surrounding intrinsic musculature; the tensor veli palatini, levator veli palatini, palitinus, and palatopharyngeus muscles. All are innervated by the pharyngeal branch of the vagus nerve except for the tensor veli palatinus muscle, which is supplied by the mandibular branch of the trigeminal nerve.[15]

Indications

Partial resection of the soft palate is indicated in certain cases of dorsal displacement of the soft palate (DDSP) or for the resection of granulomas and cysts from the caudal-free edge of the palate.[14] The etiology of DDSP is not completely understood, and it is probable that there are many inciting factors involved. DDSP may arise from a neuropathy of the pharyngeal branch of the vagus nerve or secondary to conditions that involve the vagus nerves, such as guttural pouch mycosis or retropharyngeal lymphadenopathy, and in association with a hypoplastic epiglottis.[16] The most common form of soft palate displacement is intermittent, however, and is usually associated with exercise. It is a clinical impression that the condition may also accompany generalized inflammation of the pharynx. In these cases, the soft palate displacement may resolve itself on resolution of the inflammatory problem. Both so-called paresis and elongation have been postulated as causes, but not proved. Some horses with intermittent dorsal displacement of the soft palate above the epiglottis respond to tongue-tying, which prevents complete retraction of the tongue.[17]

Partial resection of the soft palate is not a panacea for dorsal displacement of the soft palate, but it has been described as a method of treatment in horses that do not respond to conservative therapy. Surgical patients should be selected carefully. Other primary causes of the problem should be eliminated, and caution must be used because tranquilizers increase the tendency for soft palate displacement. A flexible endoscope in the caudal portion of the pharynx may interfere with the normal act of deglutition and may lead to an erroneous diagnosis. When the condition is the result of a hypoplastic epiglottis or guttural pouch mycosis with nerve involvement, soft palate surgery is not indicated.

Anesthesia and Surgical Preparation

The horse is prepared for laryngotomy as previously described. In this case, the surgery is always performed with the horse under general anesthesia and in dorsal recumbency.

Instrumentation

1. General surgery pack
2. Self-retaining retractor such as a Gelpi, Weitlaner, or Hobday's roaring retractor

Surgical Technique

Laryngotomy is performed as previously described. In some instances, the body of the thyroid cartilage may be sectioned to extend the laryngotomy incision and to provide additional exposure. If the thyroid cartilage is sectioned, one should be careful not to incise the epiglottis, which is in close association with the thyroid cartilage. Splitting the thyroid cartilage is not performed routinely in this procedure.

When laryngotomy is completed, the endotracheal tube must be withdrawn into the mouth to enable one to visualize the soft palate. The concave, U-shaped free border of the soft palate will be observed rostrally (Figure 11.3A). Allis tissue forceps are placed on each side of the soft palate, approximately 1 cm from the midline, and the positioning is checked for symmetry (Figure 11.3B). An incision into the soft palate with Metzenbaum scissors is made on the right side beside the forceps; this incision is extended toward the midline in a semicircular fashion so that, at the midline, it is about 1 cm from the central free border of the soft palate (Figure 11.3C). This procedure is repeated on the left side of the soft palate, so a piece of tissue approximately 2 cm × 1 cm is removed from the central free area of the soft palate. Hemorrhage is negligible, and no attempt is made to suture the soft palate. Alternatively, the resection of tissue can be made in a V-fashion, rather than in crescentic fashion. The cricothyroid membrane is closed with 3-0 polyglytone 6211 (Caprosyn) in a simple continuous pattern while the rest of the laryngotomy incision is left to heal by second intention.

Soft palate resection should be conservative. It is better to subject the animal to a second surgical procedure for resection of additional soft palate than to resect excessive tissue initially, because excessive resection can result in a bilateral nasal discharge of mucus and food material and, possibly, aspiration pneumonia.

Postoperative Management

The horse is confined to a stall until the laryngotomy incision is completely healed and should rest for 4 weeks before being placed into work. Antiinflammatory medication may be administered for 3 days, and systemic antibiotic therapy may be administered for up to a week. The incision site should be cleaned twice daily until it is healed.

Complications and Prognosis

The prognosis after partial resection of the soft palate is quite variable, and it is very difficult to determine the most appropriate treatment.[18] One study looked at an external device (laryngohyoid support [LHS]) that has shown some value in an experimental model, field studies are lacking.[19]

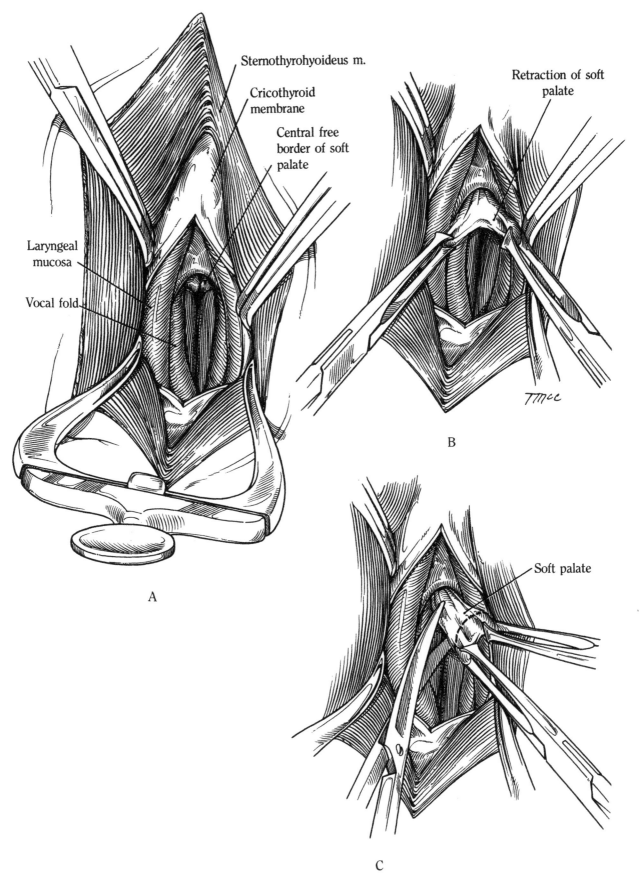

Sternothyrohyoideus m.

Cricothyroid membrane

Central free border of soft palate

Retraction of soft palate

Laryngeal mucosa

Vocal fold

Soft palate

A

B

C

Fig. 11.3. **A–C.** Partial resection of the soft palate.

Surgical Entry and Drainage of the Guttural Pouches

Relevant Anatomy

The guttural pouches exist as paired, air-filled diverticula of the eustachian tubes, which connect the middle ear to the pharynx. Guttural pouches are unique to horses and originate from the midline, dorsocaudal to the pharynx. The stylohyoid bone divides each pouch into lateral and medial portions, and a funnel-shaped opening, the pharyngeal orifice, serves to communicate with the pharynx. The mucous membrane lining of the pouch contains the facial, glossopharyngeal, vagus, spinal accessory, and hypoglossal nerves, as well as the cranial sympathetic trunk, internal carotid artery, and branches of the external carotid artery.[20,21]

Indications

Each of the three surgical approaches to the guttural pouches has particular uses, advantages, and disadvantages. Viborg's triangle approach is used mainly for drainage of the guttural pouch in cases of empyema. It may also be used for the treatment of guttural pouch tympany.[21,22] The hyovertebrotomy approach provides access through the dorsolateral aspect of the guttural pouch and is used for the removal of chondroids and inspissated pus. It is commonly combined with Viborg's triangle approach in the treatment of chronic guttural pouch empyema. A drain may be placed through both incisions postoperatively. The hyovertebrotomy approach may also be used to ligate the internal carotid artery in the treatment of guttural pouch mycosis. Further details of the technique of internal carotid artery ligation are described elsewhere.[4]

The third approach is the ventral or Whitehouse approach. (There is also a modified Whitehouse approach.) This provides the best surgical exposure to the dorsal aspect of the guttural pouch for procedures such as ligation of the internal carotid artery within the pouch in the treatment of guttural pouch mycosis associated with epistaxis. The Whitehouse approach may also be used to treat guttural pouch tympany.[21,22] Although the Whitehouse approach seems a logical choice for ventral drainage of the guttural pouch, temporary and permanent dysphagia has been experienced following the use of this procedure for the treatment of empyema. The dysphagia is presumably associated with compromise of the pharyngeal branches of the glossopharyngeal and vagus nerves that pass ventral to the guttural pouch. Because of the thickened nature of the guttural pouch in this inflammatory condition, these nerves may be difficult to identify, and the associated cellulitis may also compromise the nerves. Consequently, we are hesitant to recommend the Whitehouse approach as a drainage technique for guttural pouch empyema. (Details of the technique are available elsewhere.)[23]

If the response to medical treatment of guttural pouch empyema is poor, surgical drainage of the guttural pouch will be indicated. Surgery is also indicated when the purulent material becomes inspissated or when chondroids have formed. In such cases, ventral drainage through Viborg's triangle is the approach of choice.

Anesthesia and Surgical Preparation

The Viborg's triangle approach may be performed using local analgesia, but general anesthesia is preferred. General anesthesia is recommended for the hyovertebrotomy approach. The surgical sites, illustrated in Figure 11.4A, are clipped and prepared in a routine manner.

Instrumentation

1. General surgery pack
2. Blunt Weitlaner retractors
3. Drain or seton
4. Sponge forceps

Surgical Technique

Viborg's Triangle

Viborg's triangle is the area defined by the tendon of the sternomandibular muscle, the linguofacial (external maxillary) vein, and the caudal border of the vertical ramus of the mandible. A 4- to 6-cm skin incision is made just dorsal to and parallel with the linguofacial vein from the border of the mandible caudad. The subcutaneous tissue is separated, and the base of the parotid gland is reflected dorsad if necessary (Figure 11.4B). Care should be taken to avoid trauma to the parotid gland and duct, the lingofacial vein, and the branches of the vagus nerve along the floor of the guttural pouch. This procedure exposes the guttural pouch. Localization of the guttural pouch is facilitated by its distention when it is in a pathologic state. The guttural pouch membrane is grasped with forceps and is incised with scissors (Figure 11.4C). The wound is left open for drainage, or a drain is inserted. The surgical wound heals by granulation (secondary intention).

Hyovertebrotomy Approach

This approach, which gives access to the dorsolateral aspect of the guttural pouch, is more difficult and should probably be used only to access the arteries for ligation. Care should be taken because of the vessels and nerves within the surgical site. An 8- to 10-cm incision is made parallel and just cranial to the wing of the atlas (Figure 11.4A). The skin incision exposes the parotid salivary gland and the overlying parotidoauricularis muscle. The ventral part of the parotidoauricularis muscle is incised,

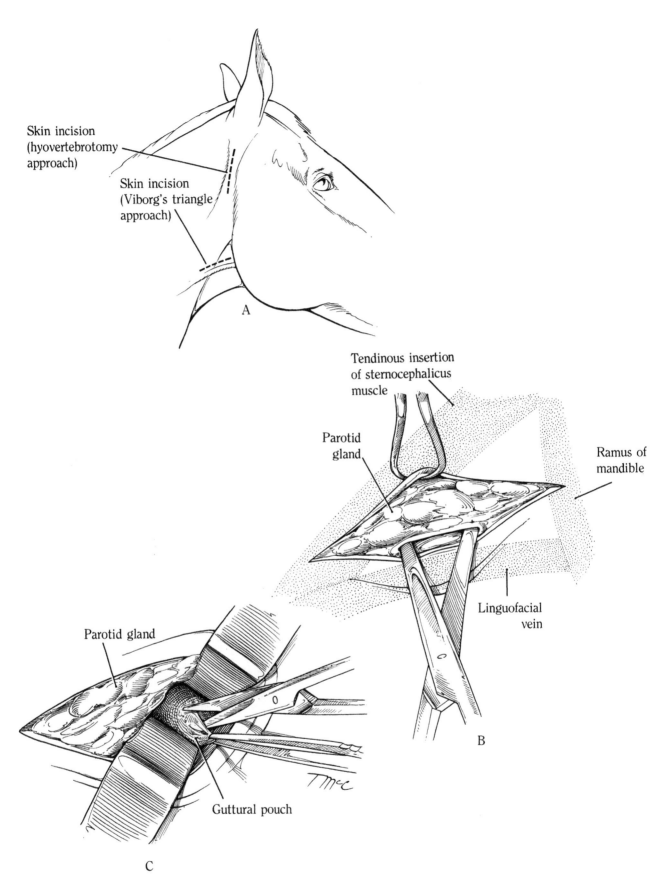

Skin incision
(hyovertebrotomy
approach)

Skin incision
(Viborg's triangle
approach)

A

Tendinous insertion
of sternocephalicus
muscle

Parotid
gland

Ramus of
mandible

Linguofacial
vein

B

Parotid gland

Guttural pouch

C

Fig. 11.4. **A–E.** Surgical entry and drainage of the guttural pouches.

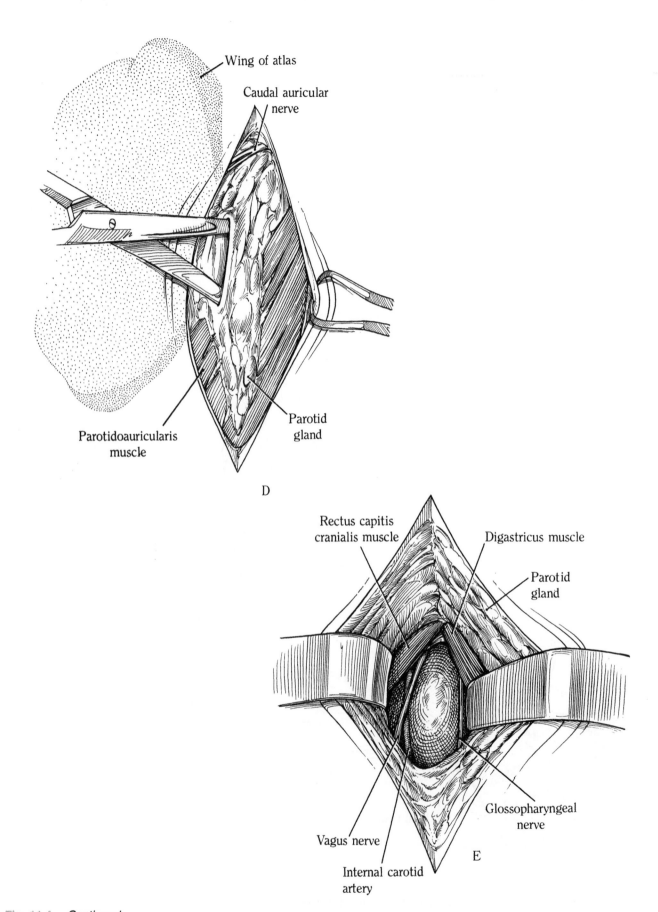

Wing of atlas

Caudal auricular nerve

Parotid gland

Parotidoauricularis muscle

D

Rectus capitis cranialis muscle

Digastricus muscle

Parotid gland

Vagus nerve

Internal carotid artery

Glossopharyngeal nerve

E

Fig. 11.4. *Continued.*

and a dissection plane for the parotid gland is established by incising the fascia on its caudal border (Figure 11.4*D*). The parotid gland is reflected craniad. The caudal auricular nerve crosses obliquely in the dorsal aspect of the surgical field and is reflected caudad if necessary. Reflection of the parotid gland reveals the occipitohyoideus and digastricus muscles craniodorsally and the rectus capitis cranialis muscle caudodorsally (Figure 11.4*E*). The mandibular salivary gland may be identified ventrally. Blunt dissection through areolar tissue exposes the dorsolateral wall of the guttural pouch. The direction of dissection is caudal and then medial to the occipitohyoideus-digastricus muscle group.

The exact site of entry into the guttural pouch may vary, depending on the anatomic placement of the nerve branches overlying the surface. The position of the nerves seems variable and may also be influenced by pathologic distortion of the guttural pouch. Entry is usually made between the glossopharyngeal nerve rostrally and the vagus nerve caudally (Figure 11.4*E*). The internal carotid artery runs beneath the vagus nerve in this region and should be avoided. The guttural pouch is incised with scissors.

The hyovertebrotomy incision may be closed primarily if contamination is not excessive and if a drain is not going to be placed in the guttural pouch. The guttural pouch membrane is closed with simple interrupted sutures of synthetic absorbable suture material. One must be careful to avoid the adjacent nerves. The fascia associated with the parotid gland is also apposed with synthetic absorbable sutures. The skin is closed with nonabsorbable sutures.

Postoperative Management

Daily flushing of the pouch may be performed postoperatively. In some instances, removal of additional particulate debris may be necessary, and this can be performed by a combination of flushing and digital manipulation. When pus and debris are evacuated completely from the pouch, flushing is discontinued, any drains are removed, and the incisions are left to heal by secondary intention.

Complications and Prognosis

Some cases of guttural pouch empyema can be treated with the insertion of indwelling catheters to provide local therapy and to assist in drainage. Irritating solutions, should not be infused into the guttural pouches because of severe inflammatory changes. We believe that the mechanical drainage of the contents of the pouch is more important than the antibacterial activity of the solutions placed in them. In one study of 91 cases of guttural pouch empyema, treatment with lavage offered a good prognosis for resolution of uncomplicated empyema, while an endoscopic snare was needed in cases presenting with

chondroids.[24] With improved techniques and materials for endoscopy, surgical intervention is less necessary.

References

1. Stick, J.A. Trachea. *In* Equine Surgery. 3rd Ed. Edited by J.A. Auer, J.A. Stick. St. Louis, MO, Saunders, 2006, pp. 608–615.
2. Chesen, A.B., and Rakestraw, P.C. Indications for and short- and long-term outcome of permanent tracheostomy performed in standing horses: 82 cases (1995–2005). *J. Am. Vet. Med. Assoc.*, 232:1352–1356, 2008.
3. McClure, S.R., Taylor, T.S., Honnas, C.M., Schumacher, J., Chaffin, M.K., and Hoffman, A.G. Permanent tracheostomy in standing horses: Technique and results. *Vet. Surg.*, 24:231–234, 1995.
4. McIlwraith, C.W., and Robertson, J.T. McIlwraith & Turner's Equine Surgery: Advanced Techniques. 2nd Ed. Baltimore, MD, Williams & Wilkins, 1998.
5. Stick, J.A. Larynx. *In* Equine Surgery. 3rd Ed. Edited by J.A. Auer, J.A. Stick. St. Louis, MO, Saunders, 2006, pp. 608–616.
6. Stick, J.A. Ventriculocordectomy. *In* Ninth Annual ACVS Veterinary Symposium, Sept. 30–Oct. 3, 1999.
7. Taylor, S.E., Barakzai, S.Z., and Dixon, P. Ventriculocordectomy as the sole treatment for recurrent laryngeal neuropathy: Long-term results from ninety-two horses. *Vet. Surg.*, 35:653–657, 2006.
8. Brown, J.A., Derksen, F.J., Stick, J.A., Hartmann, W.M., and Robinson, N.E. Laser vocal cordectomy fails to effectively reduce respiratory noise in horses with laryngeal hemiplegia. *Vet. Surg.*, 34:247–252, 2005.
9. Bohanon, T.C., Beard, W.L., and Robertson, J.T. Laryngeal hemiplegia in draft horses. A review of 27 cases. *Vet. Surg.*, 19:456–459, 1990.
10. Brown, J.A., Derksen, F.J., Stick, J.A., Hartmann, W.M., and Robinson, N.E. Ventriculocordectomy reduces respiratory noise in horses with laryngeal hemiplegia. *Equine Vet. J.*, 35:570–574, 2003.
11. Davenport, C.L.M., Tulleners, E.P., and Parente, E.J. The effect of recurrent laryngeal neurectomy in conjunction with laryngoplasty and unilateral ventriculocordectomy in Thoroughbred racehorses. *Vet. Surg.*, 30:417–421, 2001.
12. Hawkins, J.F., and Andrews-Jones, L. Neodymium:yttrium aluminum garnet laser ventriculocordectomy in standing horses. *Am. J. Vet. Res.*, 62:531–537, 2001.
13. Robinson, P., Williams, K.J., Sullins, K.E., Arnoscky, S.P., Stick, J.A., Robinson, N.E., de Feijter-Rupp, H., and Derksen, F.J. Histological evaluation of the equine larynx after unilateral laser-assisted ventriculocordectomy. *Equine Vet. J.*, 39:222–225, 2007.
14. Ducharme, N.G. Pharynx. *In* Equine Surgery. 3rd Ed. Edited by J.A. Auer, J.A. Stick. St. Louis, MO, Saunders, 2006, pp. 544–566.
15. Holcombe, S.J., Derksen, F.J., Stick, J.A., and Robinson, N.E. Effect of bilateral nerve blockade of the pharyngeal branch of the vagus nerve produces persistent soft palate dysfunction in horses. *Am. J. Vet. Res.*, 59:504–508, 1998.
16. Holcombe, S.J., Derksen, F.J., Stick, J.A., and Robinson, N.E. Pathophysiology of dorsal displacement of the soft palate in horses. *Equine Vet. J. Suppl.*, 30:45–48, 1999.

17. Franklin, S.H., Naylor, J.R., and Lane, J.G. The effect of a tongue-tie in horses with dorsal displacement of the soft palate. *Equine Vet. J. Suppl.*, 34:430–433, 2002.

18. Allen, K.J., Christley, R.M., Birchall, M.A., and Franklin, S.H. A systematic review of the efficacy of interventions for dynamic intermittent dorsal displacement of the soft palate. *Equine Vet. J.*, 44:259–266, 2012.

19. Woodie, J.B., Ducharme, N.G., Hackett, R.P., Erb, H.N., Mitchell, L.M., and Soderholm, L.V. Can an external device prevent dorsal displacement of the soft palate during strenuous exercise? *Equine Vet. J.*, 37:425–429, 2005.

20. Baptist, K. Functional anatomy observations of the pharyngeal orifice of the equine guttural pouch (auditory tube diverticulum). *Vet. J.*, 153:311–319, 1997.

21. Freeman, D.E. Complications of surgery for diseases of the guttural pouch. *Vet. Clin. North Am. Equine Pract.*, 24:485–497, 2008.

22. Honnas, C.M., and Pascoe, J.R. Guttural pouch disease. *In* Equine Internal Medicine. 2nd Ed. Edited by B.P. Smith. St. Louis, MO, Mosby, 1996, pp. 610–615.

23. Freeman, D.E. Diagnosis and treatment of diseases of the guttural pouch. Part II. *Compend. Contin. Educ. Pract. Vet.*, 2:525, 1980.

24. Judy, C.E., Chaffin, M.K., and Cohen, N.D. Empyema of the guttural pouch (auditory tube diverticulum) in horses: 91 cases (1977–1997). *J. Am. Vet. Med. Assoc.*, 215:1666–1670, 1999.

Chapter 12

EQUINE DENTAL AND GASTROINTESTINAL SURGERY

Dean A. Hendrickson, DVM, MS, DACVS

Objectives

1. Discuss a technique for removal of the 1st molar in the equine upper arcade and the 3rd premolar in the lower arcade.
2. Provide a basic discussion of exploratory laparotomy in the horse, including indications, technique, and anatomy.
3. Discuss the advantages and disadvantages of two surgical approaches—ventral midline and flank laparotomy—for abdominal exploration in the horse.
4. Describe a surgical treatment of umbilical hernias in the foal.

Repulsion of Cheek Teeth

Relevant Anatomy

The equine dental formula for permanent teeth is I(3/3) – C(1/1) – PM(3/3 or 4/4) – M(3/3). There are a total of 36–44 teeth depending upon the presence of wolf teeth (PM1) and canines. Most of the tooth is composed of a cream-colored calcified tissue, called *dentin,* which is secreted by odontoblasts and functions to protect the pulp from infection.[1] The next external layer is the *cementum,* followed by the outermost and hardest layer of the tooth, the *enamel.* The elasticity of the underlying dentin and cementum prevents the brittle enamel from shattering and chipping by absorbing shock.[1]

The pulp of the tooth contains the pulpar nerves, capillaries, lymphatics, odontoblasts, and fibroblasts that support sensory capabilities and regenerative capabili-ties.[1] The crown of the tooth refers to the portion of the tooth extending from the root and is further divided into the visible crown and reserve crown, which lie below the gum line.

Blood supply to the teeth originates from the greater palatine artery, which courses around the periphery of the hard palate (2–3 mm medial to the lingual gingival margin of the maxillary teeth) and adjoins its counterpart rostrally.[1] This artery must be carefully avoiding during tooth extraction.

Nervous supply to the teeth is provided by the infraorbital and inferior alveolar nerves. The infraorbital nerve emerges from the infraorbital foramen approximately 5 cm dorsal to the rostral aspect of the facial crest. The infraorbital canal is in close proximity to the roots of the upper 8th, 9th, 10th, and 11th cheek teeth and must be carefully avoided when repelling cheek teeth.[1] The inferior alveolar nerve enters the mandibular canal and branches to innervate the teeth in the mandibular teeth, exiting out the rostral mental foramina.

Also in the vicinity of the surgical site are the parotid duct, facial artery, and facial vein, which follow the ventral edge of the mandible and run up the lateral aspect of the face near lower cheek teeth 10 and 11.

Indications

Cheek tooth repulsion is a method of tooth removal that is indicated when tooth preservation is not possible and extraction through the mouth with forceps is not feasible. Tooth removal is indicated in cases of infundibular necrosis, fractures extending into the reserve crown, or abscesses of teeth, periodontal disease, chronic ossifying alveolar periostitis, and tumors of the teeth. Infection of the teeth of either the upper or lower arcade may be secondary to fractures of the bones of the skull (mandible and maxilla) that also involve the roots of the teeth.

Repulsion of both upper and lower cheek teeth involves either trephining a hole or creating a maxillary sinus flap

---

Turner and McIlwraith's Techniques in Large Animal Surgery, 4th Edition. Dean A. Hendrickson and A. N. (Nickie) Baird.
© 2013 John Wiley & Sons, Inc. Published 2013 by John Wiley & Sons, Inc.

to gain access to the base of the tooth and driving the tooth from its socket into the mouth using a dental punch and mallet. It is the preferred technique for removal of maxillary cheek teeth 3–6 and all cheek teeth in the lower arcade.[2] Buccotomy extraction and vertical alveolar osteotomy techniques may also be used for cheek tooth extraction but are described in detail elsewhere.[2] Buccotomy extraction involves a lateral approach and longitudinal sectioning of the tooth so that it may be removed piecemeal. Vertical alveolar osteotomy is similar to buccotomy but with a modification of the approach so that the incision is parallel to the parotid duct and linguofacial vein. This method is recommended for removal of mandibular cheek teeth 4 and 5.

All methods of tooth extraction in horses have a high documented rate of complications. Although not described here, surgical endodontic therapy is an alternative to tooth extraction that is relatively new to equine dentistry. By preserving the tooth, apicoectomy avoids problems associated with abnormal tooth wear and step formation along the occlusal table.

When the maxillary cheek teeth are involved (usually the 4th premolar or the 1st molar), signs of purulent nasal discharge are present because of secondary maxillary sinusitis. When the disease involves the mandibular teeth, swelling of or chronic drainage from the ventral border of the mandible is usually present. The teeth to be removed are ascertained by oral and radiographic examinations. In this chapter, repulsion of the 1st molar in the upper arcade and the 3rd premolar in the lower arcade are discussed.

Anesthesia and Surgical Preparation

Repulsion of teeth in the horse should be performed with the horse under general anesthesia. The horse is positioned with the affected tooth (teeth) uppermost. A mouth speculum is placed on the horse and is opened sufficiently to allow admission of the surgeon's hand. The hair is clipped over the surgical site, and routine surgical preparation is performed.

Instrumentation

1. General surgery pack
2. Mouth speculum
3. Molar forceps
4. Mallet or hammer
5. 3/4-inch and 1/2-inch trephines
6. Molar cutters
7. Straight and curved dental punches
8. Bone curettes (sizes 1, 3, and 5)
9. Umbilical tape
10. Gauze roll, dental wax, or dental acrylic
11. Mild antiseptic solution, such as chlorhexidine
12. Bone saw (for the maxillary sinus flap)

Surgical Technique

In the case of trephination for the upper teeth, a curved incision should be made through the skin, with the apex pointing dorsad. The exact location of the incision depends on which tooth is to be repelled. Radiographs can be taken with radiopaque markers to help identify the proper location. The skin flap is reflected back, and the periosteum is incised and reflected from the bone to expose sufficient area to accept the trephine. A 3/4-inch trephine should be used for the upper teeth. For the repulsion of lower teeth, a straight incision is made directly over the proposed site of trephination, and the edges of the skin are undermined to allow the trephine to be positioned on the lower border of the mandible. The periosteum is incised and reflected from the mandible. A 1/2-inch trephine should be used for the lower teeth.

The trephine hole is begun by extending the center bit of the trephine 3 mm beyond the end of the trephine and fixing it to the bone. The trephine is turned back and forth in a rotary motion until it has cut a distinct groove in the bone. The center bit on the trephine is retracted, and cutting is continued until a disc of bone is detached (Figure 12.1A).

Locating the Trephine Opening for Upper Cheek Teeth

A line from the medial canthus of the eye to the infraorbital canal that continues forward past the roots of the 1st cheek tooth is the line of maximum height at which any trephining may be done for superior cheek teeth. This line marks the course of the osseous nasolacrimal canal. The trephine openings for all superior cheek teeth should be placed just below this line. In the case of old horses in which the teeth have grown out, it is permissible to drop down nearer to the facial crest. For the 1st and 2nd upper cheek teeth, which are straight, a line is drawn through the center of each tooth, and a trephine opening is made along each line. For the 3rd, 4th, and 5th upper cheek teeth, which have a caudal curvature, the trephination is made below the nasolacrimal canal, along a line directed over the posterior margin of the table surface of each tooth.

For repulsion of the 6th cheek tooth, a trephine hole must be made through the frontal sinus 4 cm lateral to the midline on a transverse line between the cranial margins of the orbits. It is necessary to go through the frontal sinus and the frontomaxillary opening into the maxillary sinus. The dental punch is passed lateral to the infraorbital canal to the root of the tooth. It is necessary to use a curved punch because the tooth has a tendency to lie under the infraorbital canal. The punch is seated on the base of the tooth, and the tooth is repelled. If the vein that lies above the infraorbital canal is severed, the area will have to be packed. This operation is difficult in young horses because of the marked caudal curvature of the tooth. Fortunately,

Dental punch

Tooth to be removed

A

B

Fig. 12.1. **A–D.** Repulsion of cheek teeth.

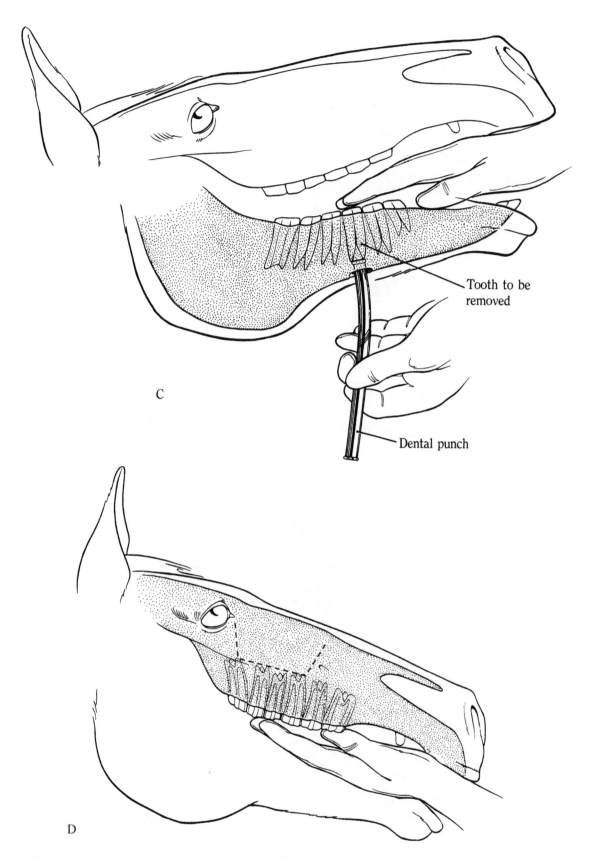

Tooth to be removed

Dental punch

C

D

Fig. 12.1. *Continued.*

this tooth does not require removal as frequently as other upper cheek teeth. Figure 12.1A,B shows trephination and repulsion of the 4th upper cheek tooth (1st molar).

Locating the Trephine Opening for Lower Cheek Teeth

The trephine holes for repulsion of the lower cheek teeth are made on the ventrolateral border of the mandible. The inner and outer alveolar plates rest directly on the tooth, so it is necessary to align the punch with the long axis of the tooth to avoid punching toward the medial alveolar plate and fracturing it. For repelling the 1st cheek tooth, the trephine is centered directly below the table surface; for the 2nd to 5th cheek teeth, the opening is made below the caudal borders of the teeth because of their caudal curvature (Figure 12.1C); for horses older than 12 years, the opening can be made directly under the center of the table surface. Exposure of the trephine site for the 4th and 5th lower cheek teeth is complicated by the parotid duct and linguofacial artery and vein, which should be identified and retracted caudad. When a dental fistula is present on the lower border of the mandible, the trephine is positioned directly over the center of it because the fistula usually occurs opposite the affected alveolus.

The location of the 6th lower cheek tooth necessitates trephination over the lateral surface of the mandible. A line is drawn from the center of the table surface of the tooth to the point of greatest curvature of the ramus of the mandible. An incision is made on this line through the skin and masseter muscle over a bulging prominence where the two plates of bone that form the mandible are separated to accommodate the tooth. The muscle is separated from the bone by spreading it with wound retractors. The trephine opening is made and is elongated dorsad with a chisel to give better direction for the punch and to lessen the chances of fracturing the medial bony plate of the mandible. The skin-and-muscle incision is terminated at least 4 cm from the border of the mandible to avoid severing the branches of the facial nerve that spread out over the surface of the masseter muscle from above, ventrad, and rostrad. Further details of this technique are available in the advanced techniques textbook.[3]

Maxillary Flap Sinusotomy for Tooth Repulsion

In some cases, a larger opening is desired. The location of the flap is outlined in Figure 12.1D. The caudal border is just rostrad to a line drawn from the medial canthus of the eye to the facial crest. The ventral border is just dorsal to the facial crest, and the rostral border just caudal to a line drawn from the rostrad facial crest to the infraorbital foramen. The skin is incised down to the periosteum. The flap is cut on the caudal, ventral, and rostral sites with

either an osteotome and mallet or an oscillating bone saw. The flap is lifted using the dorsal margin and periosteum as a hinge. The sinus is explored and lavaged.

After repulsion of the teeth, the flap is replaced and the periosteum sutured with 2-0 polyglyconate (Maxon) in a simple continuous pattern. The subcutaneous layer is closed similarly and the skin stapled. In some instances, the rostral ventral portion of the flap is left open for drainage.

Repulsion Following Trephination

The surgeon's hand is introduced into the patient's mouth, the diseased tooth is located, and the tooth's path in the sinus or jaw is determined. The punch is directed onto the root of the tooth, and an assistant begins to tap the punch with a mallet. The first few blows with the mallet should be sufficient to seat the punch into the root of the tooth. The trephine hole may have to be enlarged to allow the punch access to the diseased teeth.

Once the punch is seated, the assistant delivers steady blows to the punch. The mallet blows produce a characteristic ringing sound when the punch is seated properly, and the surgeon feels the vibrations of these blows transmitted through the tooth to his hand. If the punch slips off the tooth into alveolar tissue, it will need to be repositioned. After some time, the surgeon will feel the gradual loosening of the tooth with the hand that is in the patient's mouth. Subsequent blows with the mallet should be less forceful as the tooth is driven from the alveolus.

Following tooth repulsion, any fragments should be removed from the alveolus with forceps. The alveolus may require curettage if diseased bone surrounds the tooth. To prevent the socket from becoming packed with food, it should be filled with a suitable material until the socket is almost filled with granulation tissue. Dental wax, dental acrylic, gutta-percha, or gauze rolls may be used, depending on individual preference. The author prefers the use of Justi® hoof acrylic to fill the hole. If gauze rolls are used, a roll that will fit snugly into the hole is made and is tied around the center with umbilical tape, leaving two long ends. The ends are passed through the socket and trephine hole, the gauze is wedged firmly into the cavity, and the umbilical tape is brought to the exterior. The umbilical tape is then secured to the skin by tying it to another gauze roll. The ends should be kept long so that the gauze roll in the alveolus can be replaced without having to thread the new piece of umbilical tape back through the trephine hole.

Infected cheek teeth that are removed will usually require postoperative lavage of the associated sinuses with saline. Antibiotics can be left in the sinus after the lavage. For caudal cheek teeth, an additional 10 mm trephine hole is made into the ipsilateral frontal sinus after the maxillary bone flap is closed to facilitate postoperative irrigation.[4] For rostral cheek teeth, the maxillary septum can be fenestrated to allow accumulated serum and blood in the conchal sinus to drain to the rostral maxillary sinus and out the nares.

Postoperative Management

The horse should be placed on broad spectrum antibiotics preoperatively and for approximately 1 week following surgery. During the first few days, if a gauze pack is used, the pack is changed daily, and the sinus is flushed with a mild antiseptic solution if suppuration is present. The material used to pack the socket remains until the cavity is almost filled with granulation tissue. After a week, the material used to pack the socket can be changed every 2 or 3 days (if gauze is used). If the Justi® hoof acrylic is used, it will generally be pushed out of the socket in time and does not need to be removed.

Complications and Prognosis

Tooth repulsion is the traditional method for cheek tooth removal. However, all tooth extraction methods are associated with a high rate of complications as well as the inherent risks of general anesthesia in horses. Complication rates of maxillary cheek tooth repulsion have been near 50% in some studies with these horses requiring a second surgery.[5] Possible untoward sequelae of this procedure include punching out the wrong tooth, puncturing the hard palate by incorrect positioning of the punch over the tooth, rupturing the palatine artery, and breaking the alveolar plates of an adjacent tooth with the punch, which may lead to alveolar periostitis. Dixon et al. (2000) reported that 64% of horses treated with mandibular cheek tooth repulsion responded to a single surgical treatment.[4] Repulsion of maxillary cheek teeth was successful in 62% of horses (no continuation or recurrence of symptoms). A recent paper concluded that tooth repulsion of maxillary and mandibular cheek teeth could be performed in the standing horse.[6]

Ventral Midline Laparotomy and Abdominal Exploration

Relevant Anatomy

A discussion of relevant anatomy for this procedure is included in the description of surgical technique.

Indications

The ventral midline approach provides the greatest single incision exposure of the peritoneal cavity of the horse; it is also the quickest approach. It is particularly indicated for surgical management of acute equine abdominal disorders, although some surgeons use the paramedian technique.[7] This approach may also be used for bilateral ovariectomy or for removal of an ovarian tumor. Fears

regarding the risk of dehiscence are not justified, and it is a practical approach that avoids both muscles and blood vessels. Although the scope of this text does not extend to detailed surgical management of patients with acute abdominal disorders, a basic discussion of exploratory laparotomy in the horse is appropriate.

Anesthesia and Surgical Preparation

This surgical procedure is performed with the patient in dorsal recumbency under general anesthesia. The ventral abdomen is clipped from the area of the pubis to the area of the xiphoid process extending at least 30 cm from the midline. This may be performed prior to the induction of anesthesia. The area of incision is shaved, and routine aseptic preparation is performed. Draping includes the use of hock drapes over the limbs to prevent contamination if the laparotomy sheet is displaced. An impervious drape is also used, so the bowel can be placed over it, to minimize soaking of the cloth drapes underneath.

Instrumentation

1. General surgery pack
2. Additional sterile lap sponges and gauze
3. Long-sleeved sterile gloves

Surgical Technique

The incision begins over the umbilicus and extends craniad. Its length depends on the procedure, but it is generally 30–40 cm long (Figure 12.2A). Such an incision is used in patients with acute abdominal disorders, but cystotomies and ovariectomies require a more caudal incision. The skin incision extends through a layer of subcutaneous tissue, which is thin in most animals. When hemorrhage has been controlled, the linea alba is incised; it is preferable to maintain the incision within the linea alba (Figure 12.2B). Slight divergence from the midline will result in entry into the rectus abdominis muscle, particularly in the cranial portion of the incision, but this event is generally of no consequence. Incision of the linea alba reveals the retroperitoneal adipose tissue deeply (Figure 12.2B). The retroperitoneal adipose tissue is cleared with a sponge to reveal the peritoneum, with the round ligament of the liver demarcating the midline (Figure 12.2C). The peritoneum is picked up and is incised with Metzenbaum scissors, and the incision may either be extended with the scissors (Figure 12.2D) or torn by hand. Retractors are not used routinely in exploratory laparotomy. Any exteriorized bowel is kept moist while systematic exploration of the abdomen is performed.

Upon opening the abdomen, the problem may be immediately obvious or may be determined quickly on cursory examination. In many instances, however, a systematic examination should be performed prior to closure

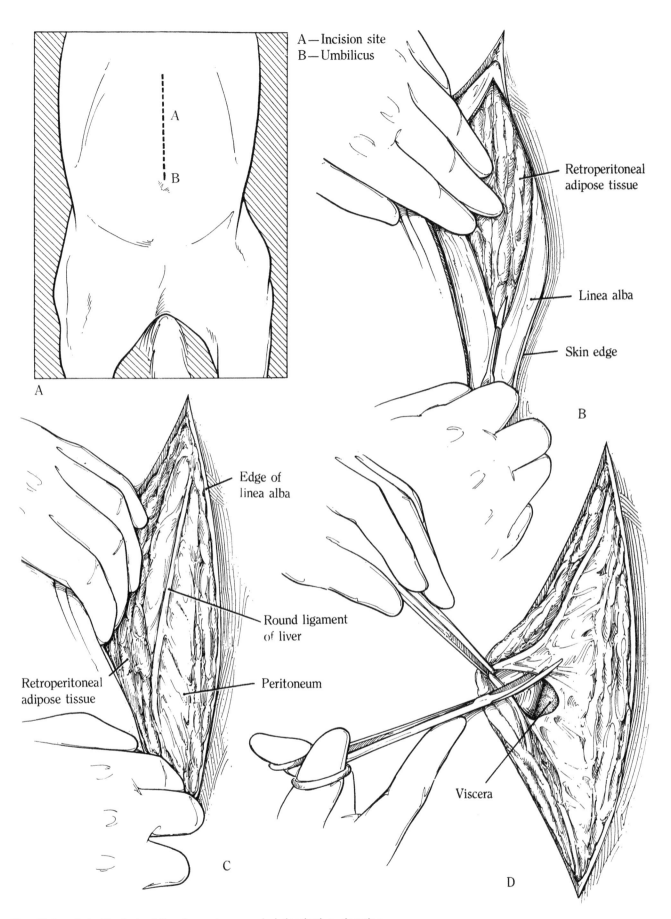

A—Incision site
B—Umbilicus

Retroperitoneal adipose tissue

Linea alba

Skin edge

B

Edge of linea alba

Round ligament of liver

Retroperitoneal adipose tissue

Peritoneum

Viscera

A

C

D

Fig. 12.2. **A–L.** Ventral midline laparotomy and abdominal exploration.

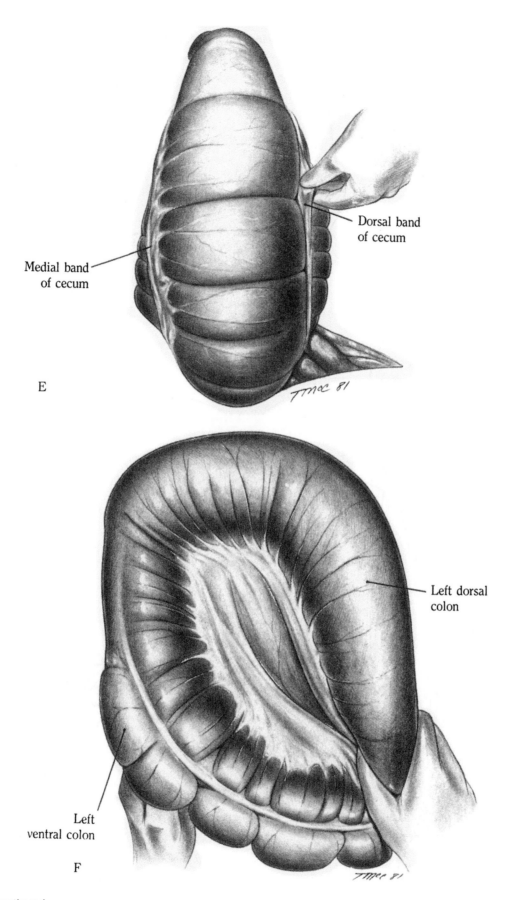

Dorsal band
of cecum

Medial band
of cecum

E

Left dorsal
colon

Left
ventral colon

F

Fig. 12.2. *Continued.*

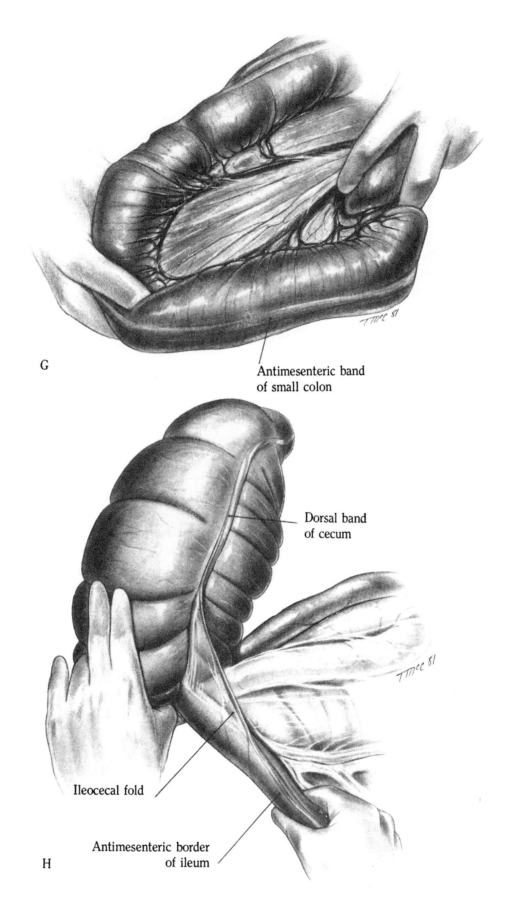

G

Antimesenteric band
of small colon

Dorsal band
of cecum

Ileocecal fold

Antimesenteric border
of ileum

H

Fig. 12.2. *Continued.*

Arcuate vasculature
of jejunum

Jejunum

Mesentery

I

J

Subcutis

K

Subcutis

L

Fig. 12.2. *Continued.*

of the abdomen. The systematic identification of normal, undisplaced viscera only is presented here.

If the cecum is not displaced (it lies ventrally, on the right side of the midline, with the apex directed craniad), it should be identified quickly after entering the peritoneal cavity (Figure 12.2E). The cecum is a reference point for systematic exploration of both the small and large intestines. The lateral band of the cecum is continuous with the cecocolic fold, which leads into the right ventral portion of the large colon. From this point, the large colon can be explored. The right ventral colon runs craniad and leads into the left ventral colon at the sternal flexure. The left ventral and left dorsal portions of the colon are the mobile parts and bend sharply at the pelvic flexure, which is located near the pelvic inlet (Figure 12.2F). The left dorsal colon passes forward from the pelvic flexure to the diaphragmatic flexure and becomes the right dorsal colon. This runs caudad in a dorsal position and, on reaching the medial surface of the base of the cecum, turns to the left, becomes narrower, and leads into the transverse colon. It joins the small colon ventral to the left kidney.

The small colon is characterized by two longitudinal bands, one within the mesentery and the other on the opposite (antimesenteric) side. It has two rows of sacculations and is attached to the sublumbar region by the colic mesentery (Figure 12.2G). The proximal small colon is also attached to the distal duodenum by the narrow duodenocolic fold of peritoneum. This fold is an identification point for the junction of the terminal duodenum and the proximal jejunum.

The small intestine is examined routinely by first locating the ileum. To do this, one retracts the cecum caudad to expose the dorsal band. This thin, avascular band runs into the ileocecal fold, which continues into the antimesenteric border of the ileum (Figure 12.2H). Using these landmarks, the surgeon can palpate the ileocecal junction deep in the abdomen; the junction cannot be exteriorized. The thin membranous fold called the antimesenteric border is 180° opposite the ileal mesentery and allows one to positively identify the ileum. Once the ileum is located, the small intestine may be examined systematically. Moving proximad, the entire length of the jejunum is explored until the duodenocolic fold, which is the junction between jejunum and duodenum, is reached. The jejunum has a mobile mesentery and is characterized by a lack of bands or sacculations (Figure 12.2I). The root of the mesentery may be palpated at this stage. The duodenum also may be explored manually, not visually, because the duodenum's lack of mobility makes visualization difficult. The duodenum leads to the pylorus.

At this stage, the epiploic foramen should be palpated. It is most easily examined by standing on the patient's left side and using the left hand. If one holds the duodenum loosely between fingers and thumb with the dorsal surface of the fingers against the caudate lobe of the liver and moves laterad, the fingertips will locate the small opening of the epiploic foramen. This opening is larger in older horses.

The stomach and the spleen, which are in the left lateral quadrant, should be palpated. In a stallion, the internal inguinal rings that are ventrolateral to the femoral canals are palpated; in the mare, the uterus and ovaries are examined.

The ventral midline incision is closed in three layers. A separate closure of the peritoneum is not necessary. The linea alba is closed with a simple interrupted or a simple continuous pattern. Simple interrupted sutures should be placed 1 cm apart (Figure 12.2J). If a simple continuous pattern is used, the suture should commence and should be tied beyond the extremities of the incision in the linea alba. Five or six throws should be used in each knot. If the incision is less than 20 cm (8 inches approximately), one length of doubled commercially available suture material is usually sufficient. If the incision is longer, two separate strands should be started beyond the commissure of the linea alba incision and directed to the center of the incision. Bites in the linea alba should be placed 0.75–1.00 cm apart and 1.5 cm from the cut edge (Figure 12.2K).[8]

The choice of suture material depends on personal preference, but we have been most satisfied with synthetic absorbable materials such as polyglyconate (Maxon) or polyglactin 910 (Vicryl). The multifilament, nonabsorbable sutures have superior strength, but suture sinuses may be formed, depending on technique and degree of contamination. The subcutaneous tissue is closed with a simple continuous layer of 2-0 synthetic absorbable material (Figure 12.2L). The main purpose of this layer is to close dead space and cover the ends of the suture material, especially when an interrupted pattern is used. A continuous closure has fewer knots to cover with the subcutaneous layer and less chance that the ends of the sutures will protrude into the skin incision. Generally, the skin is closed with skin staples (Figure 12.2L). In most abdominal surgical procedures, speed is important. Staples offer satisfactory closure as well as speed. Peritoneal drainage is not used routinely following abdominal surgery. The routine use of Penrose drains, in particular, is to be discouraged because of the risk of retrograde infection. If contamination is suspected or if bowel anastomosis has been performed, the abdomen should be irrigated and a fenestrated orthopedic drain should be inserted, mainly to drain the irrigation fluid. Generally, the drain is removed within 24 hours.

Postoperative Management

Nonsteroidal antiinflammatory drugs are administered at the end of surgery to decrease the immediate incisional (parietal) pain. Antibiotics and replacement fluids are used; the type and dosage depend on the particular surgical procedure. Additional drugs and supportive therapy may be necessary in patients with acute abdominal disorders. If a drain has been inserted, its patency must be checked regularly by applying negative suction to its end using a syringe. Bandaging is not used routinely, but a stent bandage may be indicated. Skin sutures or staples are removed in 12–14 days.

Complications and Prognosis

In the literature, incisional-related complication rates following ventral midline celiotomy range from 29% to 40%.[9,10] Incisional drainage is the most common, but other complications include peri-incisional edema, abscessation, suture sinus, and dehiscence. Ultrasonographic evaluation of the incision postoperatively can be a useful means of identifying incisional complications.[11] Reported rates of herniation following ventral midline celiotomy are relatively low (15 to 16%).[9,10] Horses that develop incisional drainage are more likely to develop incisional hernias than horses without incisional complications.[10] Other factors that are believed to contribute to the development of hernias include uncontrolled exercise, violent postoperative recovery, and early failure or weakening of suture material. While concerns have been raised about including a subcutaneous suture pattern in the closure of the ventral midline incision, there does not seem to be an increased risk of infection with a three-layer closure compared to a two-layer closure. However, there also does not seem to be any extra value in adding a third layer of closure either.[12] Antimicrobial suture does not appear to limit the likelihood of incisional complications and may actually lead to potential adverse side effects.[13] Horses that have an incisional hernia are less likely to return to use and performance, making client education regarding healing times post surgery very important.[14] There does not appear to be any increase in complications when performing a paramedian celiotomy incision.[7]

Generally, the prognosis for this procedure is good, and the complications are relatively mild. Most survival rates in the literature are a reflection of the severity of the disease that necessitated surgery.

Standing Flank Laparotomy

Relevant Anatomy

A discussion of relevant anatomy for this procedure is included in the description of surgical technique.

Indications

The standing flank approach is useful for some procedures. It is important to consider the limitations associated with a flank approach prior to beginning the approach. In general, only the ipsilateral organs are accessible through the flank, and only organs with a long blood supply or attachments can be exteriorized. The size of the approach is also limited in the horse. The approach has been used for intestinal biopsy,[15] for abdominal lavage,[16] for access to the equine reproductive tract,[17] for uterine torsion reduction,[18] and for standing exploration of the chronic colic horse. In many cases, standing laparoscopy has become the approach of choice for standing abdominal procedures.[19]

Anesthesia and Surgical Preparation

Tranquilization of the patient is optional. The paralumbar fossa area is clipped, and the immediate area of the skin incision is shaved. The surgical area is prepared for aseptic surgery in a routine manner. Local analgesia is instituted by either a line block, an inverted L block, or a paravertebral block; for these techniques, refer to Chapter 2, "Anesthesia and Fluid Therapy. The surgical area is then given a final preparation before surgery. With the standing procedure, aseptic preparation of a wide area and limited draping are preferred.

Instrumentation

1. General surgery pack
2. Long sterile gloves

Surgical Technique

A 20-cm skin incision is made midway between the tuber coxae and the last rib (Figure 12.3A). The dorsal limit of the incision is below the longissimus dorsi muscle and level with the tuber coxae. The incision is continued through the subcutaneous tissue, and any hemorrhage is controlled.

At this stage, there are two techniques for dividing the muscle layers. In the "grid" technique, all three layers may be divided along the direction of the muscle fibers. With the exception of the external abdominal oblique muscle, the fascial components of the flank muscles are weak; and splitting the muscles is preferred to transecting them. The grid technique, however, decreases the exposure. In most cases, a modified grid technique with a vertical incision through the fascia and muscle of the external abdominal oblique is used. (The two alternate incisions in the external abdominal oblique muscle are illustrated in Figure 12.3B.) The grid incision between the muscle fibers in a caudoventral direction is started with scissors and is completed with fingers (Figure 12.3C). In the modified grid approach, the fascia and muscle are incised with a scalpel (Figure 12.3D).

The remainder of the procedure is illustrated in a situation in which the external abdominal oblique muscle has been separated using the grid approach. In Figure 12.3E, the dotted line shows the line of cleavage in the internal abdominal oblique muscle where the fibers run

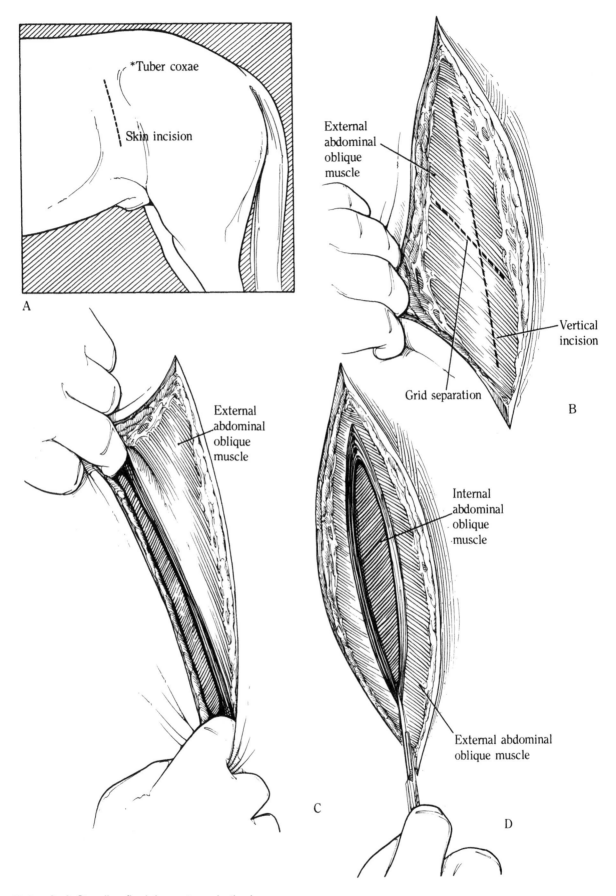

Fig. 12.3. A–J. Standing flank laparotomy in the horse.

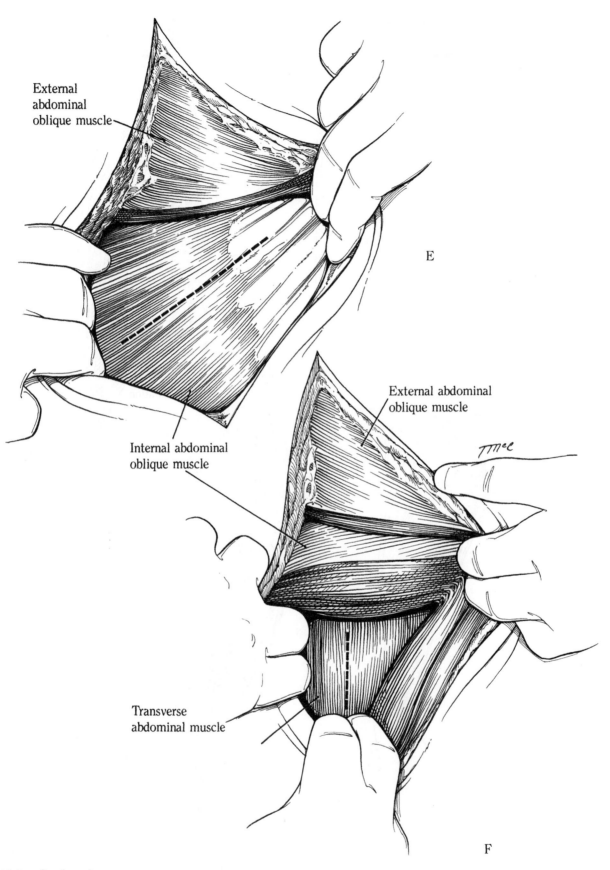

External
abdominal
oblique muscle

E

External abdominal
oblique muscle

Internal abdominal
oblique muscle

Transverse
abdominal muscle

F

Fig. 12.3. *Continued.*

204

Fig. 12.3. *Continued.*

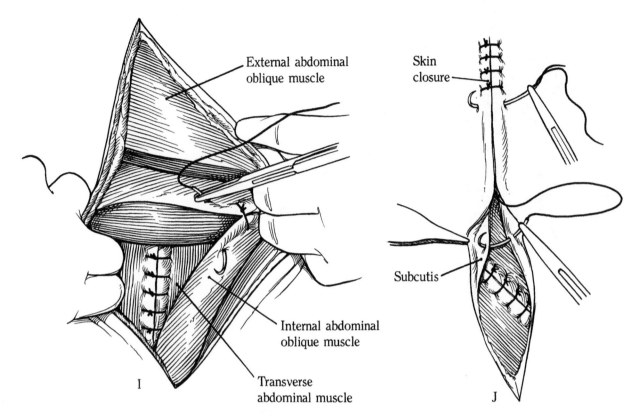

Fig. 12.3. *Continued.*

cranioventrad. This layer is split to reveal the transverse abdominal muscle deeply (Figure 12.3*F*). A vertical split is made in the layer. (The line of cleavage is indicated in Figure 12.3*F*.) For this layer, the muscle should be tented with thumb forceps and nicked with scissors. The opening is enlarged to reveal retroperitoneal adipose tissue (Figure 12.3*G*), and the peritoneum is opened to expose the viscera (Figure 12.3*H*).

The surgeon should then don a sterile plastic sleeve to explore the peritoneal cavity. It is possible to exteriorize the small intestine, small colon, and pelvic flexure of the large colon. In addition, it is feasible to palpate the spleen, kidney(s), liver, stomach, cecum, large colon, cranial mesenteric artery, rectum, pelvic inlet, bladder, aorta, and reproductive tract. The peritoneal surface is also examined.

The flank incision is closed in five layers. The peritoneum and transverse abdominal muscle are closed with simple interrupted sutures of no. 2-0 synthetic absorbable material. The internal abdominal oblique muscle is apposed with four or five simple interrupted or simple continuous sutures of no. 0 synthetic absorbable material (Figure 12.3*I*). A negative suction drain may be placed between the internal and external abdominal oblique muscles, and the last layer is closed with no. 0 or no. 1 synthetic absorbable material in a simple continuous pattern. Care is taken to ensure firm apposition of the

fascia in the external abdominal oblique muscle. A suction drain, rather than a Penrose drain, is used to prevent seroma formation. However meticulous the closure is, a drain is generally necessary.

The subcutis is closed with a simple continuous pattern using synthetic absorbable sutures. The skin is closed with nonabsorbable sutures in a simple interrupted, simple continuous, or Ford interlocking pattern (Figure 12.3*J*).

Postoperative Management

Whether antibiotics are used and which type of antibiotics are used depend on the individual case. The negative suction syringe is taped over the patient's back and is emptied regularly. The drain is removed when the volume of aspirated contents decreases (2–3 days). The skin sutures are removed in 12–14 days.

Complications and Prognosis

Complications are similar to those described in the ventral paramedian approach. The major advantage to this approach for laparotomy is that it can be performed in a standing position. This may improve prognosis by decreasing contamination and avoiding the risks associated with general anesthesia.

Umbilical Herniorrhaphy in the Foal

Relevant Anatomy

There is no further anatomy to discuss relevant to this section.

Indications

Umbilical hernias may be congenital or acquired and are seen in foals, calves, and pigs. Many small umbilical hernias may appear to resolve spontaneously, but large or strangulated umbilical hernias require surgical correction. Various methods are described in the literature for treatment of umbilical hernia—counterirritation, clamping, transfixation sutures, and even safety pins and commercially available rubber bands. The most popular of these techniques is the wooden or metal clamp technique. (The clamps are illustrated in the discussion of instruments used in large animal practice in Chapter 3, "Surgical Instruments".) This method may result in infection, loss of clamps, or premature necrosis of the hernial sac. The last complication can lead to an open wound and, possibly, evisceration or formation of an enterocutaneous fistula. These methods are obviously unsuitable for the occasional strangulated hernia.

Ideally, surgery should be performed after one is sure that apparent external resolution is not going to occur and before the animal is too big. (A typical hernia is represented in Figure 12.4A.) Generally, the hernial sac is lined with peritoneum and contains some bowel (usually jejunum or ileum) or omentum. Another factor that the surgeon should always consider is possible heritability of hernias.

If the patient has large defects in the body wall or incisional hernias from previous abdominal surgery, it may be a candidate for the insertion of a prosthetic mesh. This technique is not covered in this book.

The incidence of incarceration of an umbilical hernia in foals is low; and signs include increased swelling of the hernia, which becomes firm and warm, and a plaque of edema surrounding the hernia sac. Colic is an inconsistent sign of hernial strangulation. Incarceration of only a portion of the intestinal wall (Richter's hernia) does not produce a complete obstruction of the lumen, but a Richter's hernia may progress to an enterocutaneous fistula.[20] When entire portions of the intestine are incarcerated, resection and anastomosis of the intestine may be required unless color and motility improve when the segment is freed.

The operation described here is also suitable for umbilical hernia repair in calves and pigs. Hernias in calves and pigs can be large and may be complicated by abscess formation. In such cases, pre- and postoperative antibiotics are indicated. It is also wise to resolve the abscess before attempting repair, especially if the abscess is large. If an abscess is present, the use of braided, synthetic nonabsorbable material should be avoided. For umbilical hernia repair in male pigs, the incision should avoid the preputial diverticulum and prepuce.

Anesthesia and Surgical Preparation

Inhalation anesthesia is preferable. Anesthesia in small foals can generally be induced with halothane administered by mask. Anesthesia in yearlings is induced intravenously and is maintained with an inhalation anesthetic. The animal is placed in dorsal recumbency and is prepared for aseptic surgery in a routine manner.

Instrumentation

1. General surgery pack

Surgical Technique

A fusiform skin incision, pointed at both ends, is made around the hernial sac (Figure 12.4B). This shape avoids puckering or "dog ears" at the end of the wound at the time of skin closure. The shape of the incision should be such that sufficient skin remains at the wound edges to allow apposition without undue tension. Using either sharp dissection or blunt-tipped scissors, the surgeon dissects the subcutaneous tissue down to the hernial sac and ring (Figure 12.4C). Further sharp dissection around the base of the hernial sac delineates the hernial ring; this dissection should extend around the ring and outward for about 1 cm (Figure 12.4D). When the bowel has been incarcerated in the hernial sac, it is generally necessary to enter the sac carefully to replace the offending piece of bowel into the abdominal cavity. When opening the hernial sac, one must be careful not to cut through any adherent bowel because gross contamination of the surgical site will occur. If the surgeon cannot cut into the hernial sac without incising the bowel, the abdomen should be opened carefully along the linea alba, cranial to the hernial ring. This will allow the surgeon to identify the incarcerated portion of the bowel and to decrease the chance of inadvertent incision of the bowel.[21] There are two options available at this point for closure of the hernia. If the hernial sac has not been opened, a closed herniorrhaphy can be performed.

To perform a closed herniorrhaphy, often the hernial sac and ring have been freed of fascia, the sac is inverted into the abdomen, and the hernial ring is closed with a simple continuous pattern using a no. 1 or no. 2 synthetic absorbable suture material. It is preferable that an open approach is used. In this technique, the hernial ring is sharply dissected and the entire hernial sac is removed (Figure 12.4E). The edges are then opposed using a simple continuous suture pattern with no. 1 or no. 2 synthetic absorbable suture material such as polyglyconate of polysorb (Figure 12.4F).

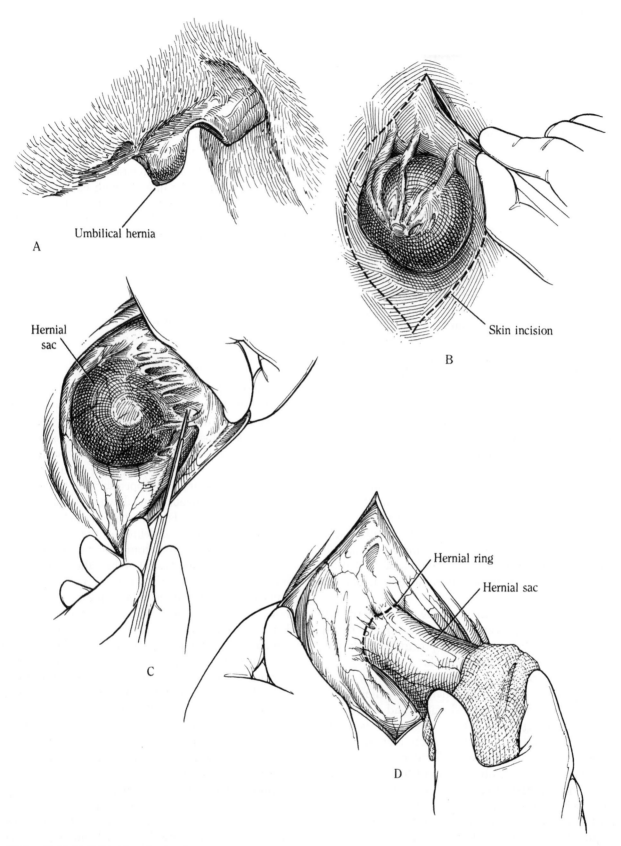

A
Umbilical hernia

B
Skin incision

C
Hernial sac

D
Hernial ring
Hernial sac

Fig. 12.4. **A–H.** Umbilical herniorrhaphy.

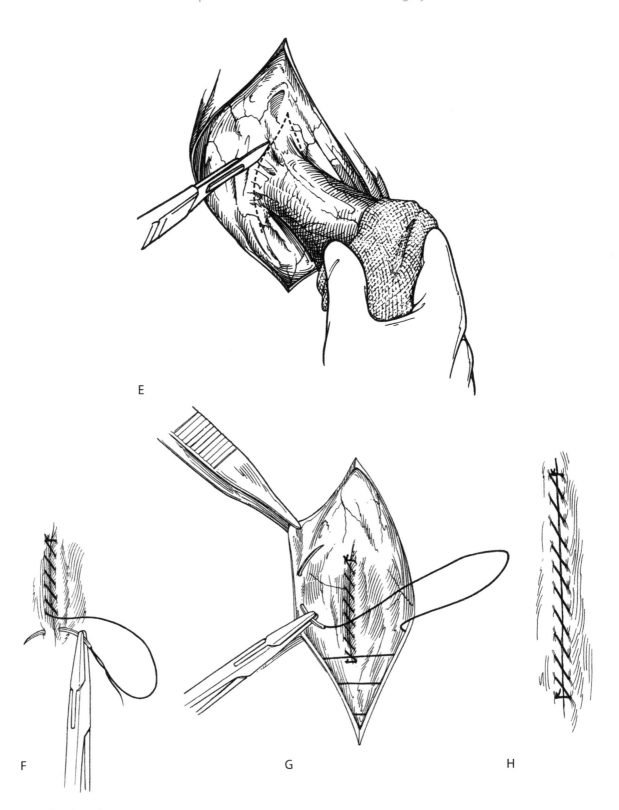

E

F   G   H

Fig. 12.4. *Continued.*

The subcutaneous tissue is closed using a simple continuous subcutaneous suture using no. 2-0 synthetic absorbable material (Figure 12.4G). Skin closure is performed with a nonabsorbable material of the surgeon's choice in either a continuous interrupted or intradermal pattern (Figure 12.4H).

Postoperative Management

The decision to use antibiotics is left to the discretion of the surgeon. If the surgery is performed under aseptic conditions, antibiotics generally are not required. Preoperative antibiotics are also indicated if strangulation is suspected or if an enterocutaneous fistula has developed. Postoperative exercise seems to minimize swelling at the surgical site. Generally, a plaque of edema appears on the second or third postoperative day and persists for 2–3 weeks. Sutures are removed 10–14 days postoperatively. Some surgeons prefer trusses or belly bands to aid in the reduction of edema.

Complications and Prognosis

Complications associated with umbilical hernias in horses vary between 8.8%[2] and 19% in foals that received herniorrhaphy.[21,22] Of these foals, short-term complications included pneumonia in one foal and mild edema adjacent to the incision in two foals. No long-term complications occurred, and all owners were satisfied with the cosmetic results. The prognosis for this procedure is good.

References

1. Pence, P. Equine Dentistry. Baltimore, MD, Lippincott Williams & Wilkins, 2002.
2. Tremaine, W.H., and Lane, J.G. Exodontia. *In* Equine Dentistry. 2nd Ed. Edited by G.J. Baker, J. Easely. Edinburgh, Saunders, 2005, pp. 267–279.
3. McIlwraith, C.W., and Robertson, J.T. McIlwraith & Turner's Equine Surgery: Advanced Techniques. 2nd Ed. Baltimore, MD, Williams & Wilkins, 1998.
4. Dixon, P.M., Tremaine, W.H., Pickles, K., Kuhns, L., Hawe, C., McCann, J., McGorum, B.C., Railton, D.I., and Brammer, S. Equine dental disease. Part 4: A long term study of 400 cases: Apical infections of cheek teeth. *Equine Vet. J.*, 32:182–194, 2000.
5. Dixon, P.M., and Dacre, I. A review of equine dental disorders. *Vet. J.*, 169:165–187, 2005.
6. Coomer, R.P., Fowke, G.S., and McKane, S. Repulsion of maxillary and mandibular cheek teeth in standing horses. *Vet. Surg.*, 40:590–595, 2011.
7. Anderson, S.L., Vacek, J.R., Macharg, M.A., and Holtkamp, D.J. Occurrence of incisional complications and associated risk factors using a right ventral paramedian celiotomy incision in 159 horses. *Vet. Surg.*, 40:82–89, 2011.
8. Trostle, S.S., Wilson, D.G., Stone, W.C., and Markel, M.D. A study of the biomechanical properties of the adult equine linea alba: Relationship of tissue bite size and suture material to breaking strength. *Vet. Surg.*, 23:435–441, 1994.
9. Kelmer, G. Update on recent advances in equine abdominal surgery. *Vet. Clin. North Am. Equine Pract.*, 25:271–282, 2009.
10. Wilson, D.A., Baker, G.J., and Boero, M.J.: Complications of celiotomy incisions in horses. *Vet. Surg.*, 24:506–514, 1995.
11. Wilson, D.A., Badertscher, R.R., Boero, M.J., Baker, G.J., and Foreman, J.H. Ultrasonographic evaluation of the healing of ventral midline abdominal incisions in the horse. *Equine Vet. J. Suppl.*, 7:107–110, 1989.
12. Coomer, R.P., Mair, T.S., Edwards, G.B., and Proudman, C.J. Do subcutaneous sutures increase risk of laparotomy wound suppuration? *Equine Vet. J.*, 39:396–399, 2007.
13. Bischofberger, A.S., Brauer, T., Gugelchuck, G., and Klohnen, A. Difference in incisional complications following exploratory celiotomies using antibacterial-coated suture material for subcutaneous closure: Prospective randomized study in 100 horses. *Equine Vet. J.*, 42:304–309, 2010.
14. Davis, W., Fogle, C.A., Gerard, M.P., Levine, J.F., and Blikslager, A.T. Return to use and performance following exploratory celiotomy for colic in horses: 195 cases (2003–3010). *Equine Vet. J.*, 45:224–229, Aug 1 Epub. 2013.
15. Mair, T.S., Pearson, G.R., and Scase, T.J. Multiple small intestinal pseudodiverticula associated with lymphoma in three horses. *Equine Vet. J. Suppl.*, 39:128–132, 2011.
16. Mair, T.S., and Sherlock, C.E. Surgical drainage and post operative lavage of large abdominal abscesses in six mature horses. *Equine Vet. J. Suppl.*, 39:123–127, 2011.
17. Carnevale, E.M., Squires, E.L., Maclellan, L.J., Alvarenga, M.A., and Scott, T.J. Use of oocyte transfer in a commercial breeding program for mares with reproductive abnormalities. *J. Am. Vet. Med. Assoc.*, 218:87–91, 2001.
18. Pascoe, J.R., Meagher, D.M., and Wheat, J.D. Surgical management of uterine torsion in the mare: A review of 26 cases. *J. Am. Vet. Med. Assoc.*, 179:351, 1981.
19. Hendrickson, D.A. A review of Equine Laparoscopy. ISRN Veterinary Science, vol. 2012, Article ID 492650, 17 pages, 2012.
20. Markel, M.D., Pascoe, J.R., and Sams, E.A. Strangulated umbilical hernias in horses: 13 cases (1974–1985). *J. Am. Vet. Med. Assoc.*, 190(692):1987.
21. Freeman, D.E., Orisini, J.A., Harrison, I.W., Muller, N.S., and Leitch, M. Complications of umbilical hernias in horses: 13 cases (1972–1986). *J. Am. Vet. Med. Assoc.*, 192:804–807, 1988.
22. Riley, C.B., Cruz, A.M., Bailey, J.V., Barber, S.M., and Fretz, P.B. Comparison of herniorrhaphy versus clamping of umbilical hernias in horses: A retrospective study of 93 cases (1982–1994). *Can. Vet. J.*, 37:295–298, 1996.

Chapter 13

BOVINE GASTROINTESTINAL SURGERY

A. N. Baird, DVM, MS, DACVS

Principles of Laparotomy

Laparotomy is commonly performed either for exploratory purposes when a clinical diagnosis is still uncertain or for a specific purpose when a clinical diagnosis has already been made. Flank laparotomy performed on the standing animal under local anesthesia is the most common technique. Flank laparotomy through the left paralumbar fossa is commonly used for exploratory laparotomy if a problem is suspected on the left side, and the procedure is specifically indicated for left-sided abomasopexy, rumenotomy, or cesarean section. The right paralumbar approach is used for exploratory laparotomy if a problem is suspected on the right side, and it is specifically indicated for surgical conditions of the abomasum, including right-sided pyloro-omentopexy or abomasopexy, small intestine, cecum, and colon. The right paralumbar approach will provide the best access to the abdomen and the most complete exploratory in the adult ruminant. A right-flank approach may also be used for cesarean section when ruminal distention or right-sided positioning of the fetus causes the surgeon to consider the right side a superior approach to the left side. Although flank laparotomy is generally performed on the standing animal, general anesthesia may be indicated when surgery is to be performed through the right flank for a small intestinal or colonic problem because the pain and shock associated with tension on the mesentery during surgery may cause the animal to go down during the procedure. Small intestinal surgery can be done in many cases via the standing flank if one is careful to minimize tension on the mesentery. When environmental or economic situations do not allow general anesthesia it is worth performing such procedures standing after informing the client of potential complications rather than destroying the animal. There are few advantages, if any, to a recumbent flank approach with local anesthesia only.

Laparotomy via a ventral midline or paramedian approach is an alternative that necessitates the animal being cast and/or sedated and placed in dorsal recumbency. The two main indications for these techniques are for right paramedian abomasopexy and ventral midline cesarean section, in which it offers advantages in the delivery of oversized or emphysematous fetuses and in complicated deliveries, including uterine tears. Another advantage of ventral midline laparotomy is less-visible postoperative scarring in feedlot heifers. This approach

Turner and McIlwraith's Techniques in Large Animal Surgery, 4th Edition. Dean A. Hendrickson and A. N. (Nickie) Baird.
© 2013 John Wiley & Sons, Inc. Published 2013 by John Wiley & Sons, Inc.

may also be useful for cesarean section in heifers that have a relatively small paralumbar fossa. The paramedian incision is parallel to the midline, between the midline and the subcutaneous abdominal vein. The incision for paramedian abomasopexy extends from the umbilicus craniad to the xiphoid process, as illustrated later in this chapter. The incision for ventral midline cesarean section extends from the umbilicus caudad to the udder and is illustrated in Chapter 14.

A third, less common laparotomy approach is the ventrolateral oblique incision, which may be performed on the right or left side and may also be indicated for cesarean section. As with the ventral midline approach, fetal and uterine debris can be removed more efficiently, with less potential contamination of the peritoneum than with a flank approach. The ventrolateral oblique incision is considered advantageous to the ventral midline incision in the high-producing dairy cow with a large udder and subcutaneous abdominal veins that have the potential for severe hemorrhage.[1] The technique may be performed conveniently with the cow in lateral recumbency. However, the closure of this laparotomy incision is more difficult than other techniques.

Flank Laparotomy and Abdominal Exploration

Relevant Anatomy

In the ruminant, the most cranial forestomach, the reticulum, lies just caudal to the diaphragm and to the left of the midline, beneath the 6th through 8th ribs.[2,3] The space left of the median, from approximately the 7th or 8th rib to the pelvis, is occupied by the rumen. On the right side of the ruminant lie the omasum and the elongated true stomach, the abomasum. The omasum lies near the ventral aspect of the 7th to the 11th ribs, and the abomasum extends from the xiphoid region to the 9th or 10th rib, occupying primarily the right side except for the fundus, which deviates to the ventral aspect of the rumen atrium.[2,3]

Autonomic innervation of these structures is accomplished by a balance of both sympathetic and parasympathetic nervous inputs, supplied by the splanchnic nerves and the dorsal and ventral vagal trunks, respectively.

Indications

The following are indications for left-flank laparotomy: general exploratory laparotomy, particularly if a problem amenable to treatment from the left side is suspected; rumentomy; left-flank abomasopexy; and cesarean section when the viable fetus is only moderately oversized and the cow is capable of enduring the surgery in the standing position. The major advantage to the left-flank approach is that the bulk and position of the rumen generally precludes the risk of intestinal evisceration.

Right-flank laparotomy is indicated in the following instances: exploratory laparotomy when a problem amenable to treatment from the right side is suspected; omentopexy or pyloro-omentopexy; surgical correction of small intestinal, cecal, and colonic conditions; and cesarean section when, because of rumenal distention or fetal positioning, removal of the calf by a left-flank approach would be difficult or when hydrops amnii or allantois is present. Right-flank laparotomy is also chosen when the problem is unknown and a full exploratory is needed.

Anesthesia and Surgical Preparation

Typically, this surgical procedure is performed with the animal standing, and anesthesia is provided by a line block, an inverted L block, or a paravertebral block. Refer to Chapter 2 for these techniques. For surgery of the small or large intestinal tract, pain and shock associated with both the condition itself and the tension on the mesentery created by surgical manipulation may cause the animal to go down during surgery, with obvious compromise to aseptic technique. In such patients, general or high-epidural anesthesia may be used. However, small intestinal procedures can be performed with care in the standing animal.

The surgical area is clipped and is prepared for aseptic surgery in a routine manner. Any bars on the stocks adjacent to the operative field are draped.

Instrumentation

1. General surgery pack

Surgical Technique

The site of the incision for left-flank laparotomy is illustrated in Figure 13.1A. A vertical incision is made in the middle of the paralumbar fossa extending from 3 to 5 cm ventral to the transverse processes of the lumbar vertebrae for a distance of 20 to 25 cm. For rumenotomy in a large cow, it may be advantageous to make the incision cranial to the midway point. For cesarean section, the incision may begin 10 cm ventral to the transverse processes and may extend 30–40 cm.

To incise the skin, reasonable pressure should be exerted on the scalpel to ensure complete penetration. This incision is continued ventrad, so the skin is opened in one smooth motion. Separation of the skin and subcutaneous tissue reveals fibers of the external abdominal oblique muscle and fascia (Figure 13.1B). This layer is incised vertically to reveal the internal abdominal oblique muscle (Figure 13.1C). A similar incision through the internal abdominal oblique muscle reveals the glistening aponeurosis of the transverse abdominal muscle (Figure 13.1D). Then the muscle is picked up with tissue forceps and is nicked with a scalpel in the dorsal part of the incision to avoid cutting the rumen. The incision through the

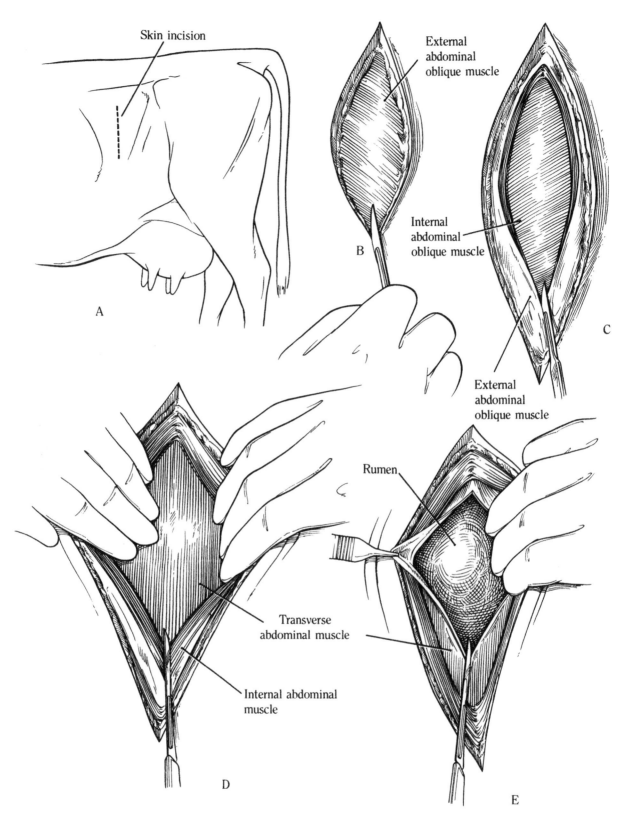

Fig. 13.1. **A–H.** Flank laparotomy and abdominal exploration.

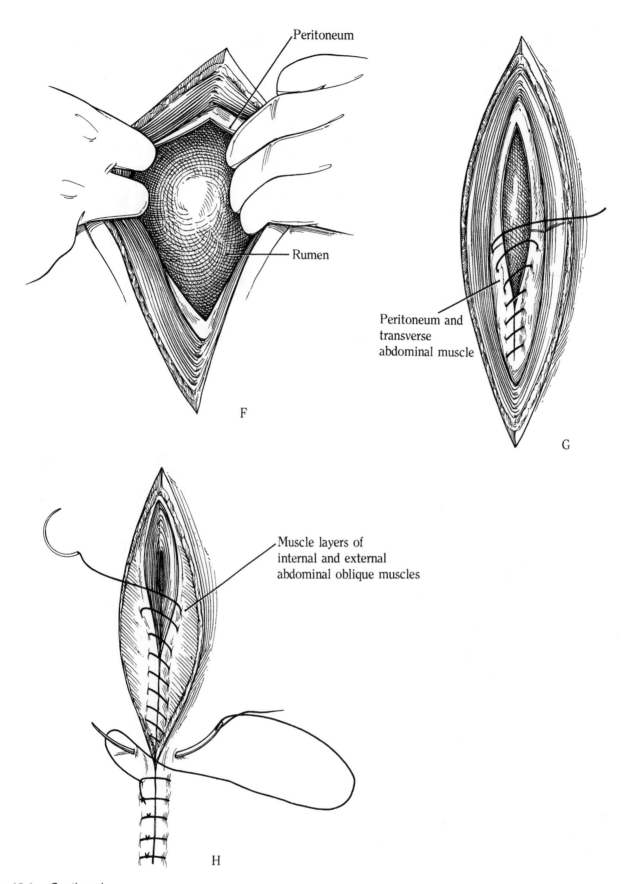

Peritoneum

Rumen

F

Peritoneum and
transverse
abdominal muscle

G

Muscle layers of
internal and external
abdominal oblique muscles

H

Fig. 13.1. *Continued.*

transverse abdominal muscle and peritoneum may be extended with scissors or a scalpel for entrance into the peritoneal cavity (Figure 13.1*E*).

A thorough, systematic examination of the abdomen should always be carried out before specific surgical manipulation is performed on a viscus. Unless a left displacement of the abomasum is present, the rumen will be visible following completion of the left-flank laparotomy incision, and the color of its serosa may be noted (Figure 13.1*F*). The rumen is palpated to determine the nature of its contents. The left kidney is pendulous and also can be palpated straight in from the incision if the rumen is empty. If the rumen is full, the kidney is located by passing a hand around caudal to the dorsal sac of the rumen. Passing a hand forward on the left side of the rumen, the spleen, reticulum, and diaphragmatic area may be palpated, and the presence of adhesions or abscesses in this area may be ascertained. Moving behind the rumen over to the right side, the viscera within the omental bursa are palpated. Further forward on the right side, it is possible to palpate the caudate lobe of the liver and the gallbladder. The pelvic region, including the uterus (in a cow) and bladder, should also be palpated. It is questionable whether routine palpation of the ovaries and fimbriae of the uterine tubes is appropriate in the cow, especially if peritonitis is present in the abdomen. It is possible that local infection and adhesions could result in problems with reproduction. Following this exploration, any specific procedures indicated, such as rumenotomy or abomasopexy, are performed.

Abdominal exploration may be similarly performed through a right-flank incision. If the viscera are in normal position, the duodenum will be encountered running horizontally across the dorsal part of the incision with the mesoduodenum dorsal and the greater omentum ventral. The pylorus and abomasum can be palpated ventrally. The greater omentum may be reflected craniad to allow examination of the jejunum, ileum, cecum, and colon. The kidneys and pelvic region can also be palpated at this stage. The rumen can be palpated as well as part of the reticulum and diaphragm feeling for adhesions between the two. The omasum, liver (the right-flank approach allows complete palpation of this organ), gallbladder, and diaphragm can be palpated cranially on the right side. The anatomic peculiarities with abomasal displacements are discussed in the sections of this chapter on abomasopexy and omentopexy.

Routinely, a flank laparotomy incision is closed in three layers. The peritoneum and transverse abdominal muscles are closed together with a simple continuous suture pattern using no. 0 or no. 1 synthetic absorbable suture (Figure 13.1*G*). Placing this suture layer in a ventral-to-dorsal direction is helpful to maintain the viscera within the incision, particularly on the right side. The internal and external abdominal oblique muscles may be closed with a second simple continuous layer using no. 1 synthetic absorbable suture (Figure 13.1*H*). This suture line

is anchored to the deeper transversus muscle at various intervals to obliterate dead space. It is also desirable to take even bites on either side with the muscle closures, so the muscles will come together without a defect and without wrinkling. If the external and internal abdominal oblique muscle layers are substantial in a large cow, closure should be performed in separate layers. Generally, skin closure is performed with a continuous Ford interlocking pattern using heavy polymerized caprolactam (Vetafil™) (Figure 13.1*H*). At the surgeon's option, 2–3 simple interrupted sutures may be placed in the ventral aspect of the incision (Figure 13.1*H*). This measure allows easy drainage if infection develops in the incision. Such an event is possible in the compromised conditions under which this surgical procedure may have to be performed. If the skin incision has been obviously contaminated, as by the delivery of an emphysematous fetus, an interrupted suture pattern may be more appropriate.

Postoperative Management

Antibiotics are administered, if indicated, depending on the procedure. Supportive management is also instituted in accordance with the animal's condition. Sutures may be removed 2–3 weeks after surgery. At 10–14 days, the incision is still vulnerable to trauma; and in cattle housed together, a popped incision may occur if sutures are removed at this time.

Complications and Prognosis

Complications such as peritonitis and adhesions may arise following abdominal exploration. Cattle in particular may be more prone to incisional dehiscence and wound infection when housed together. The incidence of incisional infection can be greatly reduced when antibiotics are given preoperatively.

Rumenotomy

Relevant Anatomy

The rumen and reticulum accommodate most of the microbial fermentation during digestion. They are divided from each other by the same mechanism that the rumen itself is partitioned, by the internal pillae formed by internal projections of the rumenal wall.[4] Externally, the pillae appear as grooves. The ruminoreticular fold demarcates the rumen from the reticulum. The rumen itself is divided into dorsal and ventral sacs by the ruminal pillars, and cranial and caudal blind sacs by the coronary pillars. A cranial pillar further divides the dorsal sac into a ruminal atrium, which is most closely associated with the reticulum.[4] The reticular-omasal and esophageal orifices are located in the reticular groove, which runs down the right internal surface of the reticulum from the cardia to the fundus.

The mucosal lining of the reticulum is characterized by honeycomb shaped ridges that house a collection of short papillae.[4] This honeycombed appearance subsides at the ruminoreticular fold as it merges into the papillated mucosa of the rumen. These projections are associated with a subepithelial capillary plexus that facilitates the absorption of the volatile fatty acid by-products of microbial fermentation.[4]

Indications

Rumenotomy is indicated for the removal of metallic foreign bodies, whose presence may cause traumatic reticulitis or traumatic reticuloperitonitis, materials such as baling twine or plastic bags that are obstructing the reticulo-omasal orifice, and foreign bodies lodged in the distal esophagus or over the base of the heart.

Rumenotomy is also indicated for evacuation of rumen contents in selected cases of rumen overload or following ingestion of toxic plants, spoiled roughages, or chemicals.[3] Finely ground feedstuffs readily pass into the omasal–abomasal region, but coarser, more fibrous material remains in the rumen for longer periods. Other indications for rumenotomy include rumen impaction and impaction and atony of the omasum or abomasum.[2]

There are several techniques described for performing a rumenotomy including suturing the rumen to the skin prior to rumenotomy (described here), the use of fixation devices such as Weingarth's ring, the use of stay sutures, or the use of towel clamps to fix the rumen to the skin.[3] Although more time consuming than the alternatives, suturing the rumen to the skin prior to rumenotomy provides the most secure seal between rumen and skin, is not easily displaced (as are the fixation devices), and has been shown to result in fewer postoperative complications.[3]

Anesthesia and Surgical Preparation

The left-flank area is prepared for aseptic surgery in a routine manner, and local anesthesia is instituted by line block, inverted L block, or paravertebral block.

Instrumentation

1. General surgery pack
2. Kingman tube to drain fluid from the rumen
3. Rumenotomy board or fixation ring if the rumen is not sutured to the skin as described here

Surgical Technique

Rumenotomy is performed through a left paralumbar incision (a 20-cm incision generally is sufficient) with the animal standing. The technique for left-flank laparotomy has been described previously. In large cows, the flank incisions for rumenotomies sometimes are made just caudal and parallel to the last rib, to place the incision closer to the reticulum. It is essential, however, to leave sufficient tissue caudal to the last rib for suturing. (The incision should be approximately 5 cm [2 inches] caudal to the last rib.)

Following opening and systematic exploration of the peritoneal cavity (no attempt is made to break down firm adhesions in the region of the reticulum), it is necessary to anchor the rumen to the incision to avoid contamination of the abdominal musculature and peritoneum during the rumenotomy procedure. A technique for suturing the rumen to the skin prior to rumenotomy is illustrated in Figure 13-2A–D. A continuous inverting suture pattern (similar to a Cushing pattern) is used, to pull the rumen over the edge of the skin incision (Figure 13-2A,B). This suture should be of heavy-gauge material such as nylon or polypropolene (Surgipro, Prolene). Two large, inverting sutures are placed at the ventral aspect of the incision so that the rumen projects well over the skin edge. This avoids contamination in the ventral region (Figure 13.2C). Alternate techniques for isolating the rumen and preventing contamination include the use of stay sutures, a rubber rumenotomy shroud, a fixation ring (Weingart's),[5] or a rumenotomy board. These alternatives are quicker than suturing the rumen, but they are also more easily displaced; the consequent contamination may be disastrous.

The rumen is incised with a scalpel taking care to leave enough room dorsally and ventrally for closure at the end of the procedure (Figure 13.2D); and the operator, wearing long rubber gloves, evacuates and explores the rumen (Figure 13.2E). A rumen shroud or a wound edge protector (3M™ Steri-Drape™) may be placed in the incision to prevent ingesta from accumulating at the incisional site and compromising wound healing.[6,7] The inside of the rumen and the reticulum are explored; and, if a foreign body is present, it is removed. A large bore stomach tube, such as a Kingman tube, may be used to siphon out liquid contents.

To reach the reticulum from the rumenotomy incision, the dorsal wall of the rumen (where a natural air pocket exists) should be followed until it becomes the ventral wall, at which point one is in the reticulum. Following a direct line from the incision, one encounters ingesta as well as the cranial pillar of the rumen and ruminoreticular fold. To help locate foreign bodies, the reticulum can be gently picked up with the hand. The area where the foreign body is located usually has extended adhesions and cannot be picked up. This is an ideal area to look for foreign bodies by carefully palpating each "honeycomb" of the reticulum, as all but the slightest remnant of a linear metal foreign body may already have exited through the wall of the reticulum. Moreover, while exploring the inside of the reticulum, one should also feel for abscesses. Abscesses are frequently found on the medial wall of the

Fig. 13.2. A–F. Rumenotomy.

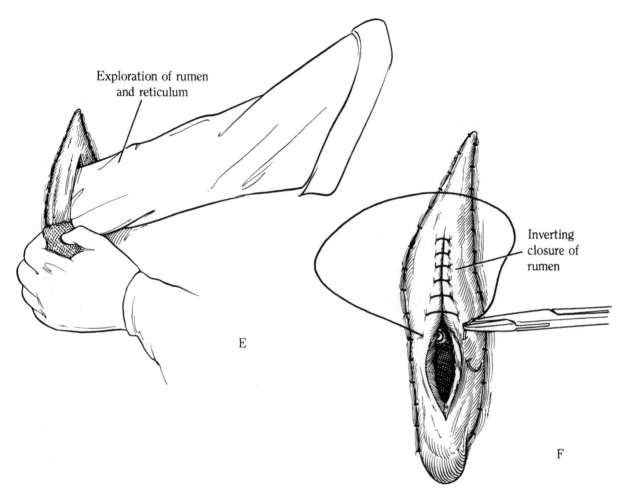

Exploration of rumen
and reticulum

E

Inverting
closure of
rumen

F

Fig. 13.2. *Continued.*

reticulum near the reticulo-omasal orifice. If abscesses are found, they should be evaluated. If the cow's economic value justifies the surgeon to proceed, abscesses that adhere to the reticulum should be lanced or drained. This is best accomplished by carrying a scalpel or scalpel blade, attached to a piece of string or umbilical tape in case it is dropped, into the reticulum and lancing the abscess into the reticulum through the adhesion. Following this exploration, the reticulum may be swept with a magnet to pick up additional metallic debris. A magnet is placed (or replaced) in the reticulum, and fresh rumen contents (if available) are placed in the rumen. Alkalinizing products may be inserted at this stage in cases of rumen overload, and mineral oil may also be instilled when indicated. The surgeon's contaminated gloves are then discarded.

The rumen incision is closed with a simple continuous pattern using of no. 1 or no. 2 synthetic absorbable material (Figure 13.2F). A single layer can be adequate,[5] but a double row is generally used with the second row an inverting pattern with similar suture material. The surgical site is thoroughly irrigated with polyionic fluid after closure of the lumen and any contaminated gloves, gowns, or drapes should be replaced prior to removal of the rumen-fixation suture and second layer closure. No

further exploration of the abdominal cavity should be done after closure of the rumen. Closure of the laparotomy incision has been described previously.

Postoperative Management

Postoperative medication varies with the indication for the rumenotomy. Although rumen overload often requires intensive fluid therapy, traumatic reticulitis requires little intensive care. Antibiotics are indicated following the removal of foreign bodies from the reticulum. Oral fluids can be administered following rumenotomy; and mild osmotic laxatives, such as magnesium hydroxide, often promote gut motility.

Complications and Prognosis

Potentially fatal peritoneal contamination may occur if a fluid-tight seal is not created between the rumen and abdominal wall. This can be avoided by thoroughly palpating between suture bites for any gaps large enough to fit an index finger through.[7] These gaps should be eliminated by additional sutures. Incisional swelling and infection may also occur.[6] Peritonitis is also likely if one performs exploration of the abdominal cavity after closure of the rumen, no matter how clean you believe the site to be.

Prognosis depends on the diagnosis of disease and the location and extent of perforations, if any, in the reticulum. Cases of traumatic reticuloperitonitis involving a perforation of the diaphragm have a very poor prognosis due to the risk of developing myocarditis, septic pericarditis, and thoracic abscesses.[6] Perforations on the right wall of the reticulum also carry a guarded prognosis due to their tendency to involve adhesions along the ventral branch of the vagus nerve, which may result in vagal syndrome.[6] Surgical treatment of perireticular abscesses secondary to traumatic reticuloperitonitis appears to be favorable in the literature.[6]

Rumenostomy (Rumenal Fistulation)

Relevant Anatomy

Anatomy relevant to this procedure is discussed in previous sections.

Indications

The techniques of rumenal fistulation have been developed for experimental purposes, as well as for the relief of chronic bloat. The experimental techniques use various types of cannulas to maintain a permanent opening, which allows direct treatment and sampling of the rumen. The therapeutic technique provides temporary, symptomatic relief of chronic bloat. Chronic bloating results from abnormal function of the parasympathetic nerve supply to the cardia of the stomach and dorsal sac of the rumen. This situation can result from reticuloperitonitis or fibrinous pneumonia-pleuritis involving the vagus nerve. Bloat may also develop secondary to enlarged lymph nodes or liver abscess. Bloat is also observed occasionally in nursing cows and is thought to be associated with disturbed rumen metabolism. Another cause of bloat, especially in feedlot cattle, is altered rumen flora secondary to a rapid change from one feed to another. We will describe both the therapeutic rumenostomy used to treat animals with chronic bloat and the permanent rumenostomy used for nutritional research or for ease of rumen fluid collection for transfaunation into ruminants with disturbed rumen flora.

Anesthesia and Surgical Preparation

This surgical procedure is performed with the animal standing. If rumenal tympany is present, it is relieved by a stomach tube. This measure will facilitate exteriorization of the rumen later. The left paralumbar fossa area is prepared surgically in a routine manner. A circular area immediately ventral to the transverse processes of the lumbar vertebrae and approximately 10 cm in diameter is infiltrated with local anesthetic.

Instrumentation

1. General surgery pack
2. Permanent fistula device

Surgical Technique for Therapeutic Rumenostomy

A circular piece of skin, approximately 4 cm in diameter, is removed to expose the underlying abdominal musculature (Figure 13.3A). The abdominal muscles and peritoneum are bluntly dissected to expose the rumen. It may be necessary to remove some of the external abdominal oblique muscle if it is thick and limits exposure of the rumen. The wall of the rumen is then grasped with forceps, and a portion of it is pulled through to the exterior. In this fashion, a "cone" of rumen is brought to the skin surface, where it is anchored to the skin with four horizontal mattress sutures of polymerized caprolactam or nylon (Figure 13.3B). These mattress sutures pass through rumen and skin. The central portion of the exposed rumen is removed (Figure 13.3B), and the incised edge of the rumen is sutured to the skin with simple interrupted sutures of nonabsorbable material (Figure 13.3C,D). The rumenal fistula that results from this procedure should be no larger than 2–3 cm in diameter. The muscle layers perform a valve-like function and help to control seepage of rumenal ingesta while relieving gas accumulation in the rumen.

Postoperative Management for Therapeutic Rumenostomy

When surgery is performed properly, antibiotics need not be administered and aftercare is not usually indicated. Many animals with chronic bloat fail to recover normal eructation, so the fistula should be permanent. If the fistula is made with the dimensions we have described, it should remain patent for a sufficient time. A smaller fistula will close earlier. With the valve-like function of the muscle layers, the fistula generally stays open as long as gas is expelled from it. However, it usually closes once the animal regains normal eructation.

Surgical Technique for Permanent Rumenostomy

A circular piece of skin 3 inches in diameter is excised. Then elliptical sections of the external abdominal oblique and internal abdominal oblique muscles are made independently in the direction of the muscle fibers approximately 3 inches long and 2 inches wide. The transverse abdominal muscle and peritoneum are incised in the

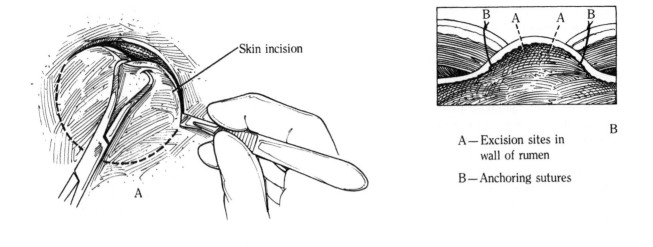

A — Excision sites in
wall of rumen

B — Anchoring sutures

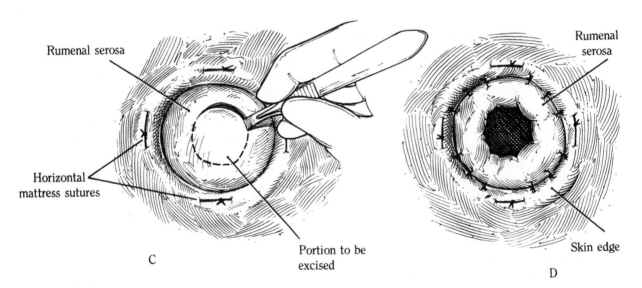

Fig. 13.3.   **A–D.** Rumenostomy.

direction of the muscle fibers. At this point the muscular body wall should easily dilate to the size of the initial skin incision. The rumen can then be grasped and pulled out of the skin incision to make a cone as described in the therapeutic rumenostomy only larger. The rumen is then secured to the skin using no. 3 polymerized caprolactam in an interrupted horizontal mattress pattern. The first 4 sutures are placed equidistant around the incision. Then others are placed until there is a fluid-tight seal between the rumen and skin as judged by the inability to easily place the tip of an instrument such as large needle holders between sutures. The rumen is then incised leaving a margin approximately 1 cm wide from the mattress sutures. The rumen incision is made from the 7 o'clock position dorsally and around to the 5 o'clock position. The ventralmost area is not incised so as to leave an island

of rumen wall still attached ventrally. The flap of rumen wall is then reflected ventrally and sutured to the skin with 2 or 3 simple interrupted sutures to create a "splashboard" effect protecting the ventralmost aspect of the rumen-to-skin suture. The commercially available 3-inch cannula is then inserted into the created rumenostomy.

Postoperative Management for Permanent Rumenostomy

The skin ventral to the ostomy is cleaned and coated with petroleum jelly to lessen scalding of the skin from leakage of ingesta. The ring of skin and rumen wall on the interior of the ring of mattress sutures will slough in 2 to 3 weeks. During this time the rumen wall will adhere to the skin at the site of the suture placement. Occasional cleaning of the site and antibiotics are indicated. One should monitor the cannula periodically over the following months to determine when the stoma has stretched enough to facilitate placement of a 4-inch cannula.

Complications and Prognosis

Ruminal fistulation has not been shown to cause permanent effects on heart rate, respiratory rate, or EKG patterns. These effects have been temporary in the literature and may last an average of 20 days postoperatively. Temporary side effects include increases in ruminal pH, total volatile fatty acids, propionic acid, valeric acid, respiratory rate, and heart rate.[8] The prognosis for the procedure is good and complications are generally few and mild. Abscesses may occur at or near the incision site.

Surgical Corrections of Abomasal Displacements and Torsion

Relevant Anatomy

In general, the exact position of the abomasum in the living animal depends on the rate and size of contractions of the rumen and reticulum, the fullness of the other stomach compartments, the abomasum's activity, the presence of a pregnant uterus, and the age of the animal.[4] The body of the abomasum lies on the abdominal floor with the cranial aspect of the fundus anchored to the reticulum, atrium, and ventral sac by muscular attachments.[4] The pyloric part of the abomasum transverses the ventral abdomen toward the right body wall.

The lining of the abomasum is comprised of thick folds of glandular mucosa. The mucosa of the body and fundus contains peptic glands while the pyloric part secretes only mucous.[4] At the flexure of the abomasum, the folds diminish to low rugae and a large, highly vascularized, thickening of the wall, called the torus, narrows the pyloric passage.

Indications

Dilation or displacement of the abomasum is considered to be one of the most common surgical conditions in bovine patients. Displacements may occur to the left or right side (LDA or RDA), although most occur to the left side and are more common during the first month after calving in Jersey, Guernsey, and Holstien-Friesan cows.[9-11] There have been cases of abomasal displacement reported in beef cattle.[12] Abomasal displacement is believed to occur secondarily to abnormally high volatile fatty acid levels and excessive fermentation that lead to gas accumulation and distention. As a result of the gas, the abomasum may float up the abdominal wall on either the left or right side. Although less common, right torsion of the abomasum (RTA) may occur to varying

degrees. If the torsion exceeds 180°, it is termed a volvulus. Abomasal volvulus is a serious condition that leads to complete obstruction of the outflow of ingesta to the duodenum. The etiology of RTA is not completely understood, but the condition is thought to occur secondary to some cases of right-sided displacement of the abomasum. Animals with RTA generally have more acute clinical signs. In addition, they may have marked electrolyte changes, particularly in the chloride and potassium levels.[13] The severity of RTA has been classified into four grades, on the basis of the volume of sequestered abomasal fluid. This classification is useful and less subjective than the common clinical means.[13]

There are several surgical techniques described in the literature for correcting abomasal displacements.[14-16] Factors such as economy, cosmetics, surgical environment, number of assistants, and the reproductive stage and systemic condition of the patient affect the decision to choose one technique over another.[17] Both LDA and RDA may be treated with right-flank omentopexy, with or without pyloropexy, and right paramedian abomasopexy.[18,19] In addition, right-flank omentopexy and right paramedian abomasopexy may be used to treat select cases of RTA. Right-flank omentopexy was developed when the only alternative was paramedian abomasopexy, which required the patient to be in dorsal recumbency. In some cows, this position was undesirable, so a surgical procedure that could be performed with the animal standing had obvious advantages. Recumbency should be avoided in animals with compromised systemic conditions, respiratory distress, distended rumens, or those that are pregnant.[18-20] The subsequent development of the flank abomasopexy techniques offered a third alternative.

Right paramedian abomasopexy has several advantages: the abomasum is brought into position more easily in most cases, and instantaneous repositioning commonly occurs; the abomasum is easily viewed for detailed examination and detection of ulcers; and strong, positive, long-lasting adhesions can be anticipated. The main disadvantage of this approach is that it is not performed in standing position like the alternative surgical treatments for abomasal displacements and requires more assistance. Another disadvantage is the possible formation of an abomasal fistula if the retaining suture penetrates the lumen of the abomasum.

Right-flank omentopexy involves suturing the superficial layer of the greater omentum in the region of the pylorus to the abdominal wall in the right flank. There are many modifications practiced to perform pyloropexy. We will describe a technique used for years by the author to secure the pyloric antrum to the body wall cranioventral to the right-flank incision with minimal complications.[15] Some surgeons believe pyloropexy may increase the risk of penetrating the lumen during fixation, however, due to the strong adherence of the submucosa to the mucosa in this region.[20] We will describe the technique to place sutures in the seromuscular layer without penetration or compromise of the lumen.

Right-flank omentopexy has a high reported success rate for the treatment of LDA.[21] A disadvantage to this approach is that the surgeon's access to a left-sided displaced abomasum is more limited than with the ventral paramedian approach. The displacement can be exceedingly difficult to correct if movement of the abomasum is inhibited by focal adhesions from a perforated abomasal ulcer or accumulations of fibrous tissue that may occur secondary to peritonitis.[22] Also, the maintenance of long-term fixation of the abomasum can be questioned, particularly with inexperienced surgeons. Adipose tissue is weak, and the trauma of a cow being knocked down could be sufficient to tear or stretch the omental attachment. The omental attachment may also stretch over time to a length that allows recurrence of left displacement of the abomasum. Right displacement of the abomasum can also occur if the abomasum pivots around an intact omental adhesion.[21]

Left-flank and right-flank abomasopexies are used to correct LDA and RDA, respectively.[9,22] Right-flank abomasopexy may also be used to treat RTA.[23] These techniques have the advantage of offering direct fixation of the abomasum to the ventral body wall and are performed with the animal in the standing position. In addition, adhesions or ulceration of the displaced abomasum can be visualized and treated. One disadvantage of these techniques is that the abomasal anchoring achieved with the flank approaches is not considered as secure as that achieved with the right paramedian technique. Furthermore, the site for abomasal fixation to the body wall can be difficult to reach in large cows or if the surgeon has short arms. Care is necessary to avoid puncturing viscera as the needle is carried to the floor of the abdomen. In some cases, the abomasum may be lying in a cranioventral position and may be difficult to expose sufficiently for placement of the suture.[22] Auscultation during the clinical examination prior to surgery should identify the situation, and another approach may be considered.

Right-flank abomasopexy is generally preferred over a paramedian approach to treat cases of RTA in the severely affected cow. Fluid can be removed from the abomasum more easily through a flank incision, and there is less risk to a patient in a compromised condition if it is operated on in the standing position. However, in cases of severe RTA in which abomasal compromise is suspected, omentopexy should be considered because suture material may pull through the abomasal wall.[24] In animals that survive the surgery, however, this problem has not been observed.[25]

There are several alternative techniques for treatment of LDA that will not be described here. Blind stitch abomasopexy and toggle pin fixation (roll-and-toggle procedure) are two closed surgical techniques that are considered quick and inexpensive for the experienced surgeon.[9,17] However, these techniques require considerable precision and accuracy as the structures to be fixed are not directly visualized. A significant disadvantage to the closed techniques is the inability of the surgeon to assess other possible complications within the abdomen (e.g., adhesions, ulcers, fatty liver). An inexperienced surgeon will most likely find that the closed techniques are just as difficult to master as the open techniques. For this reason, many surgeons opt for an alternative approach through the paralumbar fossa. Right paramedian, left paramedian, and one step laparoscopic approaches to abomasopexy have been described.[26,27] These procedures are described in detail elsewhere.[16,26,27]

Anesthesia and Surgical Preparation

Right-flank omentopexy, right-flank pyloropexy (pyloro-omentopexy), and right- and left-flank abomasopexies are performed with the animal standing. The right or left paralumbar area is clipped and is prepared surgically. Local anesthesia is instituted by performing a paravertebral block, inverted L block, or a line block. If a left-flank abomasopexy is to be performed, an area from the xiphoid process to the umbilicus and from the midline to the right subcutaneous abdominal vein is also prepared surgically. This second area is not anesthetized.

Right paramedian abomasopexy is performed in dorsal recumbency. The cow is sedated (xylazine HCl 15–30 mg IV) and is cast in dorsal recumbency. Acepromazine or butorphanol tartate are also appropriate sedatives. The cow's legs are tied, and its body is supported by a trough or weighted side frames. The patient should be tilted slightly to the right, to facilitate later closure of the incision. An area from the xiphoid process to the umbilicus is clipped and is surgically prepared in a routine manner. Local anesthesia is administered by local infiltration along the proposed incision or an inverted L block of the right paramedian area.

Instrumentation

1. General surgery pack
2. Sterile sleeves
3. 14–16-gauge needle with sterile tubing attached
4. Large, straight, cutting needle or an S-curved cutting needle for abomasopexy
5. Sterile, medium-sized stomach tube

Surgical Technique

Right-flank Omentopexy

The abdomen is entered through a 20-cm vertical incision in the right paralumbar fossa starting 4–5 cm ventral to the transverse processes of the lumbar vertebrae (Figure 13.4A). When the peritoneal cavity is entered in the case of an LDA, the duodenum will be vertical instead of in its normal horizontal position. Wearing sterile sleeves, the surgeon palpates the left side of the abdomen by

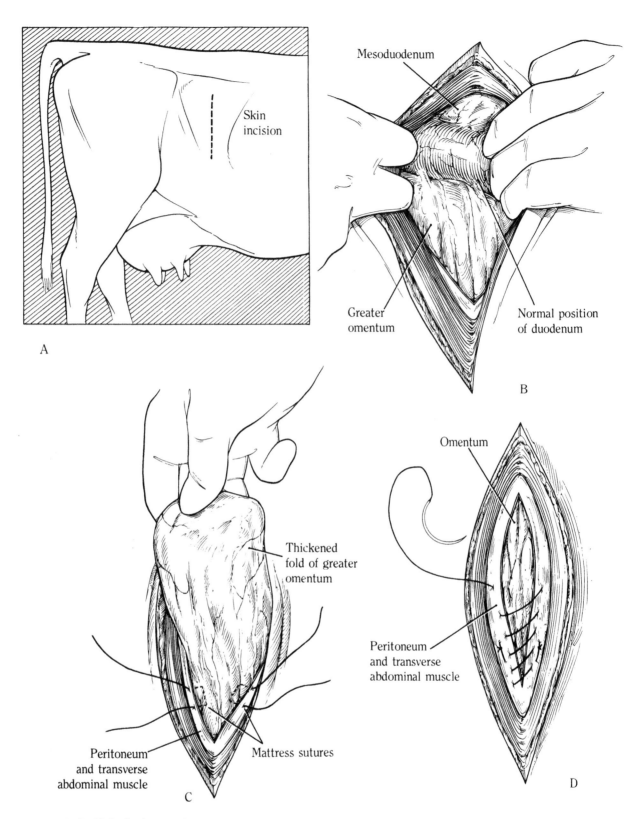

Fig. 13.4. **A–D.** Right-flank omentopexy.

Labels in image A: Skin incision

Labels in image B: Mesoduodenum, Greater omentum, Normal position of duodenum

Labels in image C: Thickened fold of greater omentum, Peritoneum and transverse abdominal muscle, Mattress sutures

Labels in image D: Omentum, Peritoneum and transverse abdominal muscle deflecting the greater omentum craniad. Then he passes his left arm caudal to the omentum and rumen to palpate the abomasum distended with gas on the left side of the rumen. This confirms the diagnosis of LDA. In addition, while palpating the displaced organ, the surgeon should feel for any evidence of adhesions.

The abomasum may be deflated using a 14–16-gauge needle with a length of sterile tubing attached. The needle is carried caudal to the rumen to the most dorsal part of the displaced abomasum and is inserted obliquely through the abomasal wall. Pressure is applied firmly with the forearm and the hand to release the gas, or the tubing may be attached to a suction device. The end of the tubing may be placed in a cup of water if suction is not available so the surgeon can appreciate the gas being removed to assure there is not obstruction of the needle or tubing. The needle is withdrawn and is carried back carefully, with the tubing folded to avoid contamination.

The abomasum is returned to its normal position by following the peritoneal surfaces ventrally with the hand between the rumen and the body wall. Once to the left of the rumen, the hand, with the fingers closed, is used to sweep the abomasum back to the right side of the abdomen. Alternatively, one may reach along the right body wall ventrally to find the muscular pylorus and pull the abomasum into the normal position. This may be done when sweeping from the left does not completely reposition the abomasum; some surgeons with short arms will prefer to use this technique after decompressing the abomasum. Gentle dorsocaudal pulling on the omentum, which has also been displaced to the left, is also helpful in this manipulation. If the rumen is full, it may be necessary to elevate the caudal ventral blind sac of the rumen with the inside of the elbow, to allow the abomasum to be pulled along under the rumen. One may also find it helpful in repositioning the abomasum to displace the rumen to the right slightly off the left body wall by using the left forearm. Once the abomasum is returned to its normal position, the duodenum resumes its normal horizontal position (Figure 13.4B) and is commonly observed to fill with gas. The greater omentum, which is observed through the abdominal incision, also feels loose (Figure 13.4B). Unnecessary handling of the duodenum during these manipulations may cause postoperative duodenitis.

If the surgery is performed for the treatment of an RDA or RTA, care should be taken not to incise the dilated abomasum when entering the peritoneal cavity. The various right-sided malpositions of the abomasum when using a right-flank approach are detailed in the section on right-flank abomasopexy. The abomasum commonly requires evacuation before the displacement can be corrected. An RTA usually has large quantities of fluid. Correct positioning of the abomasum is recognized in the same fashion as in LDA. Once the abomasum has been returned to its correct position, the technique of omentopexy (or pyloro-omentopexy) is the same whether it is an LDA, RDA, or RTA.

The omentum is grasped and pulled out through the incision. It is gently retracted dorsad and caudad until the pylorus can be visualized. This fold of omentum may be held by an assistant or attached to the upper part of the skin incision with towel forceps while the anchoring sutures are placed. Two mattress sutures of no. 1 or no. 2 synthetic absorbable suture material (one cranial to the incision and one caudal to it) are placed through the peritoneum and transverse abdominal muscle and through both layers of the fold of omentum (Figure 13.4C). The sutures are placed about 3 cm caudal to the pylorus. The peritoneum and transverse abdominal muscle are then sutured in a simple continuous pattern with no. 1 or no. 2 synthetic absorbable suture, and the omentum is incorporated into the suture line in the ventral two-thirds of the incision (Figure 13.4D). The internal and external abdominal oblique muscle layers and the skin are closed as in a routine flank laparotomy.

Pyloro-Omentopexy

There are several modifications of pyloropexy techniques used in veterinary practice.[15,28] We will describe a pyloro-omentopexy technique that the author has used successfully without complications.[15] First, the flank incision is shifted cranioventral to the middle of the paralumbar fossa. If a paravertebral block is used, this may require additional local anesthetic infusion immediately caudal to the last rib, to desensitize the more cranioventral aspect of the flank. The standard incision is made through the slightly shifted location, and the abomasum is repositioned as described. The skin is undermined for approximately 5 cm dorsocaudal and dorsocranial from the dorsal most aspect of the skin incision. This allows placement of no. 2 absorbable suture through the muscular body wall into the abdominal cavity where a bite is taken into the omentum and back through the body wall to be tied in the subcutaneous space. The first suture is placed in the dorsocaudal undermined space. A second one is placed similarly dorsocranial to the proximal aspect of the skin incision. These sutures serve to hold the omentum in place dorsally while sutures are placed to secure the pyloric antrum to the body wall. The pyloropexy is done with # 1 nonabsorbable suture. The cranial body wall is reflected cranially so that interrupted sutures can be placed near the ventral aspect of the incision approximately 5 cm cranially. The suture is placed from caudal to cranial through the peritoneum, transverse abdominus muscle, and part of the internal abdominal oblique muscle. The seromuscular layer of the pyloric antrum can then be pinched to separate it from the mucosal layer for placement of the next bite of suture from cranial to caudal into the seromuscular layer. Generally three such sutures are pre-placed before any are tied. These sutures will place the pyloric antrum immediately adjacent to the body wall. The omentum is then included in the closure of the peritoneum and transverse abdominus muscle from dorsal to ventral in a continuous pattern. The inclusion of omentum is discontinued at the level of the pyloropexy sutures. The remainder of the incision is closed in routine fashion. One recent review found a significant decrease in recurrence of abomasal displacement after pyloro-omentopexy when compared to omentopexy.[29] While one should avoid penetration of the lumen with suture, the pinching of the seromuscular layer away from the mucosa simplifies proper suture placement.

Left-flank Abomasopexy

A left-flank laparotomy is performed using a 20- to 25-cm incision in the paralumbar fossa, as previously described. Caution should be exercised when entering the abdomen because a distended abomasum may lie immediately within the incision area. Usually, the abomasum is visible through the incision. An 8- to 12-cm simple continuous or interlocking suture line of heavy polymerized caprolactam, nylon, or polypropylene, is placed in the greater curvature of the abomasum 5–7 cm from the attachment of the greater omentum (Figure 13.5A). The serosa may be rubbed with a dry surgical sponge to mildly irritate the area and enhance adhesion formation. The suture bites pass through the submucosa, and a meter of suture material should extend from each end of the suture line. Hemostats are placed on these suture ends in such a fashion that the cranial and caudal ends are easily identified. The abomasum may then be deflated using a 12-gauge needle and rubber tubing (Figure 13.5A) if this is considered necessary. The needle is placed into the dorsal portion of the abomasum and is inserted at an angle to obviate leakage when the needle is withdrawn. It is important that the abomasum not be deflated prior to the insertion of the suture; otherwise, the site for suture placement may be retracted away from the incision.

The cranial end of the suture is attached to a large, straight, cutting needle or to an S-curved cutting needle; this needle is carried along the internal body wall to a position right of midline, but medial to the subcutaneous abdominal vein and 15 cm caudal to the xiphoid process. The forefinger protects the end of the needle, and the lateral fingers reflect the viscera away from the body wall and ahead of the needle. An assistant can apply upward pressure on the abdominal wall in the area where the needles are to be inserted through the body wall. An empty syringe case works well for this purpose.

The needle is inserted quickly through the ventral body wall (Figure 13.5B). The assistant grasps the needle, and the caudal suture is placed through the body wall 8–12 cm caudal to the cranial suture. The assistant then grasps the two suture ends and applies gentle traction; at the same time, the surgeon pushes the deflated abomasum into its normal position. When the sutured area of the abomasum is lying against the floor of the abdomen, the assistant ties the suture ends together (Figure 13.5C). Care should be taken to tie the retention suture with

appropriate tension. The surgeon should be able to have one finger snuggly between the abomasum and body wall when tied. Too loose may allow intestine to become entrapped in the suture loop while too tight may lead to tearing of the suture out of the abomasum. The flank laparotomy incision is closed routinely. The suture is left in place for 4 weeks; the ends are then cut as close to the skin as possible. This time is considered necessary to allow the development of adhesions sufficient to prevent redisplacement.

Right-Flank Abomasopexy

The right-flank abomasopexy is not performed as frequently as other techniques. An RDA is probably adequately and more easily treated with pyloro-omentopexy. One may choose to use the abomasopexy technique when correcting an abomasal volvulus because the disturbance of venous return with this displacement may lead to an abomasum that is edematous and heavy so that omentopexy alone or pyloro-omentopexy may not adequately secure the abomasum. The right-flank approach to the bovine abdomen has been described previously. A 20- to 25-cm incision is made. At this stage, the particular problem needs to be recognized, and certain guidelines can be stated. In a simple RDA, the greater omentum comes into view through the laparotomy wound in the right flank as in a normal animal. The greater omentum may be looser because the distance between the abomasum and the descending duodenum is less than normal. The fundus will typically have moved caudolaterad and will appear uncovered by omentum. Abomasal torsions (volvulus may be a better term) occur counterclockwise when viewed from the rear and counterclockwise when viewed from the right flank. The omentum is usually wrapped in the torsion site, and the abomasum therefore appears at the incision without omentum covering it.

The color of the abomasal serosa is ascertained before one attempts to deflate the abomasum or correct its position. If the serosa appears viable and the organ is tightly distended, a 12-gauge needle with rubber tubing attached is inserted to relieve the gaseous pressure and to facilitate further exploration and manipulation. It is easier to remove gas and fluid before detorsion because the abomasum is closer to the incision. Early or less-severe torsion may not even require fluid removal, but severe torsion may require fluid removal before the torsion can be reduced. Placement of the suture requires careful thought, to ensure correct positioning at the completion of the procedure. An interlocking suture is placed in the middle of the greater curvature of the abomasum near the attachment of the greater omentum in the manner previously described and illustrated for left-flank abomasopexy (Figure 13.5C). If absolutely necessary, a purse-string suture can be placed in the abomasal wall, a stab incision is made, and a sterile, medium-sized stomach tube inserted into the abomasum (Figure 13.6). The fluid

Left displaced abomasum

Suction tube

A

Left displaced abomasum

Needle through ventral body wall

B

Fig. 13.5. **A–C.** Left-flank abomasopexy.

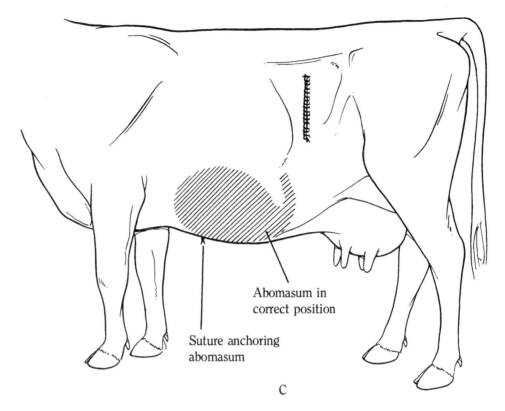

Abomasum in
correct position

Suture anchoring
abomasum

C

Fig. 13.5. *Continued.*

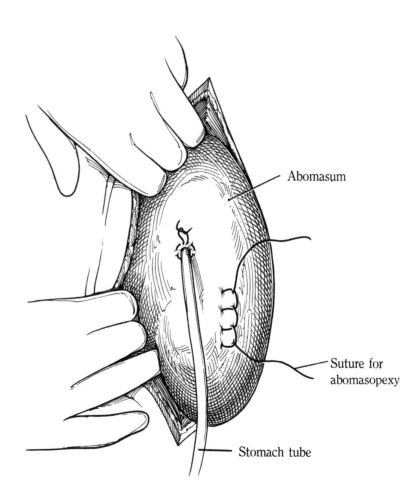

Abomasum

Suture for
abomasopexy

Stomach tube

Fig. 13.6. The fluid within the abomasum is
removed using a medium-sized stomach tube.

within the abomasum is then removed. If the fluid is difficult to drain, lavage may be performed. At the end of abomasal drainage, 2–3 L of mineral oil is instilled into the abomasum, the tube is withdrawn, and the purse-string suture is tied. The abomasopexy is completed as described for left-flank abomasopexy.

Right Paramedian Abomasopexy

A 20-cm incision is made between the midline and the right subcutaneous abdominal vein, starting approximately 8 cm behind the xiphoid process and ending immediately cranial to the umbilicus (Figure 13.7A,B). The small branches of the subcutaneous abdominal vein that are cut when incising the skin and subcutaneous tissue need to be ligated because the lack of muscle tissue in this region inhibits natural hemostasis and may result in hematoma and seroma formation. The incision is continued through the external rectus sheath (aponeuroses of external and internal abdominal oblique muscles) (Figure 13.7C) and the rectus abdominis muscle, to reveal the fibers of the internal rectus sheath (the transverse abdominal aponeurosis) running crosswise in the incision line. The transverse abdominal aponeurosis and peritoneum are incised (Figure 13.7D). The transverse aponeurosis may be cut separately with a scalpel, and the peritoneum may be entered using scissors, or both layers may be opened together with scissors.

In most cases of LDA, the abomasum will have returned to a relatively normal position during the casting procedure. If necessary, the abomasum should be returned to its normal position. Rarely, in the case of an RDA or RTA, it may be appropriate to empty gas with a 12-gauge needle and rubber tubing (Figure 13.7E). This is probably unnecessary with an LDA. Once the correct position of the abomasum has been ascertained, the lateral aspect of the greater curvature of the abomasum (where it is free of omentum) is incorporated with the peritoneum and internal rectus sheath in a simple continuous suture pattern with no. 1 or no. 2 synthetic absorbable suture material (Figure 13.7F). Care must be taken to not penetrate the abomasal mucosa. The heavy, external rectus sheath is closed with a simple continuous pattern of no. 1 or no. 2 synthetic absorbable suture (Figure 13.5G), and the skin is closed with a Ford interlocking suture using heavy polymerized caprolactam (Figure 13.5G). The patient is rolled into left lateral recumbency, followed by sternal recumbency.

Postoperative Management

Postoperative management depends on the individual case. Some animals require little or no aftercare; other animals may have septic metritis, mastitis, or ketosis and may also have been deprived of feed and water. Correction of metabolic disturbances subsequent to left abomasal displacements may necessitate the administration of electrolytes, calcium salts, and fluid therapy.

Animals operated on for RTA are in particularly critical condition and require a more gradual, cautious, return to feed and water. These patients should be monitored regularly for clinical signs, milk production, and urine ketones. Antibiotics are administered postoperatively. Many of these animals need intense fluid therapy with particular emphasis on replacement of the chloride deficit (see Chap. 2). For this purpose, 0.9% sodium chloride solution is generally appropriate; and supplementation with potassium chloride may also be indicated. With adequate fluid and electrolyte therapy in the presurgical and early postsurgical periods, the metabolic effects of RTA generally can be controlled. In severely affected cows, the abomasum's inability to regain normal function is often more important. The abomasum becomes filled and impacted if its function is not restored.[13] Typically, cases of abomasal torsion appear to improve in the first 24–48 hours and then deteriorate at 48–72 hours, with abomasal atony. Motility stimulants, such as neostigmine, have been recommended. However, neostigmine must be used repeatedly to have any effect above the pylorus; and even then, its benefit is minimal. If the animal's appetite has not returned in 2 days, a rumen inoculation may be appropriate. Oral supportive therapy, in which sodium chloride and potassium chloride are added to water, can be used in a patient capable of absorbing the fluid.

Complications and Prognosis

One of the most common complications of right-flank omentopexy is recurrence.[9] Recurrence can be due to incorrect placement of sutures during fixation—for example, fixing the omentum too far dorsal or caudal to the pylorus, or due to stretching or disruption of the omentopexy.[9] Even in the hands of experienced operators, however, redisplacement may occur in the long term. Recurrence does not tend to occur when the pyloro-omentopexy technique is used. Abomasal fistulas may occur subsequent to abomasopexy if nonabsorbable sutures are used for fixation of the abomasum. Nonabsorbable sutures that penetrate the lumen of the abomasum may potentiate bacterial colonization of the abdominal wall resulting in fistulation. Acute wound dehiscence with evisceration and redisplacements are considered rare complications of this procedure. Left flank abomasopexy in particular, is associated with an increased risk of puncturing viscera or accidentally catching omentum while carrying the needle to the floor of the abdomen. The surgeon must ensure accurate placement of fixation sutures, otherwise redisplacement may occur or other abdominal structures may be inadvertently pinned between the abomasum and abdominal wall. Again, multifilament nonabsorbable suture should be avoided due to the risk of abomasal fistulation. Other large animal surgeons have cited inadvertent damage to

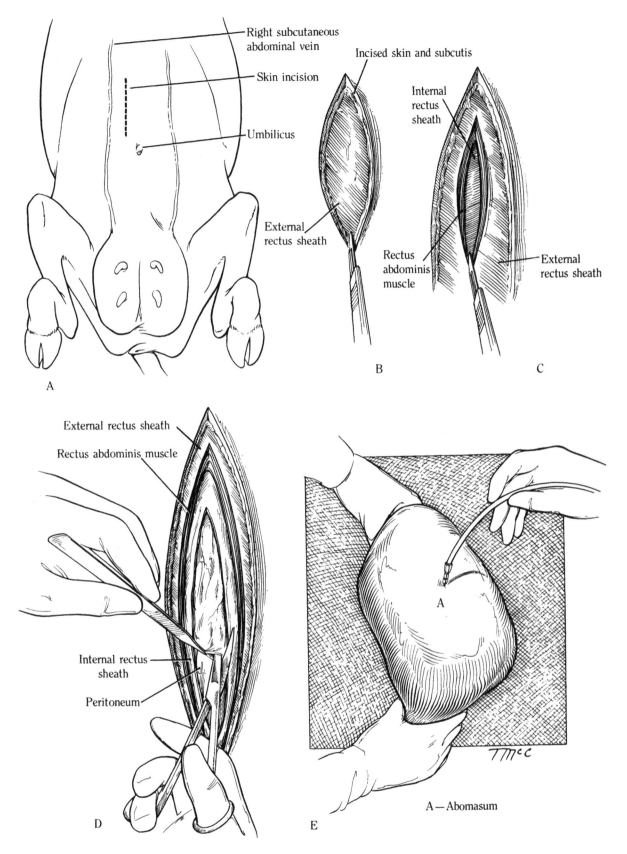

Fig. 13.7. **A–G.** Ventral paramedian abomasopexy.

Labels in figure:

- Right subcutaneous abdominal vein
- Skin incision
- Umbilicus
- External rectus sheath
- Incised skin and subcutis
- Internal rectus sheath
- Rectus abdominis muscle
- External rectus sheath
- External rectus sheath
- Rectus abdominis muscle
- Internal rectus sheath
- Peritoneum
- A — Abomasum

A
B
C
D
E

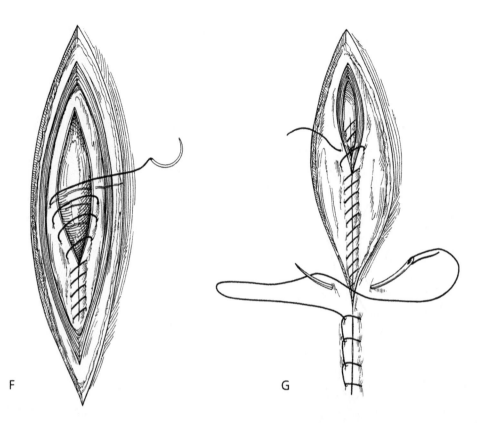

F   G

Fig. 13.7.   *Continued.*

the milk vein and partial outflow obstruction due to improper positioning of the abomasum as common complications encountered in this procedure.[20]

The reported success rate of right-flank omentopexy for the treatment of LDA is high; ranging from 87%–100% in dairy cows.[11,21,22,28] The complication rate that was reported in one of the studies was also low (3.3%) with the primary complication being peritonitis. The success rate of this procedure for cases of RDA is overall lower than that of LDA, 74.5% reported by Rohn, et al.; however, this is influenced by whether abomasal volvulus is a present or not.[30] There are few statistical evaluations of omentopexy performed in conjunction with pyloropexy in the literature.

Some surgeons believe that their success in treating cows with RTA was due largely to not opening the abomasum prior to surgery.[28] Now this claim generally is considered invalid. That acidic fluid high in chloride is easily absorbed from the abomasum following detorsion is questionable. In addition, any fluid deficit sustained by draining the abomasum can be replaced by intravenous fluid therapy; this is considered more reliable than anticipating reabsorption of the fluid from the abomasum after detorsion. The rationale for removing fluids that potentially contain endotoxins is logical, but its validity is controversial. Whether deposition of mineral oil directly into the abomasum inhibits further toxin reabsorption is uncertain, and its value is equally controversial. One

author believes that this measure has contributed to his success,[23] whereas another author does not think that this measure improved the prognosis for severely affected cows.[13]

Prognosis and survival rates for right-flank abomasopexy are not well documented. The prognosis for cases of abdominal volvulus is much less favorable than that of uncomplicated cases of RDA. Several studies have reported prognostic indicators that may be useful at the time of surgery for ascertaining outcome, such as whether or not fluid decompression is performed in addition to gas decompression, the presence of venous thrombosis, and blue or black discoloration of the abomasum.[28,31] Some surgeons believe that not performing fluid decompression is advantageous because the abomasum is allowed to resorb electrolytes and the surgical time and risk or peritonitis is decreased.[18,31] Indeed, clinical studies show higher survival rates for cows that do not receive fluid decompression. However, this may be incorrectly correlated since cows with a greater duration of torsion will not only have accrued more fluid in the abomasum, but are also more likely to have greater tissue damage and necrosis, which could account for the much lower survival rate that is observed.

The prognosis for ventral paramedian abomasopexy is comparable to that of right-flank omentopexy. In a comparison study of right-flank omentopexy and right-paramedian abomasopexy for treatment of LDA, survival rates were 81.5% and 87% at 6 months for abomasopexy and omentopexy, respectively.[28] However, this varies greatly with complicated cases or cases of RDA. In these instances, prognosis depends greatly on the extent of tissue damage and the amount and duration of volvulus. A recent study of peritoneal fluid in cows with abomasal displacement showed signs of inflammation and suggested that antiinflammatory treatment of these cows is warranted.[32]

Surgical Correction of Cecal Dilatation/Volvulus

Relevant Anatomy

The cecum is a blind-ended tubular organ that is normally approximately 12 cm in diameter. The end of the cecum extends caudally from the ileocolic junction toward the pelvic inlet. In cases of cecal dilatation, the cecum may extend into the pelvic cavity or even toward the left of the abdomen. The base of the cecum is attached to mesentery and thus less mobile.[33]

Indications

Cecal dilatation/volvulus is predominately a dairy cow condition. The cow will present with a number of clinical signs such as mild colic, decreased appetite, decreased rumen motility, and possible right-sided distention. Often the distended cecum can be detected on rectal palpation,[34] and it must be on the differential list when a ping is detected upon auscultation and percussion of the right side. Better results are reported when affected animals are surgically treated in a timely fashion.[34] The typhlotomy is the treatment of choice provided the entire cecum is viable. A recurrence rate of 10% is reported in cecal dilatation cases. The recommended treatment in repeat cases is the typhlectomy.[35,36]

Anesthesia and Surgical Preparation

The right flank is prepared as described for standing laparotomy with clipping, local anesthesia, and surgical preparation of the skin.

Instrumentation

1. General surgery pack
2. Sterile drape or towel

Surgical Technique

The skin incision is performed in the middle of the right flank approximately 20 cm in length. The distended cecum will dominate the caudal abdominal cavity as it extends into the pelvic cavity. The tip of the cecum can be exteriorized from the incision taking care not to place too much tension on the mesentery. This is where an assistant can support the cecum to prevent excessive tension or a sterile towel may be used to provide support as a sling. One may suction gas off the cecum if that is the predominant cause of the distention. If the organ is full of digesta a typhlotomy is performed at the tip of the cecum after packing sterile towels around it to prevent abdominal contamination. The typhlotomy incision may be as small as 3 cm if the contents of the cecum are mostly liquid or 6 cm or more if the organ is full of ingesta. The typhlotomy incision is closed with using no. 0 or no. 1 absorbable suture in a continuous inverting such as a Cushing or Lembert.

In the case of cecal volvulus, if the blood supply has been compromised to the degree that the organ is not viable, a typhlectomy is the required treatment. The typhlectomy would also be suggested if the cow had a previous cecal dilatation or volvulus. A typhlotomy is performed to empty the cecum prior to resection of the compromised portion. Then one may be able to place intestinal forceps across the proximal part of the cecum to allow resection and initial closure followed by a second inverting layer of suture or a Parker-Kerr pattern over the forceps. More frequently, the surgeon will choose to perform the resection in stages by making the incision through a small part of the cecum and closing that portion before continuing with incision of another portion and then continuing the closure. This method maintains traction on the cecum and helps prevent abdominal contamination. A single inverting layer of absorbable suture is often adequate for closure but some surgeons may elect to use two layers.

Postoperative Management

Perioperative antibiotics are in order for this abdominal surgery. Other management will vary with the longevity and severity of the disease.

Complications and Prognosis

The complications are minimal and the prognosis is generally good as long as the cecum is viable and no contamination occurs during the surgery.

Small Intestinal Resection and Anastomosis

Relevant Anatomy

The small intestine accessible for exteriorization in surgery is distal jejunum and ileum, which are on the outer free edge of the mesentery. The duodenum may be palpated in the dorsal area of the mesentery but is difficult to position outside the abdominal cavity. The mesentery of the proximal jejunum is too short to exteriorize. The small intestine is coiled at the free edge of relatively short mesentery. The mesentery does lengthen at the distal aspect of the jejunum. As compared to the horse, the ruminant mesentery contains more fat and the vasculature is not as easily observed.[33]

The relatively short mesentery makes manipulation and exteriorization of the small intestine challenging in the standing patient, as tension on the mesentery to exteriorize the intestine may cause pain that will lead the animal to move or even become recumbent. Therefore, one should consider general anesthesia for small intestinal surgery in cattle. However, many cases of small intestinal disease are amenable to field surgery.[37] The author has found that many cattle can safely undergo small intestinal procedures without undue stress to the patient or the staff, if one is careful to put the mesentery under minimal tension.

Indications

Intussusception or other small intestinal obstructions are the main reasons for small intestinal resection and anastomosis.[38] One may suspect a small intestinal lesion from clinical signs and rectal palpation findings. Alternatively, a small intestinal lesion may be discovered during an exploratory laparotomy.

Anesthesia and Surgical Preparation

The surgical incision is via a right flank with skin preparation and local anesthesia as described earlier. The abdominal exploratory surgery is performed in the standing cow and the resection can often be successfully completed in the standing patient. If one has a preoperative diagnosis and the cow is of high economic value, some surgeons prefer doing the procedure via a recumbent flank with the aid of general anesthesia. Alternatively, one occasionally makes the diagnosis via the standing exploratory laparotomy and determines that the resection cannot be done safely without general anesthesia. In this case, the incision is closed to be reopened after induction of general anesthesia and positioning the patient in left lateral recumbency. These options should be discussed thoroughly with the client before the start of surgery.

Instrumentation

1. General surgery pack
2. Penrose drains

Surgical Technique

The standard right-flank laparotomy incision is made. Once in the abdominal cavity the surgeon should thoroughly explore the abdomen for distended intestine. An intussusception is usually coiled and thickened with distended intestine proximally and empty bowel distal to the obstruction. One should carefully exteriorize the affected

segment to determine if it can be safely resected in the standing patient. The vasculature is difficult to isolate because of the fat in the mesentery. Some blunt dissection with sponges may help in this endeavor. The vasculature should be ligated proximal and distal to the affected bowel. The anastomosis may be done as the surgeon chooses. Most surgeons perform end-to-end anastomosis, while some opt for a side-to-side anastomosis. The end-to-end may be done in one or two layers. We do suggest the bowel be rotated slightly when doing an end-to-end anastomosis. The relatively broad area of mesenteric attachment to the intestine makes for a large area not covered by serosa. The slight rotation of the bowel allows easier leak-proof closure and better serosal coverage for healing.

After anastomosis of the intestine, the resulting mesenteric rent is closed. The site is thoroughly rinsed and returned carefully to the abdomen. The surgeon then changes gown and gloves to close the incision in a routine manner. Any further exploration of the abdominal cavity should be performed prior to intestinal resection. Regardless of cleaning the site and changing attire, the risk of contamination of the peritoneal cavity is great after resection of bowel.

Postoperative Management

The postoperative management depends largely on the condition of the animal. The ideal patient will eat after surgery and pass loose feces shortly after that. The feces will return to normal after 48 hours. The more compromised patient will require extensive postoperative care such as IV fluids, antibiotics, and anti-inflammatory agents due to endotoxemia and/or peritonitis.

Complications and Prognosis

These patients are frequently endotoxemic. They are also candidates for peritonitis from contamination with intestinal contents during the resection or due to leakage of the anastomosis. While the prognosis for individuals treated early having easily accessible lesions can be very good, cattle as a group have less than a 50% survival rate after small intestinal resection.[39]

References

1. Noorsdy, J.L. Selection of an incision site for cesarean section in the cow. *Vet. Med. Small Anim. Clin.*, 75:530, 1979.
2. Baker, J.S. Abomasal impaction and related obstructions of the forestomachs in cattle. *J. Am. Vet. Med. Assoc.*, 175:1250, 1979.
3. Dehghani, S.N. Bovine rumenotomy: Comparison of four surgical techniques. *Can. Vet. J.*, 36:693–697, 1995.
4. Dyce, K.M., Sack, W.O., and Wensing, C.J.G. Textbook of Veterinary Anatomy. 2nd Ed. Philadelphia, W.B. Saunders, 1996, p. 671.

5. Hofmeyr, C.F.B. The digestive system. *In* Textbook of Large Animal Surgery. Edited by F.W. Oehme, J.E. Prier. Baltimore, MD, Williams & Wilkins, 1974.

6. Ducharme, N.G. Surgery of the bovine forestomach compartments. *Vet. Clin. North Am. Food Anim. Pract., 6:*371–396, 1990.

7. Fubini, S.L., and Ducharme, N.G. Bovine surgery. *In* Farm Animal Surgery. St. Louis, MO, Elsevier, 2004, p. 189.

8. Rumsey, T.S., Putnam, P.A., Williams, E.E., and Samuelson, G. Effect of ruminal and esophageal fistulation on ruminal parameters, saliva flow, EKG patterns and respiratory rate of beef steers. *J. Anim. Sci., 35:*1248–1256, 1972.

9. Aubry, P. Routine surgical procedures in dairy cattle under field conditions: Abomasal surgery, dehorning, and tail docking. *Vet. Clin. Food Anim., 21:*55–71, 2005.

10. Constable, P.D., Miller, G.Y., Hoffis, G.F., Hull, B.L., and Rings, D.M. Risk factors for abomasal volvulus and left abomasal displacement in cattle. *Am. J. Vet. Res., 53:*1184–1192, 1992.

11. Seeger, T., Kumper, H., Failing, K., and Doll, K. Comparison of laparoscopic-guided abomasopexy versus omentopexy via right flank laparotomy for the treatment of left abomasal displacement in dairy cows. *Am. J. Vet. Res., 67:*472–478, 2006.

12. Roussel, A.J., Cohen, N.D., and Hooper, R.N. Abomasal displacement and volvulus in beef cattle: 19 cases (1988–1998). *J. Am. Vet. Med. Assoc., 216*(5):730–733, 2000.

13. Smith, D.F. Right-side torsion of the abomasum in dairy cows: Classification of severity and evaluation of outcome. *J. Am. Vet. Med. Assoc., 173:*108, 1978.

14. Ames, S. Repositioning displaced abomasum in the cow. *J. Am. Vet. Med. Assoc., 153:*1470, 1968.

15. Baird, A.N., and Harrison, S. Surgical treatment of left displaced abomasum. *Compendium, 23*(10):S102–S114, 2001.

16. Muller, J., Fleischer, P., and Pavlata, L. Comparison technique of laparoscopical solution left displacement of the abomasum. *Veterinarstvi, 62*(9):578–583, 2012.

17. Bartlett, P.C., Kopcha, M., Coe, P.H., Ames, N.K., Ruegg, P.L., and Erskine, R.G. Economic comparison of the pyloro-omentopexy versus the roll-and-toggle procedure for the treatment of left displacement of the abomasum in dairy cattle, *J Am Vet Med Assoc 206*(8):1156–1162, 1995.

18. Gabel, A.A., and Heath, R.B. Treatment of right-sided torsion of the abomasum in cattle. *J. Am. Vet. Med. Assoc., 155:*642, 1969.

19. Lowe, J.E., and Loomis, W.K. Abomasopexy for repair of left abomasal displacement in dairy cattle. *J. Am. Vet. Med. Assoc., 147:*389, 1965.

20. Fubini, S.L., and Ducharme, N.G. Bovine surgery. *In* Farm Animal Surgery. St. Louis, MO, Elsevier, 2004, p. 208.

21. Gabel, A.A., and Heath, R.B. Correction and right-sided omentopexy in treatment of left-sided displacement of the abomasum in dairy cattle. *J. Am. Vet. Med. Assoc., 155:*632, 1969.

22. Buckner, R. Surgical correction of left displaced abomasum in cattle. *Vet. Rec., 136:*265–267, 1995.

23. Baker, J.S. Right displacement of the abomasum in the bovine: A modified procedure for treatment. *Bovine Pract., 11:*58, 1976.

24. Boucher, W.B., and Abt, D. Right-sided dilatation of the bovine abomasum with torsion. *J. Am. Vet. Med. Assoc., 153:*76, 1968.

25. Baker, J.S. Personal communication, 1980.

26. Lee, I., Yamagishi, N., Oboshi, K., and Yamada, H. Left paramedian abomasopexy in cattle. *J. Vet. Sci., 3:*59–60, 2002.

27. Newman, K.D., Anderson, D.E., and Silveira, F. One step laparoscopic abomasopexy for correction of left-sided displacement of the abomasum in dairy cows. *J. Am. Vet. Med. Assoc., 227:*1142–1147, 2005.

28. Fubini, S.L., Ducharme, N.G., Erb, H.N., and Sheils, R.L. A comparison in 101 dairy cows of right paralumbar fossa omentopexy and right paramedian abomasopexy for treatment of left displacement of the abomasum. *Can Vet J, 33:*318–324, 1992.

29. Baird, A.N. Comparison of omentopexy versus pyloro-omentopexy for left displaced abomasum in dairy cows. Unpublished data, 2012.

30. Rohn, M., Tenhagen, B.A., and Hofman, W. Survival of dairy cows after surgery to correct abomasal displacement: 1. Clinical and laboratory parameters and overall survival. *J. Vet. Med. Assoc., 51:*294–299, 2004.

31. Constable, P.D., St. Jean, G., Hull, B.L., Rings, D.M., and Hoffsis, G.F. Prognostic value of surgical and postoperative findings in cattle with abomasal volvulus. *J. Am. Vet. Med. Assoc., 199:*892–898, 1991.

32. Grosche, A., Furll, M., and Wittek, T. Peritoneal fluid analysis in dairy cows with left displaced abomasum and volvulus. *Vet. Rec., 170*(16):413, 2012.

33. Schummer, A., Nickel, R., and Sack, W.O. The alimentary canal of ruminants. *In* The Viscera of the Domestic Mammals. 2nd Ed. Edited by A. Schummer, R. Nickel, W.O. Sack. New York, Springer-Verlag, 1979, pp. 168–169.

34. Braun, U., Beckmann, C., Gerspach, C., Hassig, M., Muggli, E., Knubben-Schweizer, G., and Nuss, K. Clinical findings and treatment in cattle with caecal dilatation. *BMC Vet. Res., 8:*75, 2012.

35. Fubini, S.L., Erb, H.N., Rebhun, W.C., and Horne, D. Cecal dilatation and volvulus in dairy cows: 84 cases (1977–1983). *J. Am. Vet. Med. Assoc., 189*(1):96–99, 1986.

36. Steiner, A., Braun, U., Lischer, C., and Iselin, U. Surgical treatment of caecal dilatation/torsion in the cow—80 cases (1988–1990). *Wien. Tierarztl. Monatsschr., 79*(2):41–46, 1992.

37. Anderson, D.E. Surgical diseases of the small intestine. Part I: Field surgery of cattle. *Vet. Clin. North Am. Food Anim. Pract., 24*(2):383–401, 2008.

38. Abutarbush, S.M., and Naylor, J.M. Obstruction of the small intestine by a trichbezoar in cattle: 15 cases (1992–2002). *J. Am. Vet. Med. Assoc., 229*(10):1627–1630, 2006.

39. Constable, P.D., St. Jean, G., Hull, B.L., Rings, D.M., Morin, D.E., and Nelson, D.R. Intussusception in cattle: 336 cases (1964–1993). *J. Am. Vet. Med. Assoc., 210:*531–536, 1997.

Chapter 14

BOVINE UROGENITAL SURGERY

A. N. Baird, DVM, MS, DACVS

Objectives

1. Discuss the indications for various urogenital surgical techniques in bovine.
2. Describe the advantages and disadvantages of different castration approaches in cattle.
3. Describe various penile, preputial, and inguinal surgical interventions including hematoma evacuation, and teaser bull preparation.
4. Describe the various surgical treatments involved with dystocia.

Calf Castration

Relevant Anatomy

The anatomy of the testes and associated structures is basically the same as in the horse (described in Chapter 10). In the bull, the scrotum is located between the cranial parts of the thighs. On the cranial face of the scrotum are small, rudimentary teats that vary in number and spacing. In contrast to the horse, the testes are situated vertically rather than horizontally within the scrotum. The epididymis runs along the caudomedial border of the testes. At the distal pole of the testes, the ductus deferens begins at the tail of the epididymis and ascends the medial border of the testes. The spermatic cord may be palpated at the scrotal neck.

Occasionally calves will present with a single scrotal testicle. The laparoscopic removal of abdominally retained testicles has been described but will not be discussed here.[1] One may use standard laparotomy techniques to remove an abdominal testicle. Often retained testicles in ruminants are actually ectopic and may be located subcutaneously between the scrotum and the preputial orifice. An ectopic testicle may be removed with the calf cast or secured in lateral recumbency on a tilt table. The line of the skin incision is infused with local anesthesia. The testicle will be located just deep to the skin incision where it can be ligated and removed. The skin incision may be closed with absorbable suture or left open to heal by secondary intention.

Indications

Castration of beef calves is a routine management procedure that is used to improve the quality of the carcass, prevent unintended births, and improve the safety and ease of herd management. There are three primary methods of castration: physical, chemical, and hormonal.[2] Chemical castration, which involves the injection of a toxic subject into the testes, is associated with a 25% failure rate and is not generally accepted as a useful technique.[2–4] Hormonal castration, which involves immunizing the bulls for gonadotrophin-releasing hormone, is not used frequently because of its limited practicality and consumer concerns.[5] All physical methods, including surgical castration, Burdizzo clamps, and latex bands, are associated with pain and discomfort to the animal as well as substantial potential complications. Generally, surgical castration is preferred because it is associated with rapid wound healing and a low failure rate although the method of castration used by beef cattle operations varies with region and is fairly subjective.[2,6]

This procedure should be performed early in a calf's life. It is recommended that nursing calves be castrated at 1–4 weeks of age. Bucket-reared calves should probably be castrated 3–4 weeks later because of their slower start nutritionally and their inferior conditions. Sometimes it may be necessary to wait longer on an individual calf.

Turner and McIlwraith's Techniques in Large Animal Surgery, 4th Edition. Dean A. Hendrickson and A. N. (Nickie) Baird.
© 2013 John Wiley & Sons, Inc. Published 2013 by John Wiley & Sons, Inc.

Some calves will be held to weaning before castration if progeny testing for weight gain is performed.

Anesthesia and Surgical Preparation

In the beef industry, it has been traditional practice to perform surgical castration quickly without anesthesia or skin preparation based on the economics, convenience, and circumstances of the procedure. The humaneness of this practice has become a significant consumer concern and has garnered further research into improving intra- and postoperative analgesia for surgical castration. In some countries it has led to revisions of welfare legislation that prohibit the surgical castration of male ruminants without local or general anesthesia, postoperative pain relief, and a veterinarian to perform the procedure.[7]

Evidence suggests that nonsteroidal anti-inflammatory drugs, such as ketoprofen, may have a more beneficial effect in alleviating postoperative pain and inflammation in surgically castrated calves than local anesthetic alone due to their systemic analgesic properties. Although local anesthesia minimizes pain related behavioral responses during surgical castration, it does not significantly reduce cortisol responses. A combination of local anesthetic and intravenous ketoprofen, however, significantly reduces both the behavioral responses and rise in mean plasma cortisol concentrations during the first 8 hours postoperatively.[2] Ketoprofen has also been shown to reduce acute-phase protein responses, and by inference, inflammation associated with the procedure.[8] While use of anti-inflammatory drugs may benefit the calf, the practitioner must remain abreast of the constantly changing environment of approved and extra-label use of any drugs in food animals.

A tranquilizer or sedative may be administered, and local infiltration analgesia is performed. Following surgical preparation of the area, the skin is infiltrated on a line 1 cm from the median raphe with 10 ml of local analgesic solution; this infiltration is continued into the subcutaneous tissue. Local analgesia can be injected directly into the testis. It is also important to infiltrate the spermatic cord in the region of emasculation with a long 18- to 20-gauge needle.

Additional Instrumentation

1. General surgery pack
2. Emasculators
3. Newberry knife

Surgical Technique

The scrotum is grasped, and a horizontal incision is made through skin and fascia at the widest part of the scrotum (junction of middle and distal thirds). The entire distal segment of the scrotum is transected (Figure 14.1A), and the common vaginal tunic is left intact. Traction is then placed on the testes, and the skin is pushed proximad so the fascia is separated from the spermatic cords enclosed in the common tunics (Figure 14.1B). The operator's hands should not touch the proximal regions of the spermatic cords.

An alternative to the horizontal incision is to use the Newberry knife. The Newberry knife makes a vertical incision from approximately the middle of the scrotum leaving cranial and caudal flaps of scrotal skin. The testes are dissected in the same manner as described in the previous paragraph. The incision heals by these flaps contracting on themselves thus allowing better drainage of the surgical site.

The spermatic cords are emasculated (site of emasculation is illustrated in Figure 14.1B). It is important that the emasculators be pushed proximad and that tension on the cord be relaxed when emasculation is performed (Figure 14.1C). Following removal of the emasculators, any redundant adipose tissue is removed (Figure 14.1D). The incision may be sprayed with a topical antibacterial powder; and at the discretion of the operator, this powder may also be put up inside the incision. In larger bulls one may wish to ligate the cords with no. 2 absorbable suture rather than trust the emasculators to adequately prevent hemorrhage. In younger bulls, most producers will rely on slow constant tension to remove the testes rather than relying on emasculators. The stretching of the cord to failure will take advantage of natural hemostasis.

Postoperative Management

The wound is left open to heal by secondary intention. Concurrent immunization for black leg and malignant edema is recommended. Prior immunization would be preferable, but it is often not practical. Exercise of the calves is important following castration. Calves should be monitored for signs of hemorrhage for approximately 24 hours.

Complications and Prognosis

The prognosis for surgical castration is good and complications are usually mild and infrequent. Potential complications include hemorrhage, excessive swelling, tetanus, and infection. Infection may occur 5–15 days following the procedure and often arises much later than would be anticipated. Infections usually manifest as acute cellulitis and require prompt treatment with drainage and antibiotics.

Urethrostomy

Relevant Anatomy

The urethra in male ruminants is described in two parts, the pelvic urethra, which lies over the pelvic symphysis,

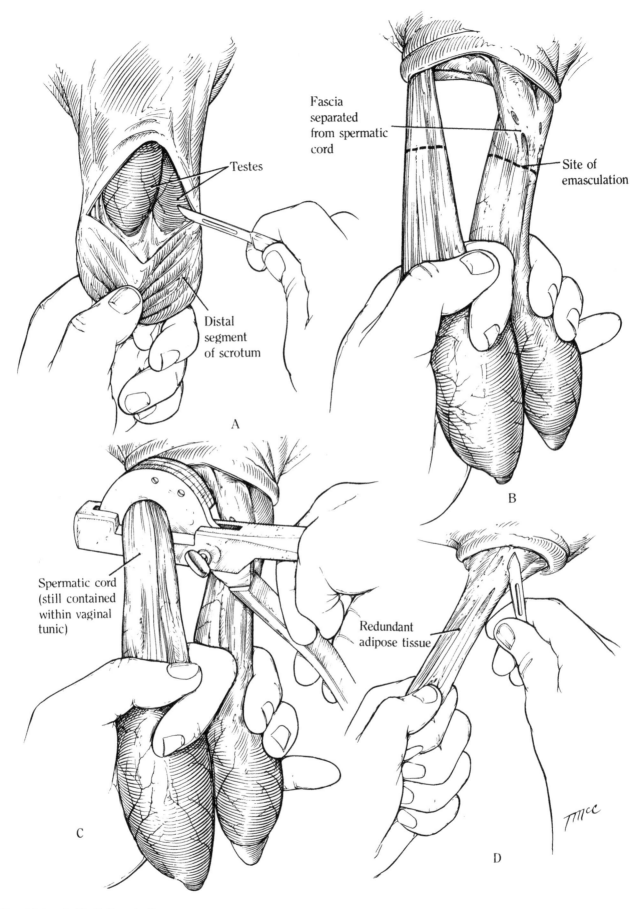

Testes

Distal
segment
of scrotum

Fascia
separated
from spermatic
cord

Site of
emasculation

A

B

Spermatic cord
(still contained
within vaginal
tunic)

Redundant
adipose tissue

C

D

Fig. 14.1. **A–D.** Calf castration.

and the penile urethra. The pelvic urethra may be fully palpated rectally. It is surrounded by the urethralis muscle with the exception of the dorsal aspect where it is replaced by the aponeurotic plate. The urethral diverticulum is located at the level of the ischial arch. Just proximal to the diverticulum is a fold of urethral mucosa that acts as a valve to prevent retrograde flow of urine into the pelvic urethra.[9,10] The excretory ducts of the bulbourethral glands empty into the urethra at the diverticulum.

The lumen of the urethra in ruminants is relatively small and is further decreased in diameter by the dorsal ridge of the bladder and longitudinal mucosal folds. The lumen of the penile urethra becomes progressively smaller and is most pronounced at the distal bend of the sigmoid flexure of the penis. Hence, urethral calculi frequently become lodged at the distal sigmoid flexure of the penis, near the attachments of the retractor penis muscles.

Indications

Urethrostomy is most commonly performed in steers because of obstruction by urethral calculi, a condition known as urolithiasis. The occurrence of urethral obstruction in steers, as opposed to bulls, is influenced by the smaller diameter of their urethra. The more frequent occurrence in steers may also be related to the higher concentrate diets to produce faster weight gain as opposed to the more reasonable maintenance diets bulls are fed. The chemical composition of the urethral calculi may vary, depending on the steer's diet. Silicate calculi, which are rough and hard, occur in steers grazing stubble and pastures consisting largely of grasses.[11] Phosphate calculi, which are soft, smooth, and often multiple, are more common in steers in feedlots.[12]

Failure to relieve the obstructed urethra can result in rupture of the bladder and subsequent uroperitoneum, or rupture of the urethra, resulting in subcutaneous infiltration of urine in the perineal region or ventral abdomen. Attending cellulitis, septicemia, and death may follow. The following technique generally is regarded as a salvage procedure to remove urine. It is usually performed to "buy time" until the animal's condition can be stabilized sufficiently to permit slaughter.

Anesthesia and Surgical Preparation

This surgical procedure is performed using caudal epidural anesthesia with the animal in the standing position or cast in dorsal recumbency. Sometimes xylazine hydrochloride (Rompun) is used for sedation. The positioning of the animal for surgery is determined by the surgeon. The animal may be cast in dorsal recumbency with its legs tied cranially and the surgeon kneeling behind it (Figure 14.2A). This method may produce unwanted, additional pressure on an already distended urinary bladder. It is preferable to operate on large steers and bulls in the standing position. When the animal is positioned, the surgical site is clipped and is prepared for surgery in a routine manner.

Urethrostomy in steers and bulls may be performed at several sites. If it is performed just ventral to the anus at the level of the floor of the pelvis (perineal or high urethrostomy), severe scalding and matting of the escutcheon and medial aspects of the limbs result; generally, the animal is penalized at market with a lower value for slaughter. The other site for urethrostomy is in the region of the distal bend of the sigmoid flexure of the penis (low urethrostomy). The advantage of the low incision, described here, is that the penis can be directed so that the urine is forced caudad, away from the medial aspects of the limbs, to reduce damage from urine scald. In addition, an incision in this region is more likely to expose the calculi because they most commonly lodge in this region.

A low urethrostomy may also be performed cranial to the scrotum or scrotal remnant.

Instrumentation

1.　General surgery pack
2.　Urinary catheter

Surgical Technique

The penis is palpated immediately caudal to the remnants of the scrotum. The scrotal remnant is grasped and is stretched craniad, and the distal bend of the sigmoid flexure is located. A 10-cm skin incision is made on the midline directly over the penis (Figure 14.2A,B), and blunt dissection is then performed to locate the penis. In Figure 14.2A–G, the patient is in dorsal recumbency. Generally, the penis is deeper than one would anticipate and is a firm fibrous structure about the thickness of the index finger. During the dissection, the surgeon encounters subcutaneous adipose tissue and several layers of elastic tissue surrounding the penis. With traction, a portion of the penis is exposed through the skin incision (Figure 14.2C). The retractor penis muscles should be identified because they serve as useful guidelines to the location of the ventral surface of the penis as they attach at the distal bend of the sigmoid flexure. Care should be taken not to twist the penis and thereby to lose the relationship of the retractor penis muscles and ventral surface of the penis. At this point, it may be possible to palpate the calculi in the urethra.

Several options exist at this point, depending on the severity of inflammation of the urethra and surrounding tissues. If inflammation of these structures is minimal and the calculi can be located, a small incision is made directly over the calculus (calculi) on the ventral aspect of the penis (Figure 14.2D). The calculus (calculi) is then removed. Prior to closure of the urethra, a catheter should be inserted into the urethra, both proximally and distally, to search for further stones and to ensure urethral patency. The urethra may be sutured if there is no urethral

Fig. 14.2. A–H. Urethrostomy.

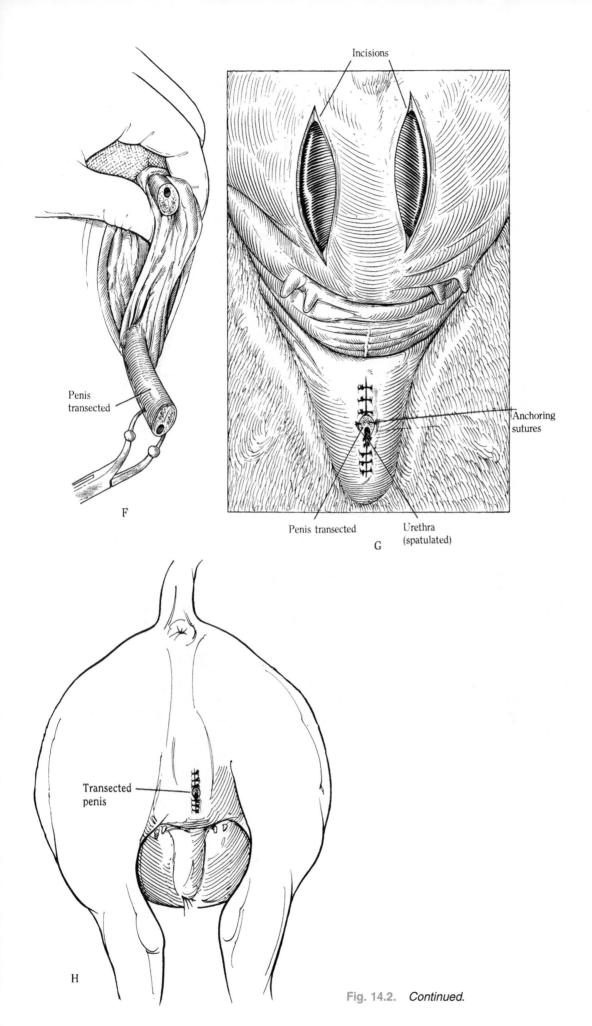

Penis transected

Incisions

Anchoring sutures

Penis transected

Urethra (spatulated)

F

G

Transected penis

H

Fig. 14.2. *Continued.*

necrosis. A catheter may be placed in the urethra to minimize stricture formation during closure. Simple interrupted or simple continuous sutures of an absorbable suture material (polyglytone 6211, Caprosyn) are inserted. The sutures should go down to, but not through, the urethral mucosa. The penis is replaced into its normal position, and the dorsal third of the skin incision is closed (Figure 14.2E). The remainder of the incision may be left open to heal by secondary intention.

If there is any necrosis of the urethra and if the urethra's ability to hold sutures is in question, the urethra and skin incisions may be left to heal by secondary intention.

If damage to the penis and surrounding tissues is extensive with rupture of the urethra, transection and extirpation of the penis are performed. The penis is dissected carefully from the dorsal arteries and veins of the penis and is transected to leave an 8- to 12-cm proximal stump (Figure 14.2F). The length of the penis varies with the size of the patient. From the surgeon's view, the arteries and veins appear ventral to the exposed stump of the penis. These vessels are ligated (some surgeons do not consider this necessary). It is a common error to isolate an insufficient amount of penile stump prior to anchoring it to the skin. The stump should be of sufficient length that when it is sutured to the skin there is no in folding of skin because of excessive tension. The stump of the exposed penis is directed caudoventrad and is anchored to the skin with two sutures. The sutures should pass through the skin, the tunica albuginea, and the corpus cavernosum penis. Care is taken to ensure that the urethral lumen is not compromised. The stump of the penis should not be bent because iatrogenic urethral obstruction may occur. The urethra at the end of the penile stump is split, and the edges are sutured to the lateral aspects of the penis (Figure 14.2G). This part of the technique is not performed routinely by all surgeons. Figure 14.2H shows a completed urethrostomy with the patient standing.

In animals with urethral obstruction and signs of subcutaneous edema and cellulitis, urethral rupture has usually occurred. The urine accumulation in the tissues causes a violent inflammatory response that may result in sloughing of the skin of the ventral abdomen. To facilitate drainage, the surgeon should make several bold, longitudinal incisions lateral to the prepuce with a scalpel, being careful to avoid the subcutaneous abdominal veins (Figure 14.2G). This procedure assists in resolution of the inflammatory process.

Postoperative Management

Unless the animal is destined for immediate slaughter, antibiotics should be administered. Other supportive measures, such as intravenous fluids, diuretics, and general therapy for shock, may also be indicated. The animal should be sent to slaughter as soon as it is judged that the carcass would be acceptable.

Complications and Prognosis

This procedure is intended to salvage the animal until slaughter. Long-term survival rates are poor. Out of 85 cattle that underwent urethrostomies, only 35% were slaughtered at normal body weight or were kept for their intended purposes.[13] The remaining 65% died or were euthanized during surgery or within 2 weeks postoperatively because of recurrence. Another study deemed urethrostomy successful in less than half of the cases.[10] The rest of the cattle suffered relapses, were sold after a low gain of body weight, or died of unknown causes. The postoperative mortality rates in cattle that undergo urethrostomy and surgical repair of a ruptured bladder are high; most cattle survive less than 2 weeks.[13]

Hematoma Evacuation of the Bovine Penis

Relevant Anatomy

The fibroelastic bovine penis is approximately 1 m long with a quarter of the total length involved in the sigmoid flexure. The body of the penis is comprised of three columns of erectile tissue, the dorsally paired crura, and the urethra. The crura arise independently from one another at the ischial arch and converge in the body of the penis. The tunica albuginea encases the cavernous tissue of the crura to form the corpus cavernosum. The urethra and its surrounding vascularized tissue, the corpus spongiosum, run in a ventral groove formed by the union of the crura.

Penile hematomas usually result from a rupture of the tunica albuginea on the dorsal aspect of the distal bend of the sigmoid flexure, opposite the insertion of the retractor penis muscles.[14,15] Swelling due to a hematoma will usually occur near the distal sigmoid flexure, which in standing bulls is located near the base of the scrotum, or in the proximal half of the sheath.[14] The size of the defect in the tunica albuginea varies and is probably related to the amount of intracorporeal blood pressure at the time of rupture. The amount of extravasated blood may be related to the length of time erection is maintained after injury or more likely the number of subsequent attempts to achieve an erection. Practitioners should be warned against using an electroejaculator to extend a bull's penis when examining the bull for swelling of the sheath. Stimulation with the ejaculator will cause an immediately recognizable increase in the swelling. While the diagnosis is apparent, the bull is not better for the process.

Indications

Penile hematomas occur during breeding when the bull fails to achieve intromission into the female prior to the copulatory thrust, resulting in a bending of the erect penis.[14] Preputial prolapse frequently accompanies penile hematomas and has been reported as one of the most common presenting complaints from owners.[14,16] Medical treatment of penile hematomas consists of hot packs, warm hydrotherapy, penicillin therapy for 2 weeks, and ultrasound therapy to speed resorption of the hematoma.[14] Generally, the decision for surgery is made on the basis of the size of the hematoma, the length of time elapsed between the accident and treatment, and ultimately the value of the bull. It is believed that, with larger hematomas, more of the peripenile fascial layers are damaged or involved (this may be obvious at surgery); consequently, the incidence of adhesions or the risk of adhesion formation is greater. With a large hematoma, the attachment region of the retractor penis muscles is also involved. If palpation reveals involvement to this extent, surgical treatment will be necessary. Mechanical interference with penile extrusion may be a problem with a large hematoma.

The ideal time for surgery is probably an hour after injury. However, this is not practical because of the fasting required to prepare the mature bull to safely undergo general anesthesia. It is believed that bleeding quickly ceases after relaxation of the penis; therefore, waiting for so-called organization of the hematoma is not necessary. After 7–10 days, extensive granulation and increased fibrosis in the peripenile areas make surgery difficult. Although organization of the fibrous tissue may make the surgery easier after 25 days, as compared to 10–25 days, difficulty can still be anticipated. Clinical studies report that the success rate of surgery decreases greatly when the injury is more than 14 days old[16] and medical treatment may be more effective. Many of these injuries occur as bulls are pasture-breeding and owners may not detect the injury for some time after it occurs. The author has operated a number of these cases in which the maturity of the blood clot did not correlate with the owner's reported time of injury. As such, we would suggest the soonest possible surgery will lead to the best chance of return to function in any bull that economically warrants surgical treatment.

Anesthesia and Surgical Preparation

The surgery is performed with the animal sedated with xylazine (see Chapter 2) and cast in lateral recumbency, and with local infiltration (line block) at the surgical site (Figure 14.3A) or under general anesthesia, if available. General anesthesia allows for a more comfortable patient and subsequently easier to maintain aseptic technique which should decrease postoperative infections.

Surgical Technique

A skin incision approximately 13 cm long is made in a cranioventral direction over the most prominent part of the swelling (Figure 14.3A, B), and this incision is continued through the subcutaneous tissues into the hematoma. Care should be taken not to incise the penis because it may be deflected by the hematoma and may be closer to the skin than anticipated. The clots of the hematoma are removed manually (Figure 14.3C). In an acute case, the rent in the tunica albuginea is easily identified. If fibrin deposition and granulation tissue formation have occurred, however, careful dissection through the fascial layers surrounding the penis may be necessary to locate the rent in the tunic (Figure 14.3D). Care should also be taken to avoid any additional damage to the dorsal nerves of the penis by dissecting through the peripenile tissue down to the tunica albugenia on the lateral aspect of the penis and reflecting this tissue dorsally with the nerve included to expose the rent in the tunica albugenia. The bull is best served if the surgeon never sees the dorsal nerve. The edges of the rent in the tunica albuginea are debrided and are sutured with simple interrupted sutures of no. 0 or 2-0 synthetic absorbable suture. Alternatively some surgeons prefer closing the rent with a continuous bootlace pattern to minimize the knots present at the surgical site. Although secondary-intention healing and fibrous union of the defect would be anticipated without suturing, it is preferable to suture the defect because vascular shunts may form between the corpora cavernosum penis and the dorsal vessels.[17] Although a rupture, if it recurs, will probably recur at the same site,[15] it is questionable whether suturing the defect will actually reduce the chances of recurrence. Some have proposed suturing of the tunica albuginea to be unnecessary.[18] However, the author has experienced a higher return to breeding success rate with closure of the rent. The fascial layers of the penis are sutured with no. 2-0 synthetic absorbable sutures in a simple continuous pattern. The skin is closed with simple interrupted or vertical mattress sutures of nonabsorbable material (Figure 14.3E).

When preputial inflammation, swelling, or prolapse is present and problems with manual retraction of the penis are anticipated postoperatively, an umbilical tape suture is placed through the dorsal aspect of the penis under the apical ligament (Figure 14.3F) and tied. Care should be taken to ensure that the tape is not passed through the tunica abugenia or urethra. This tape facilitates postoperative manipulation of the penis if required.

Postoperative Management

Penicillin is administered postoperatively to reduce the possibility of abscess formation after the injury. If extensive swelling of the prepuce is present, it should be reduced by hot packs and bandaging. If the swelling has caused a preputial prolapse, ointment should be applied to the prolapsed prepuce and a sling or bandage should be used to decrease the swelling and facilitate reduction of the prolapse.

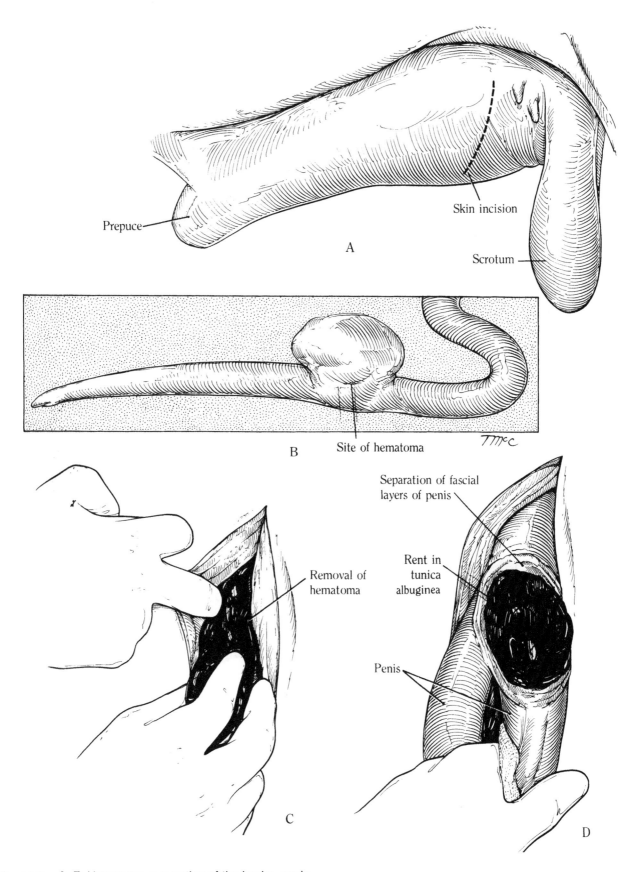

Fig. 14.3. **A–F.** Hematoma evacuation of the bovine penis.

Skin closure

E

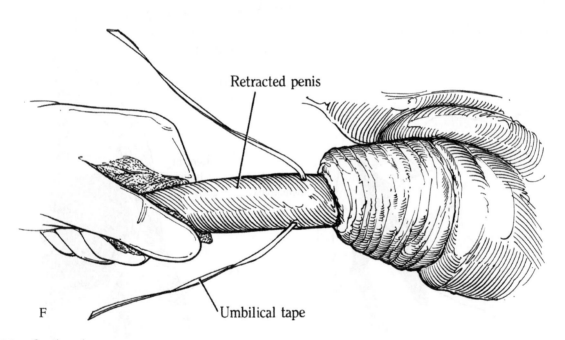

Retracted penis

Umbilical tape

F

Fig. 14.3. *Continued.*

Drainage of a seroma at the surgery site may occasionally be necessary, but seromas generally resorb spontaneously. The recommended period of sexual rest appropriate following surgery varies and ranges from 45–to 90 days. Another study reported a 40% recurrence of penile hematomas in bulls that underwent a period of sexual rest less than 2 months.[16] Most of these bulls are lost for the breeding season during which the injury occurs.

Complications and Prognosis

Hematomas may recur when the bulls are returned to service. The original injury frequently occurs in young, inexperienced (even clumsy) breeding bulls. When the rent in the tunica albuginea is closed adequately any recurrence of a hematoma is more likely due to the breeding actions of the bull than a failure of the repair. Injury of the dorsal nerves of the penis may cause failure to ejaculate or copulate, but recoveries up to 18 months later have been observed. The dorsal nerve may be damaged when the initial injury occurs or as a result of adhesions when the bull returns to breeding. Owners should observe the bull cover the first few cows when he is returned to breeding. Occasionally the bull will be seen to successfully breed 2–3 cows but then show signs of dorsal nerve damage by making searching motions with the penis but not the ejaculatory lunge. The nerve damage after successful service is probably due to a tearing of adhesions causing nerve damage when the penis is fully extended. Thrombus formation in the corpora cavernosa and formation of vascular shunts have also been proposed as causes of nonerection postoperatively,[17] although these problems likely occur more often following conservative treatment.

The literature supports a more favorable prognosis for surgical treatment of penile hematomas than medical treatment. One study reported that bulls that received surgical treatment were 2.8 times more likely to have a successful outcome than bulls treated medically.[16] Of the bulls with large hematomas (>20 cm wide), surgical treatment had an 80% success rate compared to the 33% success rate in medically treated bulls.[16] The method of treatment for small hematomas (<20 cm wide) did not differ in their respective success rates. Surgical evacuation of the hematoma may reduce the formation of adhesions and the risk of infection by removing a potential medium for bacteria.[16]

Preputial Resection and Anastomosis in the Bull

Terminology

It warrants discussion at this point that the terminology used to describe preputial resection in the bull is not used consistently in the veterinary literature. We will use the term circumcision for amputation of the prepuce with the penis retained within the preputial cavity. The term reefing will be used to describe resection of the prepuce with the penis extended with traction on the free portion of the glans penis. However, many of the leaders in the field of bovine reproductive surgery will use the term circumcision to describe preputial resection in the bull regardless of position of the penis and reefing as the equine procedure. Thus, it is crucial that the reviewer of the literature understand exactly which technique is used regardless of the terminology used to describe the procedure.

Relevant Anatomy

Anatomy relevant to this procedure is discussed in previous sections of this chapter.

Indications

Preputial amputation (circumcision) is indicated in selected cases of preputial prolapse with fibrosis and ulceration of the prepuce. The initiating factor in preputial damage is almost always a breeding injury. The preputial laceration will occur in the longitudinal direction on the ventral aspect of the penis as the bull attempts to breed a cow. The wound will contract and scar in the transverse direction. This natural process of wound healing is why the prolapsed prepuce will curve caudally or show what has been called an "elephant trunk" appearance. The breeds most often affected are the *Bos indicus* breeds (Brahman and Santa Gertrudis) and the polled *Bos taurus* breeds (notably Angus and Polled Hereford).[19] The two reasons advanced for the breed differences are a pendulous sheath and the absence of the retractor muscles of the prepuce in the polled breeds.[20,21] Protrusion of the parietal preputial lining followed by trauma or other irritation may produce inflammatory changes that ultimately prevent retraction of the prepuce.[20] Conservative treatment may be successful, but prolapse frequently recurs and eventually leads to chronic prolapse that requires surgical treatment. Prophylactic circumcision is also practiced in some areas.

Anesthesia and Surgical Preparation

Presurgical conservative treatment is usually necessary to reduce swelling and to improve the condition of the tissue. This treatment consists of hydrotherapy and some type of preputial support. One method of support is in essence a pressure bandage. The prepuce is coated with a lanolin-based ointment and covered with stockinette. A rubber tube is then placed in the preputial cavity extending from 2 cm outside of the prolapsed prepuce proximally to just above the level that the sheath starts to widen near the body wall, which will be the proximal extent of the bandage. Elastic adhesive tape is then used to very snuggly wrap from the distal aspect of the prolapsed prepuce up onto the haired sheath. One-inch standard adhesive tape can be wrapped around the distal aspect of the tube and incorporated into the elastic tape to help hold the tube in place. The free portion of the glans penis will be proximal to this wrap as will the proximal portion of the rubber tube. The bandage should be changed daily initially but then may be done every 2–3 days depending on how quickly the prepuce is responding to treatment. This is a very effective method to support the prolapsed prepuce and reduce swelling. This bandage must be monitored closely because, should the tube become displaced, the bull will pool urine in the preputial cavity. If he has a preputial laceration, there is a risk of pooled urine penetrating the laceration to contaminate the elastic tissues surrounding the penis. If this happens, sloughing of skin and uremia are probable. Alternatively, one may use a burlap snuggly connected by bungee cords (or bicycle tire inner tubes). One may use burlap off a roll or cut down one side and the bottom of a sack to have adequate size to support the sheath. The prepuce is again coated with ointment and covered with stockinette. One piece of burlap is placed over the back of the bull and the other under the ventral abdomen held together tightly enough to support the prolapsed prepuce up against the ventral body wall. This is also effective in reducing swelling. The bull can be treated twice a day with hydrotherapy and topical ointment. The sling can be rotated at each treatment so the urine-soiled ventral piece is moved dorsally to dry. If this sling fails for any reason, the effect is continued swelling only, as opposed to the catastrophic result of the tube being dislodged from the bandage.

Prior to surgery, fibrosis and edema are reduced to a minimal level, decreasing the risk of postoperative infection and failure. Feed is withheld from the bull 24–48 hours prior to surgery. Surgery is performed with the bull in right-lateral recumbency, either under general anesthesia or with a combination of xylazine HCl sedation and local analgesia. The surgical area is prepared for aseptic surgery in a routine manner.

Instrumentation

1. General surgery pack
2. Penrose drain

Surgical Technique

When performing the circumcision, the prolapsed portion of the prepuce to be resected is extended with the left hand, the index finger of which is placed inside the prepuce. (The line of amputation is indicated in Figure 14.4A.) Note that the amputation line is oblique, rather than transverse, so the resulting orifice is oval, rather than circular. This precaution reduces the danger of phimosis developing during healing. A row of horizontal mattress sutures of no. 0 or no. 1 synthetic absorbable suture is

placed around the prolapse immediately proximal to the proposed line of amputation (Figure 14.4A,B). The sutures are placed in such a manner that they overlap one another around the entire circumference and are passed from the exposed preputial skin completely through to the preputial cavity and back through both layers of the prepuce (Figure 14.4B). These sutures are tied to oppose the tissue, and the prepuce is amputated just distal to the suture line (Figure 14.4C). The preputial edges are then opposed with a simple continuous pattern suture line using a no. 0 synthetic absorbable suture material (Figure 14.4D).

It is convenient for the surgeon to perform this procedure on half of the prepuce at a time. The completed amputation (circumcision) is illustrated in Figure 14.4E.

Some cases are better treated by selected resection of affected prepuce with the penis extended. Many surgeons are more comfortable with this technique. The reefing technique in the horse is described in Chapter 10 of this text. After performing the technique in the bull, the surgeon would suture a Penrose drain over the end of the penis, with 4 simple interrupted sutures using 2-0 absorbable material, to allow urine flow to bypass the incision and to reduce the prepuce within the sheath. Then either a loose purse-string suture may be placed in the preputial orifice to maintain the prepuce and penis within the sheath or a bandage may be placed over a 6–8-inch segment of endotracheal tube within the preputial cavity as a stent with the Penrose drain exiting through the tube. The bandage is efficient in *Bos indicus* bulls with a pendulous sheath while bulls with a less-pendulous sheath will benefit from the purse-string suture.

Postoperative Management

The bull is placed on antibiotics, and the preputial cavity is infused daily with antibacterial agents until healing is complete, when a circumcision is performed. The flushing is not warranted when a reefing has been performed.

Complications and Prognosis

A study of 33 beef bulls that received circumcisions as treatment for preputial prolapse reported a 76% return to breeding soundness for 1 or more years after surgery.[22] Of the 33 bulls, 11 bulls developed one or more postoperative complications including incisional dehiscence, suture abscesses, and focal incisional hematomas.[22] In general, this technique of amputation is less successful in European breeds (*Bos taurus*) because the prepuce is too short. The loss of preputial length following surgery may prevent adequate extension of the penis to allow breeding. In less-severe cases, preputial prolapse may be treated by conservative resection of the preputial skin (reefing) and suturing the healthy internal preputial membrane near the preputial orifice. Larsen and Bellenger point out that circumcision results in the loss of equal amounts of the external

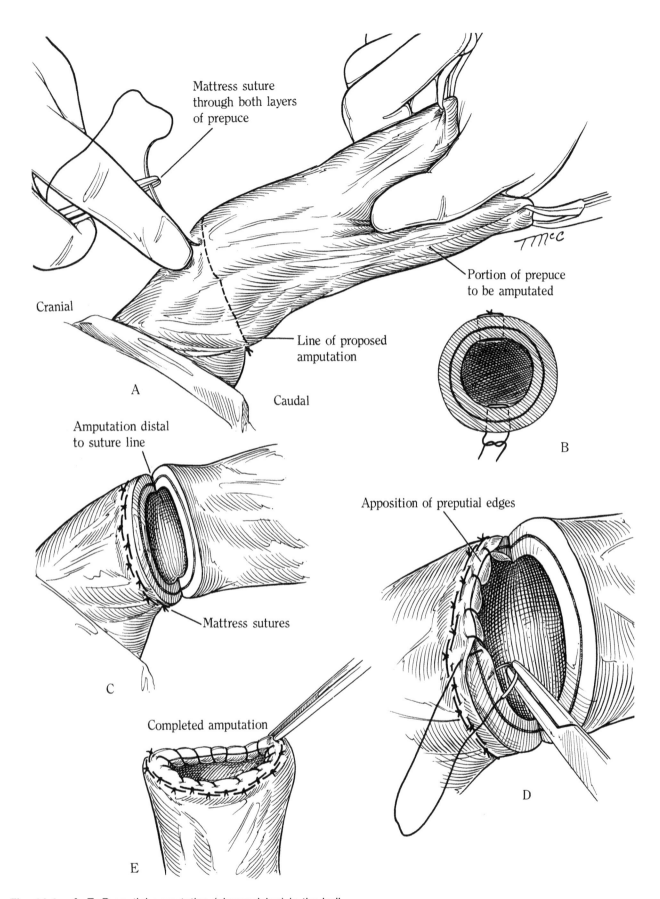

Mattress suture through both layers of prepuce

Portion of prepuce to be amputated

Cranial

Line of proposed amputation

A

Caudal

B

Amputation distal to suture line

Mattress sutures

C

Apposition of preputial edges

D

Completed amputation

E

Fig. 14.4. **A–E.** Preputial amputation (circumcision) in the bull.

and internal linings of the prolapsed portion of the prepuce even though the internal lining is frequently not seriously involved in the inflammatory process.[19] These authors advocate conservative resection, to preserve as much of the unaffected inner lining of the prolapsed prepuce as possible and thereby to increase the bull's chances of returning to service.

A technique for amputation of the prolapsed prepuce that is claimed to have advantages for the practitioner with limited facilities involves the insertion of a plastic ring into the preputial cavity.[15] The ring is fixed with sutures and a tourniquet-like effect is produced. The prolapsed portion is sloughed in 1–2 weeks. The author has seen severe strictures after this technique was used.

Surgical Techniques for Teaser Bull Preparation

Relevant Anatomy

Anatomy relevant to this section is discussed in previous procedures.

Indications

The role of teaser bulls for the detection of heat in cattle is uncertain. It is possible to use steers that have had testosterone administered to them. In addition, the increased use of prostaglandins may obviate the need for teaser bulls in an artificial-breeding program. Some producers still prefer using a teaser bull in their management system for various reasons. In the meantime, various techniques have been developed to render the bull sterile or incapable of coitus. The techniques that render the bull incapable of coitus seem to be more acceptable. In this chapter, we describe two popular techniques, penile translocation and penile fixation. We will also describe a newer technique of corpus cavernosum thrombosis which is performed on the standing bull with epidural anesthesia.[23] As a precaution, these techniques should be accompanied by a sterilization procedure, such as bilateral caudal epididymectomy, which is also described in this section.[15] One should consider making a new teaser bull every year about 30–60 days before the breeding season, considering the economics of wintering a nonproductive teaser bull and the higher libido of the younger animal.

It has been reported that teaser bulls prepared by penile translocation can occasionally serve a cow. Considering this possibility, we also describe the method of penile fixation, which produces an adhesion of the penis to the lower abdominal wall that prevents protrusion of the penis.[24]

Anesthesia and Surgical Preparation

This penile translocation procedure is performed with the animal under general anesthesia or heavy sedation and local analgesia. The bull is placed in dorsolateral recumbency and is tilted with its left side uppermost. A large area of the midline and ventral left-flank area, including the preputial orifice, is clipped and is prepared for aseptic surgery in a routine manner.

Penile fixation is usually performed with the animal tranquilized and under local anesthesia. The surgery can be done on a commercially manufactured operating table, if one is available, or it can be done with the animal cast in lateral recumbency. If done on the floor with the animal in lateral recumbency, the patient's feet must be tied for the safety of the surgeon. The ventral abdominal wall from the end of the sheath to the base of the scrotum is clipped and is prepared for aseptic surgery. A line block of local anesthesia (about 30 ml) is placed along a line where the sheath joins the body wall and about midway between the end of the sheath and the base of the scrotum (Figure 14.5A).

Corpus cavernosum penis (CCP) thrombosis is performed with the bull standing in a chute with the aid of epidural anesthesia. The perineal region is clipped and prepared for aseptic surgery.

Epididymectomy is generally performed with the animal standing in a chute. The distal area of the scrotum is clipped and is prepared for surgery in a routine manner. Local infiltration of analgesia is administered over the tail of the epididymis. Alternatively, epidural anesthesia negates the need for local anesthesia.

Instrumentation

1. General surgery pack
2. Sponge forceps
3. Sterile rubber gloves
4. Sterile obstetric sleeve
5. Sterile stomach tube for insertion within the prepuce to prevent urine contamination
6. Hoof acrylic (for CCP thrombosis)

Surgical Technique

Penile Translocation

The incision sites are illustrated in Figure 14.5A. A skin incision is made around the preputial orifice approximately 3 cm from the opening, and a ventral midline skin incision is extended caudad from this. The midline incision extends to within 5 cm of the level of the teats near the base of the scrotum (Figure 14.5A). Displace the prepuce and penis laterally when making the midline incision to avoid an unwanted incision into the preputial cavity. This incision is continued through the subcutaneous tissue; and the penis, prepuce, and surrounding elastic tissue are dissected free from the abdominal wall in preparation for translocation (Figure 14.5B). A sterile stomach tube placed within the preputial orifice helps to delineate the prepuce during dissection and may also help to

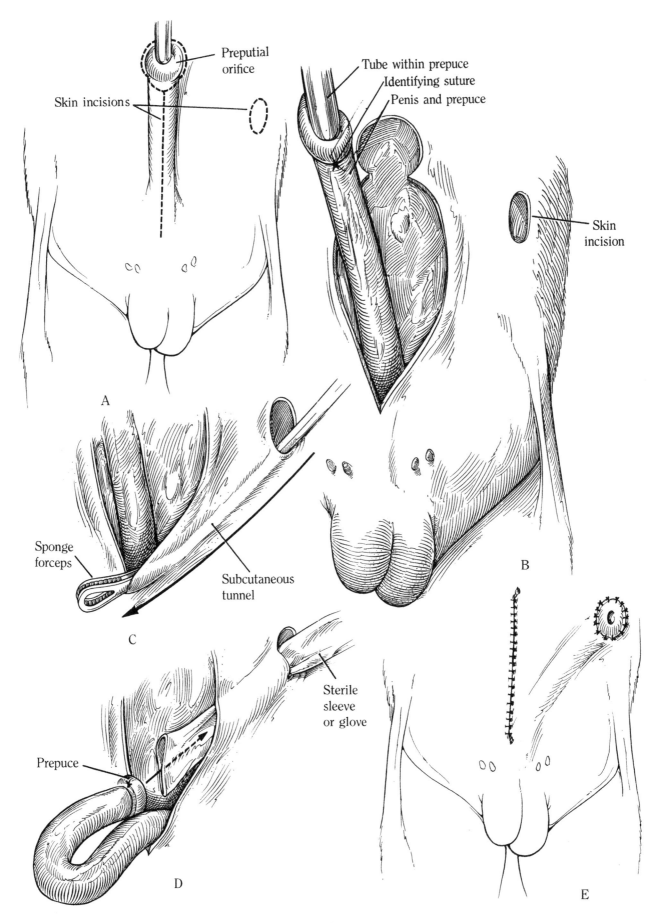

Preputial orifice

Skin incisions

Tube within prepuce
Identifying suture
Penis and prepuce

Skin incision

A

B

Sponge forceps

Subcutaneous tunnel

C

Prepuce

Sterile sleeve or glove

D

E

Fig. 14.5.   **A–E.** Teaser bull preparation by penile translocation.

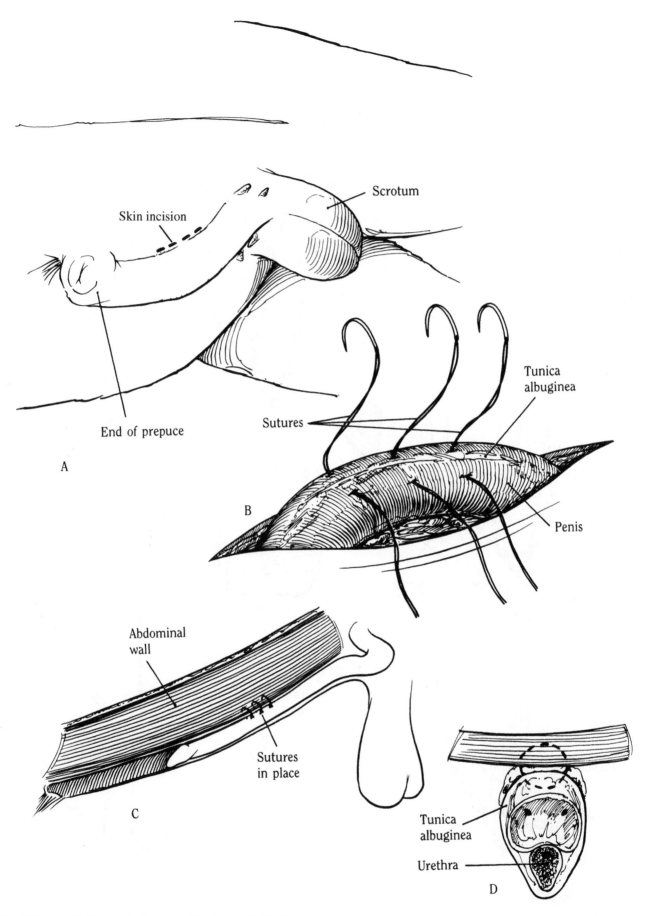

Fig. 14.6. A–D. Teaser bull preparation by penile fixation.

prevent urine contamination of the surgical area during surgery. During the dissection, it is important to maintain the integrity of the blood supply of the penis. Bleeding is controlled by ligation.

A circular skin incision is then made in the ventral left-flank area where the preputial orifice is to be moved (Figure 14.5B). Using a pair of sponge forceps, a tunnel is made from the circular incision through the subcutaneous tissues to the caudal end of the midline incision (Figure 14.5C). This tunnel must be large enough to permit the relocation of the penis and prepuce without restriction. If a tube had been positioned previously within the preputial orifice, it is removed at this stage. A sterile rubber glove may be placed over the preputial orifice. This prevents contamination of the subcutis from the preputial orifice as it is drawn through the tunnel. Alternatively, one may pull a sterile sleeve with the hand removed through the tunnel made by the sponge forceps (Figure 14.5D). Then the forceps are place inside the sleeve from the flank site to the midline incision where the preputial orifice is grasped with the forceps and pulled through the sleeve to the graft site. Then the sleeve is removed after the penis and prepuce are drawn through the tunnel and the skin of the preputial orifice is sutured to the circular skin incision (Figure 14.5E). Two layers of sutures are placed here: one in the subcutaneous tissue and one in the skin. Before suturing is performed, it is also important to ascertain that no twisting has occurred during the translocation process. This possibility can be prevented by preplacing an identifying suture in the skin of the prepuce prior to its removal (Figure 14.5B). The ventral midline incision is then closed with nonabsorbable sutures. Although closely placed simple interrupted sutures are illustrated in Figure 14.5E, an argument can be made for bringing the edges together with widely spaced sutures and allowing drainage. It is believed that the latter technique eliminates the problem of postoperative edema.

Because of the excess skin and pendulous sheath in Indian breeds of cattle, it is possible to transpose the penis and prepuce along with the encircling skin, rather than to dissect the penis and prepuce free from the skin.

Penile Fixation

A 10-cm longitudinal incision is made midway between the preputial orifice and the base of the scrotum at the junction of the sheath and the ventral body wall (about 2 cm lateral to the midline) (Figure 14.6A). This incision is made through the skin, subcutaneous tissue, and cutaneous trunci muscle. Blunt dissection through the loose connective tissue brings the surgeon to the dorsal surface of the penis. At this point, it is important to identify the urethra (urethral groove) within the penis. If the penis has not been rotated during the surgery, the urethral groove should be on the ventral surface of the penis. Because one must always be aware of the urethra during this procedure, it is often helpful to place a towel clamp

around the urethra and its adjacent portion of the penis. This serves to identify the urethra and also serves as a traction device.

The penis is exteriorized through the incision, and the preputial reflection is identified. The dorsal surface of the penis is cleared of its elastic tunics commencing at the preputial reflection and extending caudad for about 10 cm. This exposes tough fibrous tunica albuginea. Once tunica albuginea has been exposed, the linea alba is cleared of all of its loose connective tissue. The tunica albuginea of the dorsal surface of the penis is now apposed to the linea alba. Before placing the sutures, the surgeon should be sure that the glans penis and prepuce are not protruding through the preputial orifice. No. 2 nylon sutures are placed through the dorsal third of the penis (Figure 14.6B) and then through the linea alba. This suture apposes the linea alba and tunica albuginea (Figure 14.6C). Figure 14.6D illustrates in cross section the placement of the sutures. Care should be taken not to enter the preputial reflection and not to involve the urethra, to avoid iatrogenic urethral obstruction. Usually, three interrupted sutures are adequately placed about 1–2 cm apart. It is helpful to preplace these sutures and then to tie them simultaneously. The skin is closed with no. 1 or no. 2 monofilament synthetic suture.

This technique results in a permanent adhesion between the tunica albuginea and the linea alba. Ideally, the bull should have 2–3 weeks of sexual rest before use, to allow this adhesion to develop.

CCP Thrombosis

The bull is restrained in a squeeze chute and epidural anesthesia is administered. The hair is clipped over the perineal region from near the anus to the base of the scrotum at least 10 cm wide. The area is prepared for aseptic surgery. A midline incision is made 10 to 15 cm long to approach the sigmoid flexure at approximately the middle third of the prepared region. Sharp dissection of the skin, subcutaneous tissue and thick fascia of the thigh will expose the paired retractor penis muscles and the penis. The connective tissue surrounding the penis is bluntly dissected to allow retraction of the proximal bend of the sigmoid flexure through the skin incision. Identify the urethral groove at or just proximal to the proximal bend of the sigmoid flexure. Place a 14 gauge 1 ½ inch needle through the tunica albuginea from lateral to dorsal into the corpus cavernosum penis (CCP). Test inject sterile saline into the CCP to be sure it flows easily and to assure that slight filling of the CCP is detected. This direction of the needle and test injection is to help insure the surgeon does not inject the corpus spongiosum penis or urethra with acrylic. Then mix a soft acrylic which sets with a minimal exothermic reaction at setting.[a] Inject up to 10 ml of the acrylic into the

[a]Justi Products, 1200 Stellar Drive, Oxnard, CA 93033-3913.

CCP until filling of the tissue is appreciated. This creates an artificial thrombus within the CCP proximal to the sigmoid flexure which prevents the bull from achieving an erection. The penis will still extend (although not erect) when the bull mounts due to relaxation of the retractor penis muscles. To prevent this extension the distal bend of the sigmoid flexure is secured to the tough fascia of the thigh with no. 2 nonabsorbable suture by making a bite into the tunica abugenia of the penis on each lateral aspect. Take care to avoid the urethra. Also be sure when tying the suture knots not to retract the penis to the degree that urine flow is impeded. The skin incision is closed in a continuous pattern. An epididymectomy should then be performed. Skin sutures may be removed in 14 days. The bulls treated with this technique usually maintain libido and can be used for multiple breeding seasons if the owner so desires when taking into consideration the cost of feeding a nonproducing animal and the cost of creating another teaser bull the following year. The potential complications of this procedure include the occasional bull that will still achieve an erection, as well as acrylic leakage out of the CCP causing an abscess. The complication/failure rate is estimated to be less than 5%. Even the bulls that develop an abscess usually function well as teaser bulls after local treatment of the abscess.

Epididymectomy

The testis is forced manually to the distal segment of the scrotum, and a 3-cm skin incision made over the tail of the epididymis. This incision is continued through the common vaginal tunic until the tail of the epididymis is extruded (Figure 14.7A). The tail of the epididymis is dissected free from its attachment to the testis using scissors (Figure 14.7B). The ductus deferens is identified and clamped with forceps; and a ligature of nonabsorbable suture material is placed proximal to the forceps (Figure 14.7C). The ductus deferens is then transected at the level of the clamp. This procedure is repeated in the body of the epididymis so that the tail of the epididymis may be removed (Figure 14.7C).

The common vaginal tunic is closed in a separate layer using simple interrupted sutures of absorbable material, so the remaining part of the epididymis is retained within the tunic, but the transected end of the ductus deferens protrudes through the suture line (Figure 14.7D). The technique is an added precaution against reanastomosis of the reproductive tract. The skin is closed with 2–3 interrupted sutures of nonabsorbable material. The procedure is repeated on the other testis.

Some practitioners make this approach and simply clamp and guillotine cut to remove the tail of the epididymis, leaving the incisions open to drain and heal by secondary intention. The reanastomosis rate with this technique is likely higher than expected.

Postoperative Management

If penile translocation is performed, antibiotics may be administered at the discretion of the surgeon, and the skin sutures are removed in 10 days. Sutures may be removed 2–3 weeks following penile fixation. The animals are not put into work for 4–6 weeks. Skin sutures are removed in 14 days when the CCP thrombosis technique is used. These bulls can be used almost immediately although 2 weeks for skin incision healing before being placed into work is advised. Antibiotics are not administered routinely following epididymectomy. The bull may be placed into work in 3 weeks if epididymectomy is the only procedure performed. If placed in work earlier, however, the bull should be ejaculated prior to this for semen evaluation, to ensure the bull is sterile before use. Such measures are advised as liability precautions.

Complications and Prognosis

The long-term results of most techniques for teaser bull preparation have been criticized. The various charges against different techniques generally have not taken into account the probability of varying libido among bulls, however. Paraphimosis has been associated with the technique of penile translocation.[25] Successful results for penile fixation have been reported.[26] Potential complications include suture breakdown (if catgut is used), seroma formation, and insufficient retraction of the penis. Weight loss is also observed.[26] In the past, epididymectomy was commonly used as a sole procedure. It has been claimed, however, that these bulls often develop seminal vesiculitis or infections of the accessory genitalia, and they still ejaculate fluid from these glands during copulation. At present, the technique is used more often as insurance for one of the techniques that renders the bull incapable of copulation. If one chooses to use the epididymectomy alone, precautions should be taken to assure the bull does not have any venereal diseases that may be transmitted to the cows. Also, allowing the teaser bull to achieve intromission introduces contaminants into the vagina and likely decreases conception rates with artificial insemination.

Inguinal Herniorrhaphy in the Mature Bull

Relevant Anatomy

The inguinal canal is an opening in the caudal abdominal wall in between the internal oblique muscle and the pelvic tendon of the external oblique aponeurosis.[27] In the bovine, the canal itself is considered to be nearly absent compared to other domestic species. In the normal male, the inguinal canal contains the testicular artery and vein, ductus deferens, and nerves of the spermatic cord. The vaginal tunic that encloses these structures and the testes

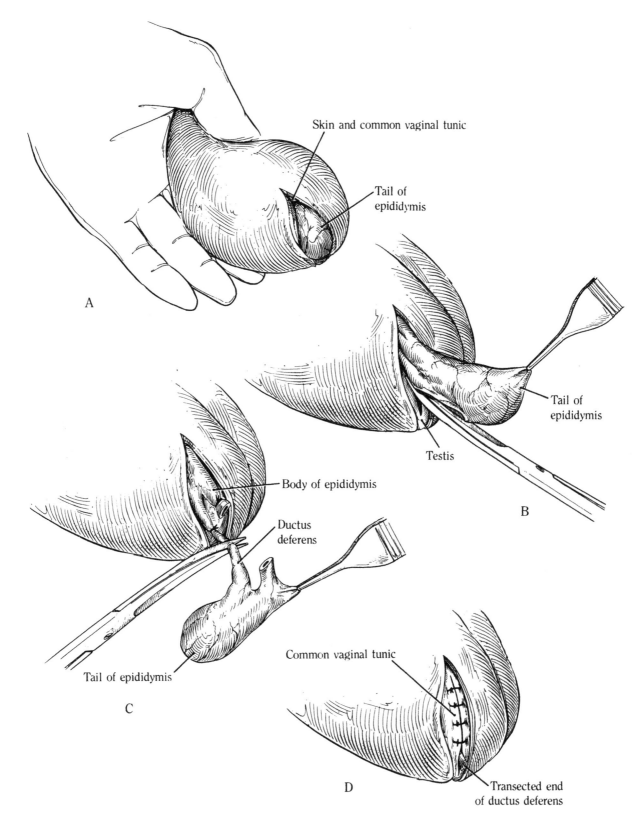

Skin and common vaginal tunic

Tail of
epididymis

A

Tail of
epididymis

Testis

B

Body of epididymis

Ductus
deferens

Tail of epididymis

C

Common vaginal tunic

Transected end
of ductus deferens

D

Fig. 14.7.   **A–D.** Epididymectomy.

is formed by an evagination of the peritoneum through the inguinal canal.

Indications

Inguinal herniation occurs when a loop of small intestine, occasionally omentum, or both, passes through the vaginal ring and into the canal and may be verified by rectal palpation. If the intestine and/or omentum protrude all the way into the scrotum, it is termed a scrotal hernia. Inguinal hernias may be further classified as direct and indirect. An indirect hernia occurs when the intestinal loops are contained within the tunica vaginalis, whereas a direct hernia occurs when the hernial sac is separate and cranial to the vaginal ring. Most hernias in the bull are indirect, but direct hernias are also seen. Unlike the stallion, an inguinal hernia in a bull seldom causes intestinal obstruction or vascular compromise, so the bull usually does not show clinical signs of discomfort. One exception is when the tunica vaginalis ruptures, allowing intestine within an indirect hernia to escape the tunic and fill the subcutaneous area of the scrotum. The intestine can fill the scrotum distending it 5 times or more the normal size. The intestine does become incarcerated, and the bull will show signs of abdominal discomfort as well as metabolic deterioration.

Inguinal hernias in the bull occur with greater frequency on the left side and are generally unilateral. (Figure 14.8A shows the external appearance of a left-sided inguinal hernia.) The inguinal canal of bulls in good condition is occupied by a substantial amount of adipose tissue, and this must be distinguished from an inguinal hernia.[15] A definitive diagnosis of inguinal hernia cannot be made simply by palpating the scrotum, because many bulls have external deposits of adipose tissue in this region. Sometimes, deposits of adipose tissue are seen with an inguinal hernia, and the hernia itself is initiated by a protrusion of subperitoneal adipose tissue through the inguinal ring.[28] Some form of trauma may also be responsible for initiation of an inguinal hernia.

Another method of repair of inguinal hernia in the bull involves a flank laparotomy.[28] The hernia is reduced by the removal of viscera from the vaginal ring; and long, sterile, nonabsorbable suture material, such as umbilical tape, is introduced into the abdominal cavity and placed in the inguinal ring. Care is taken not to strangulate the spermatic cord as it passes through the vaginal ring. If adhesions are present, this method will not be successful. Moreover, placing sutures is awkward because of the constant presence of abdominal viscera at the surgical site.

A third method of treating inguinal hernia in the bull is unilateral castration which will be described later in this text. This technique allows closure of the inguinal ring without worry of leaving it too large so that herniation recurs or leaving it too small so that vascular compromise to the testicle occurs. Bulls will produce roughly 75% of the sperm with one healthy testicle that was produced with two. This is not always the case but should be part of the decision-making when treating a bull with an inguinal hernia.

Instrumentation

1. General surgery pack
2. Sterile umbilical tape, no. 2 nylon suture, or no. 2 polypropolene suture

Anesthesia and Surgical Preparation

This surgical procedure is best performed with the animal under general anesthesia and in lateral recumbency, with its hind quarters slightly elevated to aid in reduction of the hernia (Figure 14.8B). The uppermost hind limb is secured in an upward direction and caudad, to improve exposure of the surgical area. A less-satisfactory alternative is sedation with xylazine hydrochloride supplemented with local anesthesia (see Chapter 2). The inguinal area is clipped and is prepared for aseptic surgery in a routine manner. The surgical site is draped.

Surgical Technique

A 15- to 25-cm horizontal incision is made through the skin and subcutaneous tissue over the external ring at the base of the scrotum, and hemostasis is maintained by ligation of blood vessels. A blood-free field assists progression of the surgery. Blunt dissection is performed down to the external inguinal ring, to free the common vaginal tunic from the surrounding tissue. The boundaries of the ring are isolated.

If the hernia has reduced itself when the bull is positioned for surgery, then it is not necessary to incise the common vaginal tunic (Figure 14.8C). If adhesions of the viscera have occurred within the scrotum, then it is necessary to incise the common vaginal tunic to reduce the hernia. An incision is made through the common vaginal tunic parallel to the spermatic cord and cranial to the external cremaster muscle. The hernial contents are examined, and any adhesions are broken down. Occasionally, adhesions are so severe that circulation to intestines has been compromised and intestinal resection is required. These bulls are usually presented to the surgeon on an emergency basis for intestinal obstruction. The bowel is replaced into the abdominal cavity once the surgeon has ensured that no adhesions are present at the external inguinal ring.

If the hernia is direct, located cranial to the neck of the scrotum, the subcutaneous tissue is separated, revealing the hernial contents. Adhesions are broken down to enable reduction of the hernia.

The hernial ring is repaired using no. 2 nylon or polypropolene suture or sterile double 1/8-inch umbilical tape in a simple interrupted pattern. The aim of suturing is to reduce the size of the external inguinal ring so

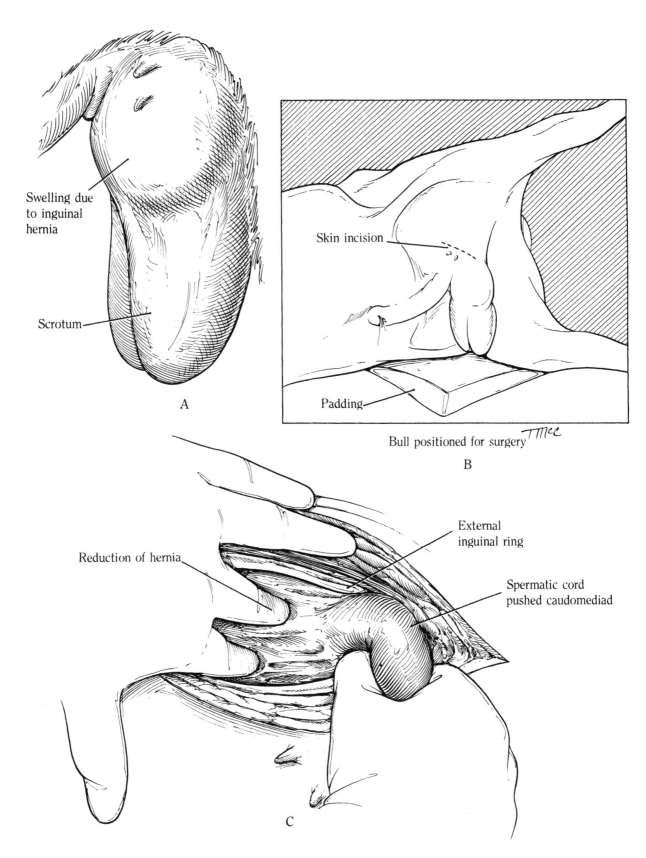

Fig. 14.8. **A–G.** Inguinal herniorrhaphy in the bull.

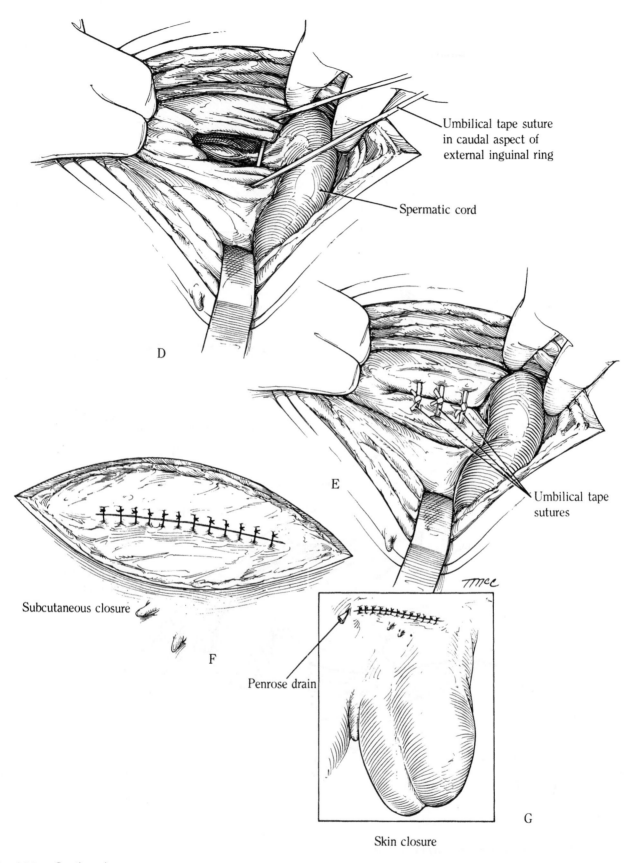

Umbilical tape suture in caudal aspect of external inguinal ring

Spermatic cord

D

E

Umbilical tape sutures

Subcutaneous closure

F

Penrose drain

Skin closure

G

Fig. 14.8. *Continued.*

reherniation does not occur. Generally, 2–3 sutures in the cranial aspect of the ring are required. The sutures are tied, but are not placed under excessive tension. The spermatic cord should be positioned in the caudomedial part of the canal. The remaining ring should be of sufficient size to allow the contents of the spermatic cord to pass freely, yet prevent recurrence of the hernia. As a rule of thumb, there should be enough room for the spermatic cord and one finger. Naturally, hooking any portion of the spermatic cord with the sutures should be avoided. The first suture to be placed is the one closest to the spermatic cord, and it is generally placed about 1 cm from the spermatic cord through the medial and lateral edge of the external inguinal ring (Figure 14.8D). The sutures, which do not penetrate the peritoneum, are all preplaced by leaving the ends long and clamping the free ends with forceps. Then the sutures are tied (Figure 14.8E).

If the common vaginal tunic is entered to reduce the hernia, it is closed using fine (0 or 00) absorbable suture material in a simple continuous pattern.

Subcutaneous closure is performed using no. 0 or no. 1 synthetic absorbable suture (Figure 14.8F). The use of a Penrose drain is indicated because of the considerable amount of dead space. The skin is closed using a synthetic monofilament suture in a simple interrupted pattern (Figure 14.8G).

Postoperative Management

Generally, antibiotics are not indicated unless there is a break in aseptic technique or an intestinal resection is performed. Considerable postoperative swelling generally occurs within 24 to 48 hours. Swelling is more severe if adhesions were present. This swelling usually responds to hydrotherapy (warm) and exercise.

The bull is confined to a clean stall for 4 weeks following surgery, and exercise should be limited for about 8 weeks. The bull should not be used for breeding for 3–6 months, pending the result of semen evaluation.

Complications and Prognosis

The most outstanding advantage of this method is that, if adhesions are present, they can be broken down and the affected bowel freed. A small survey of nine bulls admitted to the Colorado State University Veterinary Teaching Hospital for inguinal hernia repair showed that five of the nine had adhesions. These five bulls required incisions into their common vaginal tunics to reduce the hernias.

Unilateral Castration

Relevant Anatomy

The anatomy of the bull scrotum and testes has been described earlier in this text.

Indications

Unilateral castration of a mature bull may be indicated in any case of unilateral scrotum abnormality. Such cases would include inguinal hernia, hydrocele, hematocele, testicular trauma, or tumor such as mesothelioma.[29] Any unilateral condition that will negatively impact the thermoregulation and thus sperm quality produced by both testicles is an indication for unilateral castration. Removal of the abnormal testicle should allow resolution of the associated inflammation and then normal sperm production from the remaining testicle, if it has not been permanently damaged.

Instrumentation

1. General surgery pack

Anesthesia and Surgical Preparation

Unilateral castration is best performed with the bull under general anesthesia in lateral recumbency on the contralateral side from the affected testicle. The upper hind limb may be held in abduction or caudally to allow easier access to the scrotum. The scrotum and inguinal region is clipped and prepped for sterile surgery. Strict attention should be paid to aseptic technique as any postoperative infection or incisional complication may be detrimental to the remaining testicle.

Surgical Technique

An elliptical incision is made over the length of the testicle on the lateral side of the scrotum. One may make the initial incision a single linear cut then modify it to an elliptical one prior to closing the incision. The incision is made through the skin and subcutaneous tissue to expose the testicle leaving the common vaginal tunic intact. One must take care not to incise the median raphe or cause any damage to the contralateral testicle. The affected testicle is bluntly freed from the scrotum. Then the spermatic cord and tunic may be double ligated as proximal as possible. If the disease process has caused inflammation and fibrosis of the vaginal tunic, the surgeon may open the vaginal tunic in order to securely ligate the spermatic cord. Many surgeons prefer to use an emasculator distal to the ligatures to crush the cord before removal of the testicle. If the procedure is being done because of an inguinal hernia, the incision is extended proximally so the external inguinal ring may be visualized and closed with 3–4 interrupted sutures after the testicle has been removed.

The skin incision may be modified to remove more scrotal skin before closure begins. The subcutaneous tissue is closed using no. 0 absorbable suture in a simple continuous pattern. Several layers of subcutaneous tissue closure, usually three, are used to adequately ablate the dead space left by removal of the testicle. The skin is closed using no. 3 supramid in a continuous interlocking pattern. Some surgeons place a drain in this site and leave the distal end of the incision open. We do not believe the drain is necessary if one avoids any break in aseptic technique and adequately obliterates the resulting dead space. In fact, use of a drain and partial closure may prove to cause more complications from ascending contamination than is avoided by providing drainage.

Postoperative Management

The bull may receive perioperative antibiotics. Skin sutures should be removed in 14 days. The animal should be monitored closely for any incisional complications. One should also be sure the remaining testicle moves freely in the scrotum. If too much skin is removed via the elliptical incision, free movement of the testicle may be inhibited. If this occurs, one must manipulate the testicle into the distal scrotum occasionally until the scrotal skin heals and stretches enough to facilitate normal movement of the testicle.

A semen evaluation should be performed no less than 90 days after surgery. Note the bull will not pass a breeding soundness exam because of the single testicle and scrotal circumference. However, if the semen quality is good, the bull should not have fertility problems.

Complications and Prognosis

The postoperative period is usually uneventful. Certainly, surgical infections and incisional complications are concerning and must be treated if they occur. If the remaining testicle has not suffered any permanent damage during the disease process that led to the unilateral castration, it should produce approximately 75% of the total sperm produced by both healthy testicles.

Cesarean Section in the Cow

Relevant Anatomy

The anatomy of the bovine uterus is very similar to that of the mare, which is described in Chapter 10. Compared to the mare, the uterus of ruminants has a relatively short body and long horns. The body appears deceptively longer because the horns travel together for approximately a third of their length before actually bifurcating externally.[30] The uterine artery, a branch of the internal iliac artery, is the main blood supply to the uterus. The uterus is also in part supplied by the ovarian artery at the tubal ends of the horns and by the vaginal artery in the caudal portion of the body. Branches of these vessels also form anastomoses with the uterine artery.

Indications

Cesarean section is indicated in various types of dystocia (including those caused by relative fetal oversize when the pelvic inlet in young heifers is too small to allow delivery), deformities of the maternal pelvis, fetal monsters, induration of the cervix, fetal malposition, hydrops amnii and allantois, uterine torsion, and emphysematous fetuses. Cesarean section may be performed as an elective procedure in some situations, such as prolonged gestation or, in the case of a potentially valuable calf, when a dystocia is anticipated. In many cases, the choice between fetotomy or cesarean section may depend on the clinician's relative experience with either technique. Case selection is also important. The cow that has suffered a long period of fetal manipulation or attempts at fetotomy and is systemically compromised is not a candidate for cesarean section.

Different approaches are indicated in various dystocia situations.[31,32] The left paralumbar or flank approach is the standard incision for a viable or recently expired, uncontaminated fetus and a cow capable of tolerating surgery while standing. In some situations, right-flank laparotomy is indicated if there is marked distention of the rumen or when clinical examination dictates that removal from the right side would be more convenient. For example, an oversized fetus situated in the right side of the abdominal cavity would be difficult to remove by left-flank incision. In the routine case, however, the left-flank incision is more convenient because fewer problems with encroaching bowel are encountered.

In the case of a dead and emphysematous fetus, a ventral approach should be used. A ventral paramedian incision, the most common ventral approach, requires the cow to be placed in dorsal recumbency. Still some surgeons prefer a ventral midline approach with the cow tilted 30–40 degrees off straight dorsal. Another alternative is the ventrolateral oblique approach, which may be performed with the animal in lateral recumbency. All three techniques reduce contamination of the peritoneum, which may occur during removal of the emphysematous, contaminated fetus and its associated debris. The ventral approaches are also indicated if the animal is recumbent and is considered incapable of standing during surgery or if the animal is so unmanageable that it is too dangerous for the operator to stand beside the patient during surgery.

Anesthesia and Surgical Preparation

Cesarean section in the cow is performed with the animal under local analgesia. If the flank approach is used, a paravertebral block, inverted L block, or a line block may be used. For the paramedian approach, a high epidural, inverted L block, or line block may be used. A line block is used for the ventral midline approach. Casting with a rope, with or without sedation, is a supplementary restraint for cows in which a ventral approach is used. The surgical area is clipped and is prepared for aseptic surgery in a routine manner.

Instrumentation

1. General surgery pack

Surgical Technique

Cesarean section in the cow may be performed in standing, if a chute is present, or in recumbency. Both approaches for flank laparotomy and ventral paramedian laparotomy are described in Chapter 13. The ventral midline approach simply allows an incision and closure of the linea alba avoiding the rectus abdominus muscle. The exact location of the incision is adapted for performing cesarean sections. For example, the incision is more ventral for the flank approach (Figure 14.9A) and farther caudad for the ventral paramedian or midline approach. The ventral paramedian incision is made midway between the midline and the subcutaneous abdominal vein and extends from the umbilicus caudad to the mammary gland (Figure 14.9B) (as opposed to the ventral paramedian incision for abomasopexy, which extends from the umbilicus craniad to the xiphoid process). The left and right flank standing approaches have inherent risks, such as rumen prolapse with the left flank approach and small intestine evisceration through the right flank approach. The recumbent approach is preferred in many instances because it allows the uterus to be completely exteriorized, is more advantageous for extracting oversized fetuses, and is associated with a lower incidence of abdominal contamination than in standing.[31] A left oblique flank approach in the standing cow has been described that may be useful for extracting large calves or for when the uterine contents are contaminated. This specific approach is described in detail elsewhere.[33] Following entrance into the peritoneal cavity, the surgeon manipulates a portion of the uterine horn containing the fetus and attempts to exteriorize an area for hysterotomy. Exteriorization is often not possible. Many times, it is helpful to grasp a leg within the uterus and to use it as a handle to lift the uterus. The uterine incision is usually made over a limb, but in certain malpositions, the area over the head may be incised. The uterus should not be incised over a limb that is in the body of the uterus, but rather, as close to the tip of the horn as possible. This technique allows the uterine horn to be exteriorized for suturing. Incisions near the body of the uterus must be sutured within the abdominal cavity.

Figure 14.9C depicts exteriorization of an appropriate part of the uterus through a flank incision. Such exteriorization would not be possible with a swollen, emphysematous fetus. In these cases, the need for a ventral approach in which the uterus can be apposed more closely to the incision is obvious. When the uterus is positioned satisfactorily, it is incised (Figure 14.9C). The incision needs to be long enough to allow removal of the fetus without further tearing or extending the uterine incision. The incision should be made parallel to the long axis of the uterus and on its greater curvature because this area has the fewest large vessels. An attempt should also be made to avoid incising caruncles. The fetus is then removed. The surgeon attempts to retain the uterus so the fetal fluids do not fall back into the peritoneal cavity (Figure 14.9D). Although not depicted in Figure 14.9D, chains are commonly attached to the limb(s) of the calf to assist in its delivery from the uterus. These chains should be placed around the cannon bone just proximal to the fetlock and a half hitch placed over the pastern to minimize orthopedic trauma to the fetus.

The fetal membranes should only be removed if they can be separated from the uterus without undue traction or if they are lying free within the uterus.

The uterus is closed with a continuous inverting pattern and absorbable suture material. The Utrecht method of uterine closure is presented here and is illustrated in Figure 14.9E–N. This technique was developed at the University of Utrecht, the Netherlands, as part of a study to improve the fertility of cattle following cesarean section.[34] It was noted that adhesions often developed between the uterus and visceral organs and originated most often at the ends of the incision where exposed knots were tied. Adhesions also developed along the suture line when suture patterns were exposed. Moreover, uterine healing occurred across the wound edges, rather than on the apposed peritoneal surfaces, and the inflammatory response varied with the suture material. The Utrecht method of suturing was developed as a result of these findings.

The starting knot is made using oblique bites (Figure 14.9E, F), to bury the knot within the inverted suture (Figure 14.9G). Similarly, the continuous suture pattern is inserted using oblique bites (Figure 14.9H–J), so there is minimal exposure of suture material but close apposition of the wound edges. Figure 14.9K–N depicts the insertion and tying of the final knot so that it is not exposed. Using the Utrecht method, fertility rates improved from 75–92%. One surprising feature was that no. 6 nonchromic catgut produced the best results.[34] With this technique, it is important that each suture be pulled tightly following its insertion. Otherwise, the wound edges may gap, and the contents of the uterus may leak. Regardless of the suture pattern used, the rapidly shrinking uterine wall will leave less tissue in each bite of the suture material and may thereby loosen the suture.

We have questioned the rationale behind the use of large-diameter plain catgut suture material because it is more reactive than chromic catgut or one of the synthetic absorbable materials. One of the reasons that adhesions may be fewer with this material is the time factor. With the abundant blood supply to the involuting uterus, the suture material is probably absorbed so quickly that adhesions have less chance to form than when suture materials

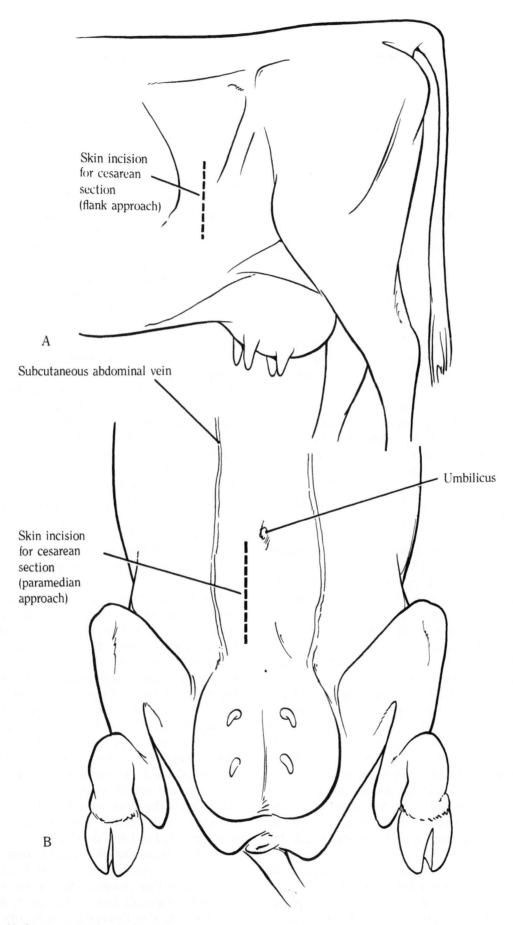

Skin incision for cesarean section (flank approach)

A

Subcutaneous abdominal vein

Umbilicus

Skin incision for cesarean section (paramedian approach)

B

Fig. 14.9. **A–N.** Cesarean section in the cow.

Flank incision

Uterus

C

D   Uterus

Fig. 14.9.   *Continued.*

E

F

G

H

Utrecht method of uterine closure

Fig. 14.9. *Continued.*

I

J

Fig. 14.9. *Continued.*

K

L

M

TMCC 81

N

Fig. 14.9. *Continued.*

remain in situ for long periods of time. Newer sutures, such as polyglytone 6211 (Caprosyn), that have rapid absorption patterns with less inflammation are even better.

The knots are the last portion of the suture line to be absorbed, probably because cellular invasion is more difficult. Therefore, burying the knots at each end of the incision should always be the goal with this suture pattern.

Once the uterus is closed, it is replaced in position. The laparotomy incision is closed as described in Chapter 13.

Postoperative Management

Antibiotics are administered, and oxytocin may be administered anytime after uterine closure, to enhance uterine involution. Fluid therapy may be indicated in certain cases.

Complications and Prognosis

In dairy cattle, there is some evidence that temporary reductions in milk production may occur postoperatively.[35] Adhesions between the uterus and the surrounding tissue have been shown to occur in roughly half of all cesarean sections, regardless of whether catgut or Vicryl suture was used for closure of uterus.[36]

Retention Suturing of the Bovine Vulva (Buhner's Method)

Relevant Anatomy

The female bovine external genitalia is basically the same as described for the horse in Chapter 10.

Indications

Vaginal or cervical prolapse occurs with the greatest frequency during the last trimester of gestation in cows. The condition may also occur during early postpartum or estrus, however. Prolapses are usually classified by the duration of the condition and the extent of the prolapse. For example, first-degree vaginal prolapse involves only intermittent exposure of the vaginal floor, usually occurring when the cow is lying down. Second degree vaginal prolapse infers that the vaginal floor is continuously exposed. The urinary bladder may or may not be retroflexed to be included in the prolapsed tissue but urination may be impeded if the urethra becomes occluded. Third-degree vaginal prolapses involve a continuous exposure of the vaginal floor and the cervix through the vulva. Third degree prolapses in *Bos indicus* and *Bos taurus* breeds have been differentiated based on the observation that third-degree prolapses in *Bos indicus* are usually primary prolapses of the cervix that have not progressed from a first- or second-degree vaginal prolapse. The *Bos taurus*

breeds, however, usually will progress from a first- or second-degree prolapse to a third-degree prolapse. Of the prolapsed tissue, the cervical os is usually located most dorsally and an extremely edematous vaginal floor most ventrally. A fourth-degree prolapse is described as either a first- or second-degree prolapse of a long enough duration that the prolapsed tissue has become necrotic.

The buried purse-string suture (Bühner method) is a simple and effective way to retain vaginal or uterine prolapse in the cow.[37,38] The method consists of a deeply placed circumferential suture that effectively simulates the action of the constrictor vestibular muscle.[37] The purse-string suture may be permanent or temporary. It is strong and does not tear out as frequently as externally placed suture patterns (lacing, Halsted, and quill). These methods promote infection along the suture line, although this infection generally is of minor significance. Bühner perivaginal suture tape, or umbilical tape, is commonly used for the purse-string suture. When the tape has been removed or has disintegrated, the fibrous connective tissue produced by the cow in response to the tape is often sufficient to prevent future prolapse. Infrequently, the scar tissue may be strong enough to result in dystocia.[37] The Bühner perivaginal tape is more expensive than umbilical tape, but is made of nylon and so lies flat and is better tolerated by tissues. Umbilical tape tends to become twisted and form a string, and it is more likely to cut through the edematous tissues of the vulva. Bühner perivaginal tape can remain as a permanent suture, whereas umbilical tape may disintegrate if left in the tissues.

There are several alternative methods for retention following a vaginal or cervical prolapse that are described in detail elsewhere.[39] The Minchev technique is used to anchor the anterior dorsal vagina to the gluteal area by passing heavy suture through the anterior dorsal vaginal wall, the sacrosciatic ligament, and the skin in the gluteal area. This technique does not restrict the vaginal opening like the Bühner method but may still permit prolapse of the vaginal floor or result in necrosis of the dorsal wall in which the sutures are passed.[39]

Anesthesia and Surgical Preparation

The cow should be restrained in a chute or crush, and some cows may be recumbent during the procedure. The surgery is performed with the animal under caudal epidural analgesia (see Chapter 2). Following administration and onset of the epidural analgesic, the perianal area and prolapsed tissues are cleaned and treated with an antiseptic. Osmotic agents and massage may then be used to reduce the size of the prolapse. Some cases with significant edema in the prolapsed tissue will benefit from a short-term pressure wrap and dorsal support to help alleviate the edema. If the bladder is included in the prolapsed vagina such that the urethra is obstructed, one should lift the prolapsed vagina dorsally which will straighten the urethra and allow the bladder to empty thus decreasing the size of the prolapse.

Instrumentation

1. General surgery pack
2. Bühner or Gerlach perivaginal needle
3. Perivaginal suture tape or sterile, 1-cm (half-inch) umbilical tape

Surgical Technique

A typical prolapse is depicted in Figure 14.10A. The prolapse is reduced, the vagina is returned to its correct anatomic location, and the perianal area is scrubbed once again. A transverse skin incision about 1 cm long is made midway between the dorsal commissure of the vulva and the anus. Another horizontal incision is made about 3 cm below the ventral commissure of the vulva. The perivaginal needle is introduced into the ventral skin incision and is driven perivaginally through the deep subcutaneous tissues parallel to the vulva. One hand is placed in the vagina to guide the needle. The needle should be driven as deep as possible (about 5–8 cm) and directed out the dorsal skin incision (Figure 14.10B). A piece of sterile perivaginal suture tape (or sterile umbilical tape) soaked in a suitable antibiotic solution, is threaded through the eye of the needle and is drawn down to emerge through the ventral skin incision (Figure 14.10C). At the same time, the tape is held at the dorsal incision, so the end is not lost in the tissue. The tape is then removed from the needle, and the needle is threaded up the contralateral side of the vulva (about 5–8 cm) to emerge through the dorsal incision. The tape is threaded into the eye of the needle once again (Figure 14.10C), and then the needle is withdrawn ventrally, resulting in two free ends of tape emerging from the ventral skin incision.

The two free ends of the tape are tied, ensuring that the loop of tape at the dorsal incision is buried (Figure 14.10D). The tape is tied so the resulting suture encircling the vulva will admit 2–3 fingers. If a square knot is used to anchor the tape, the knot will bury itself. This minimizes the chances of contamination of the suture material and thereby avoids a wicking effect with the suture and secondary infection. The dorsal and ventral incisions may be closed with a simple interrupted suture of nonabsorbable material, to further decrease the chances of secondary infection around the umbilical tape. If the cow is close to calving, we recommend that the tape be secured in the ventral incision with a bow knot. This knot allows the suture to be removed or, at least, undone to reduce tension at the time of parturition. One of the other methods to retain the prolapse may also be used. One should also consider two separate stab incisions ventrally for placement of the needle if the cow is pregnant so the suture is not buried and can be easily untied or cut. In pregnant

cows that will be returned to the range or pasture to calve, we use a double strand of gut suture instead of Bühner tape. The gut suture will break at parturition while the Bühner tape will not. The disadvantage of using the gut suture for this situation is that the suture may fail prior to calving.

Postoperative Management

The cow requires close observation to time removal or loosening of the suture correctly in relationship to parturition. The knot should be untied, and the vulva should be gently dilated to reduce tension on the suture.[37]

Complications and Prognosis

The Bühner method of repair for vaginal prolapse offers secure retention of the vagina and cervix with the convenience of quick release during calving. Calving through Bühner sutures is one of the most severe complications of this procedure and can result in severe lacerations and damage to the vulva and perineal area. Certain cattle that have a pendulous vulva may be predisposed to edema, swelling, and even necrosis of the vulva following Buhner method of repair due to the increased tension required to retain the vagina and cervix.

Cervicopexy for Vaginal Prolapse (after Winkler)

Relevant Anatomy

The external genitalia of the female bovine is basically the same as in the horse described in Chapter 10. During this procedure, the attachment of the prepubic tendon just cranial to the pelvic symphysis may be palpated through the floor of the vagina. It extends ventrad and craniad from its attachment at an angle of about 90° to the horizontal plane (Figure 14.11A).

Indications

Another method for retaining a prolapsed vagina in the cow is a technique in which the external os of the cervix is sutured to the prepubic tendon. The main advantage of the technique is that postoperative treatment is minimal.[40,41]

Anesthesia and Surgical Preparation

This procedure is performed using epidural anesthesia. Following restraint of the cow in a chute or crush, an epidural anesthetic is given, and the prolapsed tissues are cleaned, treated with the appropriate medication, and replaced.

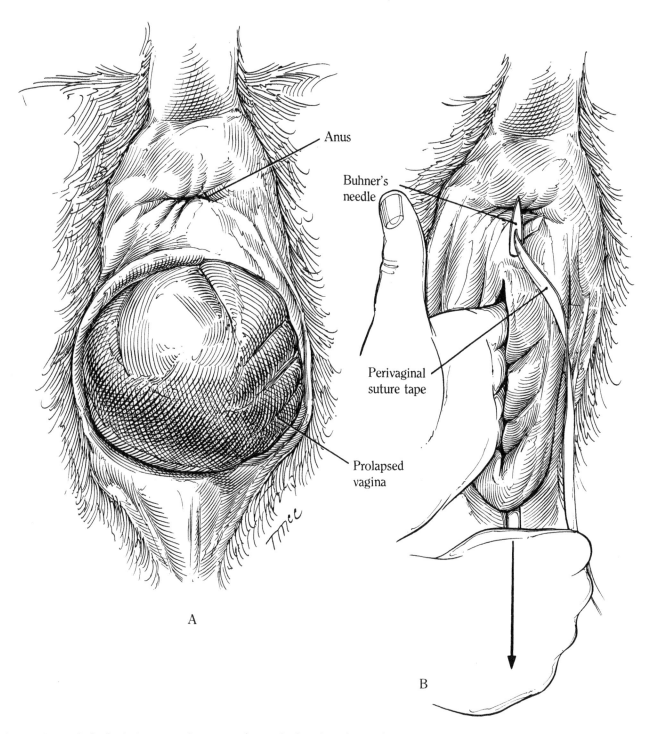

Fig. 14.10.   **A–D.** Buried purse-string suture for vaginal and uterine prolapse.

Fig. 14.10. *Continued.*

Instrumentation

1. General surgery pack
2. 8.0-cm, half-circle cutting needle that has been bent into a U-shape
3. At least 1.2 m of nonabsorbable suture material

Surgical Technique

The prepared needle is carried into the vagina by hand. The urethra and bladder are located (preferably by inserting a urinary catheter, rather than by simple palpation),

to ensure placement of the suture lateral to these structures.

The point of the needle is directed through the floor of the vagina below the vaginal end of the cervix. As originally described, the needle is directed through a triangular area toward the midline back up through the tendon and vaginal floor. This triangular area is formed by a short band of the prepubic tendon that extends caudolaterad, attaching to the iliopubic eminence of the pubis (Figure 14.11B). To decrease the possibility of breaking the needle, however, it is recommended to pass the needle down through the prepubic tendon and up through the

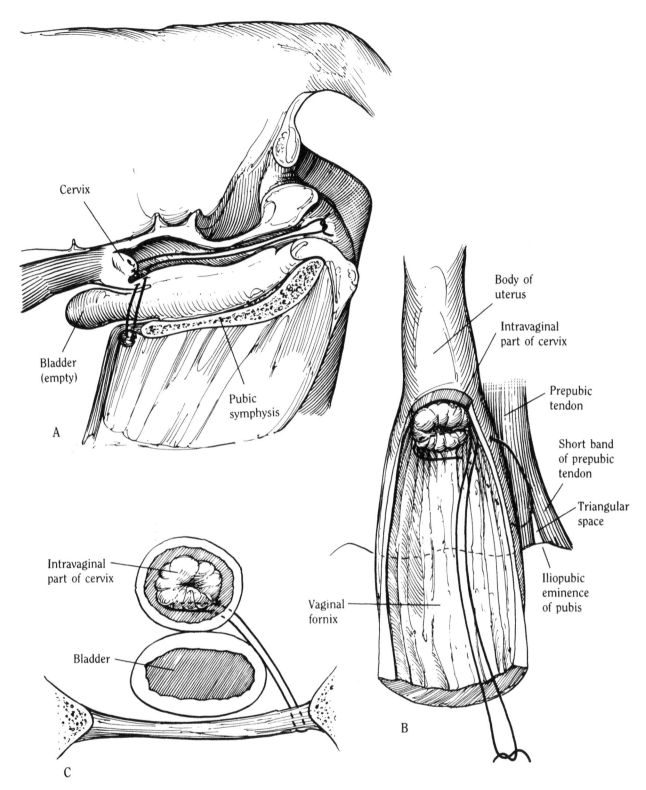

Fig. 14.11. **A–C.** Cervicopexy for vaginal prolapse.

triangular space in a medial-to-lateral direction. A bite of 1.8 cm in the prepubic tendon and 3.5–5.0 cm in the vaginal floor is usually adequate. The needle and suture are pulled through the prepubic tendon and vaginal wall sufficiently to continue the suture through the intravaginal part of the cervix. Tension should be applied to the suture to see whether it is adequately anchored in the prepubic tendon. A urinary catheter should be reintroduced into the bladder to ensure that the bladder and urethra have not been included in the suture. The needle is then directed across the lower half of the cervix at least 1.2 cm (0.5 inch) cranial to the caudal limits of the intravaginal part of the cervix. The suture ends are exteriorized, and the first throws of a surgeon's knot are performed and are then advanced craniad, tight enough to prevent caudal movement of the cervix (Figure 14.11C).

A modification of the Winkler technique is a two-person procedure in which one person works with a hand within the vagina while a second person makes a caudal right flank laparotomy incision.[39] The first person passes the curved needle through the floor of the vagina into the abdominal cavity where the second uses the needle to make the bite into the prepubic tendon. The needle is then passed back through the floor of the vagina where the first person places the bite into the cervix as described and ties the knot. The knot should be tied within the vagina for ease of removing the suture if needed. This modification allows for certainty in placement of the prepubic suture bite and minimizes the potential for including intestine or other unwanted tissue in the suture. It also decreases the chance of the U-shaped needle breaking or being lost in the abdominal cavity.

Postoperative Management

The cow should be given appropriate antibiotic therapy.

Complications and Prognosis

This procedure can be used in cows in which external retention techniques have been unsuccessful. Postoperative tenesmus has been minimal or completely absent with this technique. Embryo collection from cows treated in this manner is more difficult than in normal cows but can be done successfully. The retention suture will frequently tear out of the cervix at calving if a treated cow is allowed to carry a pregnancy and vaginally deliver. The suture will usually remain in position for an extended time if cows are not allowed to vaginally deliver. In one cow, the suture was still present when the cow was slaughtered (for unrelated reasons) 7 years after repair of the prolapse.[39]

Peritonitis has been associated with this technique when umbilical tape is used, and a suture of less capillarity is recommended. Care must be taken not to deviate too far from the midline when placing the suture through the

tendon; otherwise, inadvertent penetration of arteries of the pelvic cavity may result.

References

1. Zacharias, J.R., Baird, A.N., and Hawkins, J.F. Theriogenology question of the month. Unilateral abdominal cryptorchidism. *J. Am. Vet. Med. Assoc.*, *229*(6):937–939, 2006.
2. Stafford, K.J., and Mellor, D.J. The welfare significance of the castration of cattle: A review. *N. Z. Vet. J.*, *53*:271–278, 2005.
3. Coventry, J., McEwan, D., and Bertram, J.D. Sterilization of bulls with lactic acid. *Aust. Vet. J.*, *66*:156–157, 1989.
4. Hill, G.M., Neville, W.E., Richardson, K.L., Utley, P.R., and Stewart, R.L. Castrations method and progesterone-estradiol implant effects on growth rate of suckling calves. *J. Dairy Sci.*, *68*:3059–3061, 1985.
5. Finnerty, M., Enright, W.J., Morrison, C.A., and Roche, J.F. Immunization of bull calves with a GNRH analog-human serum albumin conjugate: Effect of conjugate dose, type of adjuvant and booster interval on immune, endocrine, testicular and growth-responses. *J. Repro. Fertil.*, *101*:333–343, 1994.
6. Fisher, A.D., Knight, T.W., Cosgrove, G.P., Death, A.F., Anderson, C.B., Duganzich, D.M., and Matthews, L.R. Effects of surgical or banding castration on stress responses and behavior of bulls. *Aust. Vet. J.*, *79*:279–284, 2001.
7. Thuer, S., Mellema, S., Doherr, M.G., Wechsler, B., Nuss, K., and Steiner, A. Effect of local anesthesia on short- and long-term pain induced by two bloodless castration methods in calves. *Vet. J.*, *173*:333–342, 2005.
8. Earley, B., and Crowe, M.A. Effects of ketoprofen alone or in combination with local anesthesia during the castration of bull calves on plasma cortisol, immunological, and inflammatory responses. *J. Anim. Sci.*, *80*:1044–1052, 2002.
9. Dyce, K.M., Sack, W.O., and Wensing, C.J.G. Textbook of Veterinary Anatomy, 3rd Ed. Philadelphia, Saunders, 1996.
10. Gasthuys, F., Martens, A., and De Moor, A. Surgical treatment of urethral dilatation in seven male cattle. *Vet. Rec.*, *138*:17–19, 1996.
11. Blood, D.C., Henderson, J.A., and Radostits, O.M. Veterinary Medicine, 5th Ed. Philadelphia, Lea & Febiger, 1980.
12. Walker, D.F. Penile surgery in the bovine: Part I. *Mod. Vet. Pract.*, *60*:839, 1979.
13. Gasthuys, F., Steenhaut, M., De Moor, A., and Sercu, K. Surgical treatment of urethral obstruction due to urolithiasis in male cattle: A review of 85 cases. *Vet. Rec.*, *133*:522–526, 1993.
14. St. Jean, G. Male reproductive surgery. *Vet. Clin. N. Am.: Food An. Pract.*, *11*:55–91, 1995.
15. Walker, D.F., and Vaughan, J.T. Bovine and Equine Urogenital Surgery. Philadelphia, Lea & Febiger, 1980.
16. Musser, J.M.B., St. Jean, G., Vestweber, J.G., and Pejsa, T.G. Penile hematoma in bulls: 60 cases (1979–1990). *J. Am. Vet. Med. Assoc.*, *201*:1416, 1992.
17. Young, S.L., Hudson, R.S., and Walker, D.F. Impotence in bulls due to vascular shunts in the corpus cavernosum penis. *J. Am. Vet. Med. Assoc.*, *171*:643, 1977.
18. Pearson, H. Surgery of the male genital tract in cattle: A review of 121 cases. *Vet. Rec.*, *91*:498, 1972.
19. Larsen, L.H., and Bellenger, C.R. Surgery of the prolapsed prepuce in the bull: Its complications and dangers. *Aust. Vet. J.*, *47*:349, 1971.

20. Arthur, G.H. Wright's Veterinary Obstetrics, 4th Ed. Philadelphia, Lea & Febiger, 1975.

21. Long, S.E., and Hignett, P.G. Preputial eversion in the bull: A comparative study of prepuces from bulls which evert and those which do not. *Vet. Rec.*, *86*:161, 1970.

22. Baxter, G.M., Allen, D., and Wallace, C.E. Breeding soundness of beef bulls after circumcision: 33 cases (1980–1986). *J. Am. Vet. Med. Assoc.*, *194*:948–952, 1989.

23. Riddell, M.G. Prevention of intromission by estrus-detector males. *In* Large Animal Urogenital Surgery, 2nd Ed. Edited by F.W. Dwight, H.D. Moll. Baltimore, MD, Williams & Wilkins, 1998, pp. 335–343.

24. Belling, T.H. Preparation of a "teaser" bull for use in beef cattle artificial insemination program. *J. Am. Vet. Med. Assoc.*, *138*:670, 1961.

25. Baird, A.N., Wolfe, D.F., and Angel, K.L. Paraphimosis in a teaser bull with penile translocation. *J. Am. Vet. Med. Assoc.*, *201*:325, 1992.

26. Hoffsis, G., and Maurer, L.M. Evaluation of the penis tie-down method to prepare teaser bulls. *Bovine Pract.*, *11*:78, 1976.

27. Dyce, K.M., Sack, W.O., and Wensing, C.J.G. Textbook of Veterinary Anatomy, 3rd Ed. Philadelphia, Saunders, 2002.

28. Frank, E.R. Veterinary Surgery, 7th Ed. Minneapolis, Burgess, 1964.

29. Heath, A.M., Baird, A.N., and Wolfe, D.F. Unilateral orchidectomy in bulls: A review of eight cases. *Vet. Med.*, *91*(8):786–792, 1996.

30. Wenzel, J.G.W. Anatomy of the uterus, ovaries, and adnexa. *In* Large Animal Urogenital Surgery, 2nd Ed. Edited by D.F. Wolfe, H.D. Moll. Baltimore, MD, Williams & Wilkins, 1998, pp. 375–380.

31. Noorsdy, J.L. Selection of incision site for cesarean section in the cow. *VM/SAC*, *75*:530, 1979.

32. Schultz, L.G., Tyler, J.W., Moll, H.D., and Constantinescu, G.M. Surgical approaches for cesarean section in cattle. *Can. Vet. J.*, *49*(6):565–568, 2008.

33. Parish, S.M., Tyler, J.W., and Ginsky, J.V. Left oblique celiotomy approach for cesarean section in standing cows. *J. Am. Vet. Med. Assoc.*, *207*:751–752, 1995.

34. Ball, L. Personal communication, 1979.

35. Newman, K.D., and Anderson, D.E. Cesarean section in cows. *Vet. Clin. North Am.: Food Anim. Pract.*, *21*:73–100, 2005.

36. De Wit, F., Raymakers, R., Westerbeek, J., Mijten, P., and De Kruif, A. A study of uterine adhesions following suturing of the uterus with catgut or vicryl in cesarean sections in cattle. *Tijdschr. Diergeneeskd.*, *118*:478–479, 1993.

37. Hudson, R.S. Genital surgery of the cow. *In* Current Therapy in Theriogenology. Vol. 2. Edited by D.A. Morrow. Philadelphia, W.B. Saunders, 1986, p. 348.

38. Sloss, V., and Duffy, J.H. Handbook of Bovine Obstetrics. Baltimore, MD, Williams & Wilkins, 1980.

39. Wolfe, D.F., and Carson, R.L. Surgery of the vestibule, vagina, and cervix. *In* Large Animal Urogenital Surgery, 2nd Ed. Edited by D.F. Wolfe, H.D. Moll. Baltimore, MD, Williams & Wilkins, 1998, pp. 397–412.

40. Hudson, R.S. Genital surgery of the cow. *In* Current Therapy in Theriogenology, Vol. 2. Edited by D.A. Morrow. Philadelphia, W.B. Saunders, 1986, p. 350.

41. Winkler, J.K. Repair of bovine vaginal prolapse by cervical fixation. *J. Am. Vet. Med. Assoc.*, *149*:768, 1966.

Chapter 15

BOVINE GENERAL SURGERY

A. N. Baird, DVM, MS, DACVS

Objectives

1. Describe some surgical procedures used in treatment of common disorders in cattle including septic arthritis and diseases of the digit, extensive neoplasia of or trauma to the eye, pericarditis, and teat lacerations.
2. Provide a technique for cosmetic dehorning.

Digit Amputation

Relevant Anatomy

In ruminants, the lateral and medial digits of each limb are connected through tough skin and interdigital ligaments until the level of the coronary band, where the distal phalanges of each digit are encased within the hoof. The distal (interdigital) collateral ligament spans the interdigital space at the level of the distal sesamoid bones and travels over the tendons of the deep digital flexor muscle to the abaxial surfaces of the middle phalanges.[1] The proximal interdigital ligament connects the axial surfaces of the proximal phalanges.[1] The distal interphalangeal joint (DIP) of each digit is formed by the articulation of two distal sesamoid bones, the distal phalanx, and the middle phalanx. There are two bursas associated with the DIP joint. The dorsal bursa lies deep to the tendon of the common digital extensor muscle, and the palmar (plantar) bursa lies deep to the tendons of the deep digital flexor and the distal sesamoid bones and associated ligaments.[1] Sepsis of the DIP joint in particular is a common pathological condition of the bovine foot and frequently necessitates surgery. Penetrations of the interdigital cleft by a foreign object, termed an interdigital phlegmon, and extensions of sole diseases, such as ulcers, are common causes of septic arthritis. The lateral digit bears more weight than the medial digit in the hind limb while the medial digit bears more weight in the forelimb. Unfortunately, in clinical studies, most cases requiring digit amputation occur in the lateral digit of the hind limb for reasons that are not fully understood.

Indications

The following are indications for amputation of the bovine digit: severe foot rot unresponsive to antibiotics and complicated by osteomyelitis; abscess formation with osteoarthritis of the distal interphalangeal joint, tenosynovitis, or infectious arthritis and sepsis of the proximal or distal interphalangeal joints; severe phalangeal fractures; and dislocations of the phalangeal joints.[2,3]

This surgical procedure is indicated to relieve pain and to return the animal to soundness and production, as well as to prevent ascending infection of the limb. The prognosis for digit amputation is good and most cattle return to productivity rapidly; however, the survival period is not as favorable as some other techniques. Facilitated ankylosis is described elsewhere as an alternate technique to digit amputation and is successful in many cattle.[4,5] Ankylosis produces a longer survival period; however, digit amputation is still used for economical reasons and rapid recovery.[3]

The following are contraindications for digit amputation: sepsis of the fetlock joint; involvement of both digits of the same foot; and heavy bulls or cows (these animals generally break down the remaining claw). Cows with amputated digits are usually culled sooner than herdmates and have a lower market value.

The same basic technique of digit amputation is applicable to pigs and small ruminants.

Anesthesia and Surgical Preparation

The animal is usually placed in lateral recumbency by means of ropes and chemical restraint, or it is secured to a surgical table, with the affected claw uppermost. The procedure may be performed with the animal standing, but this is not generally recommended. The limb is clipped from the midmetacarpal region or midmetatarsal region distad, and the area is prepared surgically prior to administering local anesthesia. The claw and interdigital space are cleared of all fecal material and debris; a scrub brush and hoof knife are useful for this initial preparation. Intravenous local analgesia is the preferred method of local desensitization (see Chapter 2), but regional nerve blocks or a ring block may also be used. Following administration of the local anesthetic, the surgical site is given a final surgical scrub. If the intravenous analgesic technique is not used, a tourniquet (rubber tubing) is applied at this stage. The limb is draped so the foot is exposed, and a sterile glove may be applied over the claw, so it can be handled by the surgeon during surgery.

Instrumentation

1. General surgery pack
2. Obstetric wire saw or Gigli wire saw

Surgical Technique

The technique illustrated in Figure 15.1 uses a skin flap and attempted closure. The skin incision is made along the abaxial and axial surface of the coronary band; then vertical incisions are made cranially and caudally (Figure 15.1A). The skin and subcutaneous tissues are incised to the bone. The skin incision on the axial surface is made first so as not to obscure the surgical field with blood. The skin is then dissected free from the underlying digit, and one attempts to save as much of the skin flap as possible. Some prefer a different skin incision in which only one vertical incision is made on the abaxial surface of the digit after the horizontal incision along the coronary band. The cranial and caudal flaps made by this incision are undermined and retracted by towel clamps while the Gigli wire is crossed near the dorsal aspect of this incision to remove the digit as described later. The corners of these two flaps can then be excised to allow partial closure of the skin incision. Alternatively, a circumferential skin incision can be made in a similar plane to the wire cut illustrated in Figure 15.1B,C.

The amputation may be performed in two locations. A low amputation is performed when only the coffin joint and distal phalanx are diseased; this amputation is directed through the middle phalanx. We describe the technique of high amputation, which is used in cases with involvement of the coffin joint, distal phalanx, pastern joint, and middle phalanx. This amputation is directed through the junction of the middle and distal third of the proximal phalanx.

An obstetric saw is placed in the incision in the interdigital space. An assistant is needed for the sawing procedure (Figure 15.1B). The amputation is commenced with the wire saw directed parallel to the long axis of the limb until the wire is located at the distal end of the proximal phalanx. The saw is directed perpendicular to the long axis of the proximal phalanx to seat the wire in the bone, and then the position of the wire is directed so it is approximately 45° to the long axis of the proximal phalanx (Figure 15.1C). The sawing motion should not be too rapid because heat necrosis of tissues, including bone, may occur, leading to excessive sloughing during the healing period. Care should be taken to avoid invading the fetlock joint capsule. Once the digit has been removed, excess interdigital adipose tissue and all necrotic tissue, especially that involving the tendons and tendon sheaths, should be dissected sharply from the wound. If the digital artery can be located, it should be ligated.

Some of the skin flap may be sutured down, but when the surgical site is swollen from infection and when some skin necrosis is present in the region, this is not usually possible. Complete closure is contraindicated because infection will resolve more rapidly if the skin flap is not completely sutured, to allow better ventral drainage (Figure 15.1D).[6] The value of skin flaps and of any attempt at closure has been questioned.[7] An antibiotic powder is applied to the area and is followed by sterile gauze sponges. A tight bandage is applied to prevent hemorrhage when the tourniquet is removed (Figure 15.1E), and some form of impervious covering may be indicated.

Postoperative Management

The bandage should be changed 2–3 days after surgery. The limb is kept bandaged until the wound has healed. The length of time the wound will need to be bandaged depends on the individual case and to what degree the wound was left open. Some cases of digit amputation may require only 10–14 days to heal, whereas others may require several more weeks for the wound to heal by secondary intention.

In the initial stages of healing, the animal should be housed in dry conditions where food and water are easily accessible to avoid overuse of the remaining digit. Penicillin or another broad spectrum systemic antibiotic may be administered.

Digit Amputation via Disarticulation

More recently a technique of digit amputation via disarticulation has been described.[8] The indications, anesthesia and preparation are as described above.

Instrumentation

1. Scalpel or sterile postmortem knife

Skin incision

Gigli (or obstetric) wire saw

A

B

C

D **Skin flap**

E

Fig. 15.1. **A–E.** Digit amputation in cattle.

Surgical Technique

A horizontal skin incision is made at the level of the proximal interphalangeal joint. The incision is continued to the bone and joint capsule to sever the collateral ligament and tendons. As traction is placed on the digit the incision is continued to the axial collateral ligament. Care is taken not to disturb the contralateral digit. The fat pad is excised, and large vessels are ligated, if identified. The advantages of this procedure include the lack of need for assistance in using the obstetrical wire and the quickness of the procedure.

Postoperative Management

A pressure wrap is placed on the site before releasing the tourniquet. The bandage is changed in approximately 3 days, and the wound is left open to heal by secondary intention unless there is some hemorrhage present when the bandage is changed. In that case the patient is out of a bandage as soon after the procedure as possible.

Complications and Prognosis

The most common complications of digit amputation are reduction in milk production in dairy cattle for the first 60 days postoperatively, ascending tendonitis, and development of disease on the remaining digit.[9]

In one study, in the authors' opinions, a good recovery from surgery was achieved in 51% of cattle that underwent digit amputation. Poor recovery was deemed in 22% of cattle with the remainder of the cattle having a fair recovery.[3] The mean survival time of cattle recovering from digit amputation ranges from 68 days to 20 months.[3,9] Heavy cattle (greater than 680 kg) generally have a much poorer prognosis for digit amputation.[5]

Eye Enucleation

Relevant Anatomy

The anatomy of the eye can be divided into the structures of the eyeball (globe) and the adnexa. In the procedure described here, the adnexal structures are emphasized as the eyeball itself is removed. Structures of the adnexa include ocular muscles, orbital fasciae, the eyelids, conjunctiva, and the lacrimal apparatus. The eyelids have three basic layers; the outer skin, a fibromuscular layer, and the palpebral conjunctiva. The palpebral conjunctiva, together with the bulbar conjunctiva, comprises the conjunctival sac. The dorsal and ventral distal extremities of the sac are called fornices. The third eyelid attaches to a T-shaped plate of cartilage on the medial aspect of the eyeball. Between the dorsolateral wall of the orbit and the eyeball is the lacrimal apparatus.[1] Several accessory glands of the lacrimal apparatus exist but are detailed in other anatomy texts.[1]

The muscles responsible for moving the eye are all located near the optic foramen behind the eyeball, except for the ventral oblique muscle. The ventral oblique muscle originates on the ventromedial wall of the orbit and passes laterally below the eyeball. The four rectus muscles all insert anterior to the equator of the eye at a dorsal, ventral, medial, and lateral site. The retractor bulbi muscle inserts posteriorly on the eyeball and envelopes the optic nerve.

The locations of the ophthalmic and maxillary nerves are also relevant to this procedure for local anesthesia of the eye. These nerves enter the orbit with the extraocular muscles through the foramen orbitorotundum, which is a combined round and orbital foramen that is unique to bovine species. This is the site of injection for anesthesia during eye extirpation.

Indications

Although the operation is called an enucleation of the eye, it is, for all practical purposes, an extirpation because everything within the orbit is generally removed; there is no demand for cosmetic repair as in other species. Enucleation involves the removal of the globe, leaving adipose tissue and muscles, whereas extirpation involves removal of everything within the orbit: globe, muscles, adipose tissue, and lacrimal gland. Extirpation in cattle is indicated for neoplasia (usually squamous cell carcinoma) of the upper and lower eyelids, third eyelid, and cornea that is too extensive to be removed by other, less-radical operations such as lid resections, H-plasties, or superficial keratectomies. Septic panophthalmitis, severe trauma beyond repair, and severe trauma with loss of globe contents are also indications for enucleation.

Anesthesia and Surgical Preparation

The animal, which is wearing a halter, should be adequately restrained in a chute and its head secured to one side. Prior to administering the retrobulbar block, the surgeon clips the hair around the animal's eyes and prepares the surgical site aseptically. Local anesthesia is administered by infiltration of the retrobulbar tissues. The four-point retrobulbar block is performed by injecting through the eyelids, both dorsally and ventrally, and at the medial and lateral canthi (Figure 15.2A). A slightly curved, 8- to 10-cm, 18-gauge needle is directed to the apex of the orbit where the nerves emerge from the foramen orbitorotundum. About 40 ml of local anesthetic are injected, divided into 10 ml per site. Exophthalmos, corneal anesthesia, and mydriasis indicate a satisfactory retrobulbar block.[10] Other surgeons use the Peterson retrobulbar eye block for this procedure. The four-point retrobulbar technique is quick and easier to administer.

Because this particular surgical procedure is performed for large, necrotic, ocular neoplasms or severe trauma, proper aseptic preparation of the surgical site may be impossible. Generally, draping is not performed for this procedure. If there are large amounts of necrotic, neoplastic tissue, then some of it may be trimmed prior to the surgical scrub.

Instrumentation

1. General surgery pack

Surgical Technique

Following surgical preparation, the patient's eyelids are grasped with towel clamps and are closed to minimize contamination of the surgical field. A recommended alternative is to suture the eyelids together and to leave the suture ends long. Sutures provide a better seal from necrotic debris than towel clamps. Using these methods, the instruments or ends of the sutures can be used to put traction on the eye throughout surgery. A transpalpebral incision is made around the orbit, leaving as much normal tissue as possible (Figure 15.2B). The incision is generally 1 cm from the margin of the eyelid. The ventral incision and subsequent dissection are done first. Sharp or blunt dissection is used for 360° around the orbit continuing down to the caudal aspect of the orbit, but avoiding entrance through the palpebral conjunctiva (Figure 15.2C). All muscles, adipose tissue, the lacrimal gland, and fascia are removed, along with the eyelids and eyeball. If the indication for enucleation is neoplasia, then one must make sure that all neoplastic tissue is removed. If the eye is enucleated for a non-neoplastic condition, such as irreparable trauma, then the surgeon can afford to leave some of the retrobulbar tissue, to reduce the amount of dead space and intraoperative hemorrhage.

The optic artery may be ligated; but most surgeons would consider that unnecessary as hemorrhage is controlled by tight skin closure and subsequent pressure as the orbit fills with blood in the dead space, which is impossible to obliterate. The cavity fills with a blood clot that will organize during the healing period and will leave a large depression in the orbit.

Closure consists of a layer of continuous interlocking sutures in the skin using synthetic nonabsorbable suture material (Figure 15.2D). Sutures are removed 2–3 weeks postoperatively. The tight seal with a skin suture seems to allow pressure to build up within the orbit and to create hemostasis through a tamponade effect. Some surgeons prefer to use an absorbable suture in the skin, to obviate the need for suture removal; this would be useful on the range, where it may be impractical to round up the animal for suture removal.

Postoperative Management

Antibiotics are indicated if sepsis is present. If dehiscence occurs, granulation tissue will generally fill the wound satisfactorily. If healing is delayed, the surgeon may suspect a recurrence of the neoplastic process if it was the original indication for enucleation. Much hemorrhage occurs at the time of surgery, and it may alarm the inexperienced surgeon. We believe that, if the surgery progresses quickly, blood loss will be minimal. Thus, a continuous interlocking pattern is used for closure of the skin incision and no vessel ligation is required.

Complications and Prognosis

Complications of this procedure include extensive hemorrhage from the optic artery, infection, dehiscence, recurrence of disease, and convulsions due to inadvertent injection of lidocaine into the meningeal reflection of the optic nerve while performing the retrobulbar block.[11] Orbital infections following enucleation in a field setting may be common but recurrence of squamous cell carcinoma has not been found to occur frequently.[12] The prognosis for this procedure is generally good but varies with the presenting disease.

Cosmetic Dehorning

Relevant Anatomy

At the junction of horn and skin lies the corium, which consists of the cells that facilitate growth of new horn. If these cells are not removed during dehorning, regrowth will occur and a scur may form at the poll. The horn itself is attached to the porous, boney, cornual process that is covered by a papillated dermis.

Nervous supply to the dermis of the horn is primarily through the cornual nerve, which arises from the orbit and travels in the ridge of the temporal line.[1] The nerve splits and wraps around the horn beneath the frontalis muscle. Complete desensitization of the cornual nerve prior to dehorning is not always successful due to variations in branching and the location of the nerve with respect to the temporal ridge.[1] Additionally, the horn may also be innervated partially by the supraorbital or infratrochlear nerves or nerves from the frontal sinus may extend into the cornual diverticulum.

The blood supply to the horn arises from the superficial temporal vessels which branch and advance up the cornual process. Once severed, these branches retract and are difficult to reach with hemostats. Significant hemorrhage can occur if the vessel is not cut close to the skull so the artery remains embedded within soft tissue.

Indications

Dehorning is performed in cattle to reduce injuries and carcass damage caused by fighting. Cosmetic dehorning permits closure of the skin over a normal defect created by the amputation of the horn at its base. Ideally, this results in primary-intention healing, a lower incidence of frontal sinusitis, and less hemorrhage. It is generally

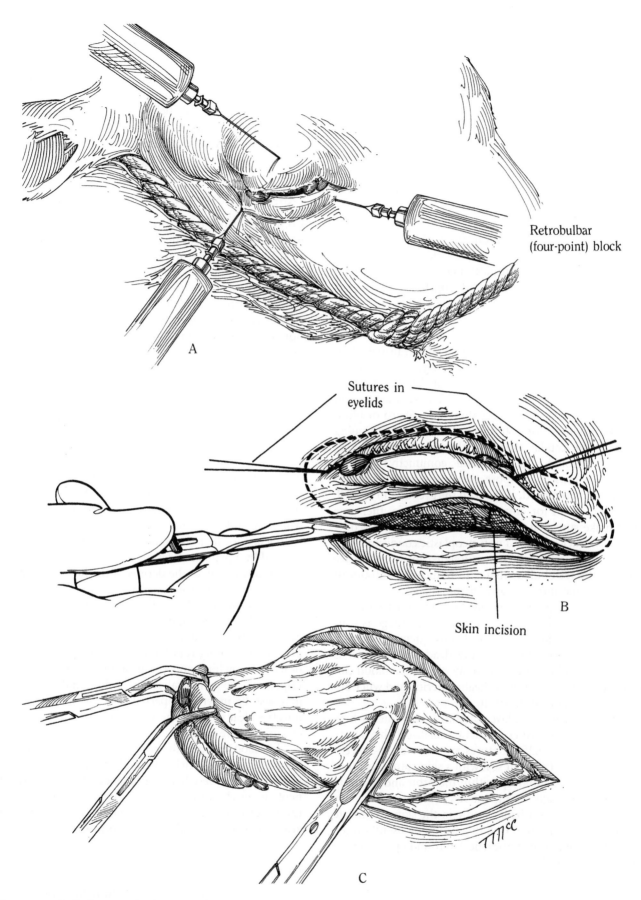

Retrobulbar
(four-point) block

Sutures in
eyelids

Skin incision

A

B

C

Fig. 15.2. **A–D.** Eye enucleation in cattle.

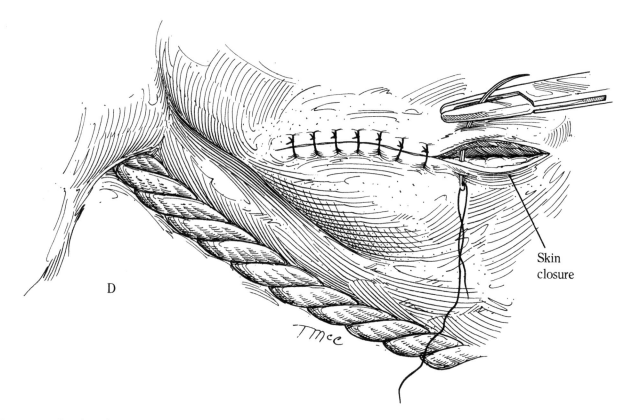

D

Skin
closure

Fig. 15.2. *Continued.*

reserved for show animals and expensive breeding live-stock in which postoperative appearance of the poll is important.[13] The method is best suited for cattle under 1 year of age because there may not be enough skin to close the defect after horn removal in older animals.[14]

Anesthesia and Surgical Preparation

The animal is restrained in a squeeze chute with its head secured to one side with a halter. The hair is removed from the poll, the base of the ears, and the face as far as the eyes; the ears can be wrapped with adhesive tape and secured to the halter to pull them back out of the way (not illustrated). Tranquilization of the animal with intravenous xylazine or another analgesic discussed in Chapter 2 will decrease stress to the animal. The tail vein is generally the most accessible route of administration and causes the least distress in this instance.[15] If tranquilizers are used, the animal should be withheld from slaughter for the recommended period of time.

The area is then scrubbed and prepared for cornual nerve block, but it is not draped. A cornual (zygomatico-temporal) nerve block is performed using an 18-gauge, 4–5-cm needle. In some of the larger breeds, an 8-cm needle is more satisfactory.[14] The needle is inserted through the skin at a point midway between the lateral canthus of the eye and the base of the horn (Figure 15.3A). The needle is directed through the frontalis muscle and under the lateral aspect of the temporal portion of the

frontal bone. At this point, 5 ml of local anesthetic are injected in a fan-like manner, and another 2 ml are deposited under the skin as the needle is withdrawn. Then the needle is directed subcutaneously toward the base of the horn, and an additional 2–3 ml of local anesthetic are deposited below the skin. The injection sites are massaged to disperse the local anesthetic. The block is repeated on the other side of the head. Generally, the head is swung around to the other side of the squeeze chute and is restrained to permit access to the sites that are to be blocked for the contralateral horn. Alternatively, due to the variations in normal anatomy, one may choose to simply ring block the horn to dependably provide adequate anesthesia to the area. When performing the ring block, one should appreciate that the skin on the rostral aspect of the horn is much thicker than that caudal to the horn. Therefore, care should be taken to ensure subcutaneous injection of local anesthetic. Having the needle too shallow will lead to intradermal injection while too deep may be subperiosteal. Either misplacement will be difficult to inject and may lead to dislodgement of the needle from the syringe. The surgical site is given a final scrub prior to commencing surgery.

Instrumentation

1. General surgery pack
2. Obstetric wire and handle or sterilized Barnes dehorner

Surgical Technique

An incision is made from the lateral limit of the nuchal eminence (poll) in a lateral direction toward the base of the horn. The incision curves rostroventral around the base of the horn and along the frontal crest for about 5–7 cm. The incision should be no more than 1 cm from the base of the horn. A second incision is begun from a point about 5–8 cm from the origin of the first incision, near the nuchal eminence. This incision is carried around the caudal aspect of the horn, about 1 cm from the base, to unite it with the first incision ventrally. The limits of the incisions are illustrated in Figure 15.3B. The incisions are deepened until bone is encountered, and the edges of the incision are undermined using sharp dissection. The rostral incision must be undermined in an area bounded by the ends of the incision (Figure 15.3B, shaded area). The caudal incision is undermined just enough to allow placement of the wire saw ventrally and deep to the base of the horn on the frontal crest. Care should be taken when the incisions are deepened not to divide the auricular muscles (located caudally and ventrally). Generally, bleeding is controlled by torsion of the cornual artery located rostroventral to the bony stump. Hematomas may occur if this is not done.

The stump is then removed using either an obstetric wire as a saw, a dehorning saw, or a Barnes dehorner, which is used like a rongeur. Many surgeons prefer the Barnes dehorner because it facilitates small, precise, cuts of bone to be removed after the horn is excised to reach the desired shape. If the saw or wire is used, the rope securing the head is untied, and the head is swung around to the other side of the chute to facilitate positioning of the wire saw. The saw must seat itself in the frontal bone at an adequate distance from the base of the horn to allow removal of sufficient bone. If this is not done, the approximation of the skin edges will be under excessive tension, and closure may be impossible. If more horn must be removed, the surgeon may use a hammer and chisel or a Barnes dehorner, so the cut will be flush with the frontal bone. The remaining horn is removed in an identical manner. Once the horns and attached skin are removed, the head is repositioned in preparation for the closure of the wound.

The surgical sites are flushed with a suitable physiologic solution, such as Ringer's solution, to rinse out any bone dust. Skin closure is usually performed in one layer using a heavy, nonabsorbable material in a simple continuous (Figure 15.3C) or continuous interlocking pattern. If there is still moderate tension on the closure after undermining the skin one may use towel clamps or a near-far-far-near suture to hold the skin edges in apposition for closure with the continuous interlocking suture pattern.

Postoperative Management

The skin sutures are removed 3 weeks postoperatively. The animal should be housed in a dry environment and perioperative antibiotics may be indicated.

Complications and Prognosis

The following are the three most common errors of the inexperienced surgeon: removal of too much skin at the base of the horn that subsequently will be removed with the horn; improper seating of the wire saw at the base of the horn, resulting in a stump of bone; and failure to undermine the skin edges adequately. These errors result in the surgeon's inability to appose the skin edges. If this happens, a varying degree of sinusitis, along with wound healing by secondary intention, is the end result. The animal may also have a sinusitis secondary to bone fragments left in the sinus. Complications are generally mild, however, and the prognosis is good.

Rib Resection and Pericardiotomy

Relevant Anatomy

Due to the large width of the ribs and the subsequently narrower intercostal space, resection of one or more ribs may be necessary to access the thorax in the bovine.[1] The thorax is shorter than in the horse and the diaphragm is positioned more vertically. Most of the heart lies on the left side of the thorax extending from the second intercostal space to the fifth intercostal space. The pericardium is a closed, serous sac comprised of a visceral layer that is closely adhered to the heart and a fibrous parietal layer.[1] A distance of less than 10 cm separates the pericardium from the reticulum, which lies caudal to the diaphragm and cranial to the rumen, occupying the space beneath the sixth to eighth ribs.[16] Cattle that ingest sharp metal objects may develop traumatic reticulitis if the object is forced through the reticular wall by the normal contractions of the organ. Due to the relatively close proximity of the heart, it is also feasible that a large foreign object may be forced through the diaphragm and puncture the pericardium as well, resulting in purulent and constrictive pericarditis and chronic pericardial effusion.

Indications

Rib resection and pericardectomy in cattle are performed primarily to treat pericarditis resulting from penetration of the pericardial sac by a foreign body from the reticulum (traumatic reticulopericarditis). Generally, congestive heart failure due to pericardial and myocardial pathologic changes ensues, along with weight loss, ill thrift, and eventually, death. Drainage is indicated because the process is a closed-cavity infection, similar to an abscess, which seldom responds to antibiotic therapy alone. Drainage using a Foley catheter introduced through a large trocar may be unsuccessful because of fibrin accumulation and pocket formation in the pericardial sac.[17]

Generally, pericardiotomy is considered a salvage operation to buy time before the animal can be slaughtered.

A

Cornual (zygomaticotemporal) nerve block

Gigli (obstetric) wire saw

Skin incisions

Undermined areas

B

Fig. 15.3.   **A–C.** Cosmetic dehorning in cattle.

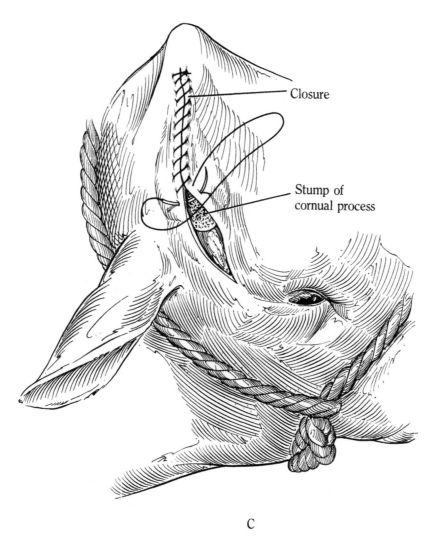

C

Fig. 15.3. *Continued.*

Although the aim of the surgery may be to allow time for a cow to calve, many cows with pericarditis abort from the stress of the disease process or the stress of the disease combined with surgery. When pericarditis is confirmed by clinical signs or pericardiocentesis, or when rumenotomy gives evidence of pericardial involvement, pericardiotomy is indicated.

Most animals with advanced pericarditis are in poor physical condition and have congestive heart failure, which makes them poor surgical risks. Animals under 5 years of age that can ambulate normally and are relatively normal in body function and condition can usually withstand the operation.[18] The surgery should be performed before the animal's body condition deteriorates to a point where there is no chance for survival. Advanced pregnancy and stress from other diseases hinder success.

Anesthesia and Surgical Preparation

Generally, preoperative antibiotics are indicated. *Corynebacterium pyogenes* is commonly the offending organism

and is usually sensitive to common antibiotics. Mixed bacterial infections from the reticulum may be present, however; and it is preferable to culture the exudate from the pericardium and to obtain specific antibiotic sensitivities. Fluid therapy during and after surgery is beneficial in counteracting the effects of surgical and septic shock.

Because most candidates for pericardectomy are poor anesthetic risks, the surgery is generally performed with the animal under local anesthesia. Sedation may also be required. General anesthesia should be avoided if possible. The intravenous sedation techniques combined with local anesthesia are generally accompanied by struggling, but they are usually safer in an animal in poor condition.

The surgery can be performed in the standing or laterally recumbent animal. Prior to casting, a large area over the left thorax and elbow region is clipped. The surgery is performed with the animal placed in right-lateral recumbency, with the aid of casting ropes or a tilt table. If a tilt table is available, it is advantageous to operate at a 30–40° tilt, to allow any exudate to drain from the surgical site. This position also seems less stressful than full-lateral recumbency with the animal in the horizontal position. Generally, sedation is commenced prior to placing the patient on the tilt table. Once the patient is positioned, the clipped area over the left ventral chest wall is prepared for aseptic surgery. The left thoracic limb should be pulled craniad to help expose the area over the fifth rib, and local analgesia is instituted by direct infiltration of a local analgesic agent along the incision line (line block).[18] The analgesic solution is infused initially into the subcutaneous space, into the underlying muscle, and onto the surface of the fifth rib. The operating time should be kept to an absolute minimum to reduce stress on an already compromised patient. The surgical site is given a final scrub, during which time the local anesthetic will be taking effect. Performing the surgery in the standing animal will reduce stress on the animal, but it may become recumbent during the procedure.

Instrumentation

1. General surgery pack
2. Obstetric wire saw or Gigli wire saw and handles

Surgical Technique

The skin incision extends from the costochondral junction to a point 20 cm dorsally on a line over the fifth rib (Figure 15.4A). The pericardial sac can also be approached through resection of the sixth rib. The latissimus dorsi and serratus ventralis muscles are incised to expose the rib. The periosteum is incised and is reflected from the rib (Figure 15.4B). Following exposure of 12–14 cm of the fifth rib, a wire saw (Gigli or obstetric) is inserted under the rib with forceps and is positioned at the dorsal commissure of the incision. The rib is transected dorsally and then is grasped and broken at the costochondral junction (Figure 15.4C). This portion of the rib is discarded. Some surgeons prefer to let the patient stand at this point in the operation before the parietal pleura is opened, to assist drainage.[19] If the animal is restrained on a tilt table, it can be positioned at a steeper angle to aid drainage of exudate. The incision is then continued through the exposed periosteum and parietal pleura for about 12 cm, using a pair of blunt-tipped scissors (Figure 15.4D).

The initial opening of the pleura should be small because a sudden influx of air may cause respiratory distress. Usually, however, the pericardium is adherent to the parietal pleura, and pneumothorax does not occur. To avoid opening the pleural cavity, some surgeons suture the periosteum, the parietal pleura, and the pericardium together using no. 0 or no. 1 synthetic absorbable suture in a simple continuous pattern prior to opening the pleura. If the pericardium is not adherent to the parietal pleura or if suturing is not performed, leakage of pus into the pleural cavity will result in contamination and pleuritis.[17]

An incision is then made between the suture lines. Once the pericardium is visible, it is opened sufficiently to allow the introduction of the surgeon's hand. A variable amount of pus will escape from the incision. Suction, if available, should be used to aid evacuation of the exudate. The pericardial sac should be explored for a foreign body. Any foreign body should be removed, but often all that is found is a firm fibrous tissue mass in the caudal aspect of the pericardial sac. As much fibrinous exudate as possible should be removed (Figure 15.4E). Adhesions should be broken down gently at this stage by passing the hand around the heart. It is unwise to proceed with a dissection that is too extensive, however, for fear of rupturing coronary vessels.[18] Following drainage, exploration, and the removal of any foreign object, the cavity is lavaged copiously with warm isotonic electrolyte solution. The inclusion of antibiotics or antibacterial agents in the lavage solution is believed to be beneficial. Drains are sometimes indicated if postoperative flushing is to be done. The wound may be closed or left open to allow drainage.

Closure consists of simple continuous sutures of no. 0 or no. 1 synthetic absorbable suture. The parietal pleura, adherent pericardium, and deep periosteal layer are included in the first row. Periosteum and intercostal musculature are closed in a second row, and nonabsorbable suture material is used for the skin closure. No attempt is made to evacuate air from the pleural cavity because normal lung function returns in about 7–10 days.[18] If the wound is to be left open, the combined edges of the periosteum, parietal pleura, and pericardium are everted and are sutured to the subcutaneous tissue to create a pericardial fistula.

In some cases, a rumenotomy will be indicated if a wire foreign body is still protruding through the reticulum and was not retrieved through the pericardiotomy.

Postoperative Management

Postoperative antibiotics are administered. If drains have been placed in the wound, they are flushed daily with a mixed antibiotic-isotonic solution. These treatments are continued until it is judged either that the animal is overcoming the infectious process or that the animal should be sent to slaughter.

Complications and Prognosis

The prognosis for traumatic reticulopericarditis is poor. Long-term recovery is unusual because the resulting constrictive pericarditis is generally fatal.

Repair of Teat Lacerations

Relevant Anatomy

There are five primary layers to the lining of the teat: the inner most layers of mucosa and submucosa, a layer of

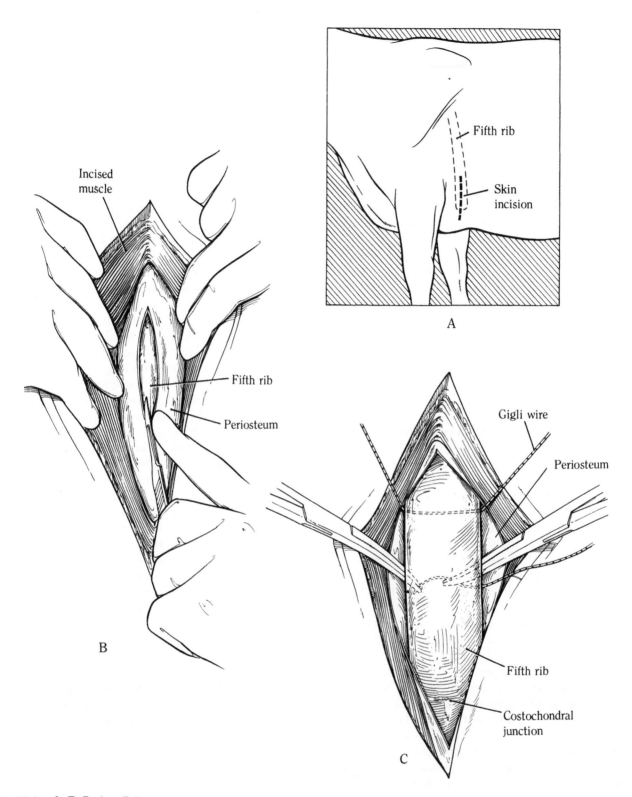

Labels in illustration:

- Fifth rib
- Skin incision
- A
- Incised muscle
- Fifth rib
- Periosteum
- B
- Gigli wire
- Periosteum
- Fifth rib
- Costochondral junction
- C

Fig. 15.4. A–E. Pericardiotomy.

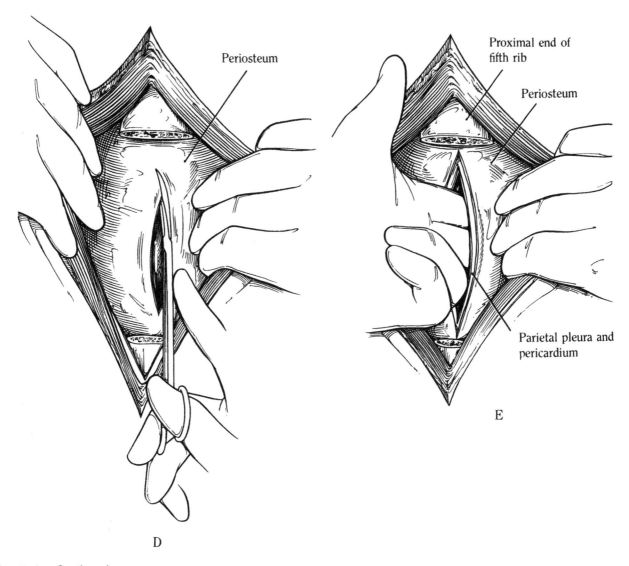

Fig. 15.4. *Continued.*

highly vascularized conjunctive tissue, the muscularis, and then the outer most layer of skin.[20] Proximally, the glandular cisterna collects the milk–gathering ducts. A narrowed portion of the cisterna, the annular relief, separates the glandular portion from the more distal papillary part.[1,20] The papillary part of the cisterna is comprised of longitudinal folds of mucosa that allow the cistern to expand to accommodate increases in volume. At the distal extremity of the teat, the internal opening of the papillary duct, called the Furstenberg rosette, probably functions to close the papillary duct in between milking and may also play an immune role in preventing infection.[1,20,21] The papillary duct, or teat canal, is the last portion of the mammary gland's excretory system which is held closed by a muscular sphincter.

The primary blood supply to the mammary gland of the cow is the pudendal artery, which enters the mammary gland through the inguinal canal and runs longitudinally down the teat. The artery divides into a large mammary artery that courses ventrocranially and a smaller mammary artery that runs caudally.[1] The pudendal vein drains the mammary gland and arises as a plexus from a vein encircling the sphincter and terminates at the base of the teat.[20]

Indications

Teat lacerations are common in dairy cows and can cause severe deficits in milk production. Lacerations that do not penetrate the mucosa of the teat generally heal rapidly by secondary intention with the aid of topical medication and bandaging. Teat lacerations that penetrate the mucosa of the teat require suturing to maintain normal teat function for milking and to prevent the development of teat fistulae or acute mastitis and loss of the quarter. As with any lacerations, early attention to the condition improves the success rate.

Diagnosis and treatment of teat disorders has advanced greatly since the first edition of this text. The most ideal suturing pattern for teat repair has been researched; radiography, ultrasound, and theloscopy have improved diagnostic capabilities; and surgical approaches have been refined to improve precision and reduce invasiveness. Obviously, not all of this equipment is readily available to many practitioners, but the changes in technique are applicable and useful.

Anesthesia and Surgical Preparation

The methods of restraint and anesthesia are important in any teat surgery because the repair must be meticulous. A tilt table, ideal for restraint, generally is not available to most practitioners who must deal with teat lacerations in the field. Xylazine hydrochloride (Rompun) is a useful means of restraining the cow in lateral recumbency for teat surgery. Many surgeons prefer positioning the cow in dorsal recumbency for teat procedures. Butorphanol (0.5 mg/kg) may be added for very fractious animals.[20] If the cow's disposition is good, teat surgery may be attempted with the cow in the standing position using local anesthesia, but results are more predictable if the cow is tabled or cast and is neither uneasy nor kicking. Local anesthetic injected around the base of the teat (circle or ring block) is the most common technique for anesthesia (Figure 15.5A). Epinephrine should not be used with the local anesthetic. Topical anesthetic can be infused directly into the teat canal to supplement ring block anesthesia. For topical anesthesia, 2% lidocaine (not procaine) should be used. Epidural anesthesia is an effective alternative for teat surgery (see Chapter 2).

To control hemorrhage and milk flow, a rubber tourniquet may be applied to the base of the teat. Doyen forceps clamped across the base of the teat can also be used successfully. When lacerations involve the base of the teat, suturing has to be performed without the benefit of a tourniquet.

The udder and surrounding teats should be washed thoroughly. Harsh disinfectants should be avoided because they can cause further tissue necrosis if they contact the lacerated tissue. The affected teat can be draped with a slit drape, so it protrudes from the opening in the drape. Once the borders of the laceration have been assessed carefully, a prognosis can usually be given.

Instrumentation

1. General surgery pack
2. Teat cannula (Larson's teat tube)

Surgical Technique

The wound edges should be freshened to remove any devitalized tissue and foreign material. Debridement is one of the most important procedures in repairing lacerated teats. Hemorrhage should be controlled because

blood clots in the lumen of the teat delay healing by making milking painful and difficult for the animal.

The wound edges should be apposed under as little tension as possible. There have been many different closure techniques described in the literature for closure of teat lacerations. Evidence suggests that closure in three layers—the mucosa, muscular-submucosa, and the skin—yields the most satisfactory healing.[20,21,22] The first layer closed is the mucosa. A simple continuous pattern using no. 3-0 or no. 4-0 synthetic, monofilament, absorbable suture material is generally preferred (Figure 15.5A).[20,21,22] When the mucosa has been closed, a teat cannula should be inserted through the teat sphincter, and the suture line should be gently probed to check its integrity. The second layer closed should be the submucosa. Again, this layer can be closed in a simple continuous pattern, using no. 3-0 or no. 4-0 synthetic, monofilament, absorbable suture material, and should support the delicate mucosal closure (Figure 15.5B). The remainder of the teat and the skin may be closed with a near-far-far-near or simple interrupted suture of nonabsorbable suture material, no. 0 or no. 2-0. This suture is placed so the deep bite is adjacent to the previously placed submucosal suture and the superficial layer is shallow (Figure 15.5C, D). The tourniquet should be removed following closure of the laceration; and, with gentle hand pressure applied to the teat, the suture line should be checked for milk leakage. Milk in the suture line will almost certainly result in a teat fistula.

Postoperative Management

Traditionally, a self-retaining teat tube, such as a Larson's teat tube, is inserted for about a week. The cap of the tube can be removed to permit the quarter to drain while the other quarters are being milked; this procedure takes advantage of the "let-down" phenomenon at the time of milking, or it can be left off permanently. The teat should not be hand-milked, but regular drainage is necessary to take the pressure off the suture line. If closure has been meticulous, as previously described, then immediate machine-milking appears to have no adverse effects on healing.[20,22]

Intramammary antibiotics should be infused into the affected teat, and systemic antibiotics should be used as indicated. If the laceration is of some duration, mastitis will be present. This can be verified with the aid of a California Mastitis Test. Bacterial cultures and sensitivity testing are indicated in some cases.

The sutures are removed after aseptic preparation at about 8–10 days postoperatively to avoid inflammation and suture tract infection.[20]

Complications and Prognosis

Complications include excessive teat swelling and fibrous reaction that can impede milking. If the sutures are left

Fig. 15.5. **A–D.** Repair of teat laceration.

Continous pattern in mucosa

Simple continuous pattern in submucosa

Near-far-far-near sutures

Skin

Submucosal layer

Mucosal layer

A

B

C

D

in too long or if the teat is handled excessively postoperatively, inflammation and infection may result.

Vertical lacerations have a better prognosis than do horizontal teat wounds because circulation to the wound edges is better. For the same reason, a V-shaped flap attached proximally has a better prognosis than a V-shaped flap attached distally. Lacerations at the distal end of the teat are considered to have a poorer prognosis because fibrosis in this area can interfere with milking. Similarly, lacerations at the base of the teat have a less favorable prognosis because they are susceptible to extensive hemorrhage due to their proximity to the pudendal venous ring.[20] Like other areas of the body, the prognosis for healing also depends greatly on the type of the injury (crushing injuries versus linear lacerations) and the degree of contamination present.

Third Eyelid Resection

Relevant Anatomy

The third eyelid of the ruminant is composed of a T-shaped cartilage covered with mucosa visible at the medial canthus of the eye. The third lid moves over the cornea dorsolaterally. It has glandular tissue that secretes material similar to the lacrimal glands.[23]

Indications

Resection of the third lid is indicated when it is affected by squamous cell carcinoma while no other structures of the eye are affected. Therefore, resection removes the diseased tissue and saves the vision in the eye.

Anesthesia and Surgical Preparation

The animal is restrained in a squeeze chute or at least in some head restraint with the head secured to the side. An auriculopalpebral nerve block may be performed to decrease the mobility of the eyelids. Local anesthetic is applied topically to the third lid and then injected across the base of the third lid.

Instrumentation

1. General surgery pack

Surgical Technique

The third lid is grasped with tissue forceps or a towel clamp taking care not to tear the tissue. Then two hemostatic forceps are placed deep to the squamous cell carcinoma lesion from dorsal and ventral directions to meet so that the entire third lid is clamped. A scalpel blade or scissors is then used to resect the third eyelid superficial

to the hemostats. The hemostats are left in place for a short period of time for hemostasis. The hemostats are removed and the animal is released.

Postoperative Management

These animals do not require any specific postoperative management related to the surgery. One should examine the cow closely for other squamous cell carcinoma lesions and owners should observe the animal in the future for new lesions.

Complications and Prognosis

Complications following this procedure are minimal and the prognosis is generally good unless the tumor has affected deeper tissues such that complete resection is not possible.

Tracheotomy

Relevant Anatomy

The trachea consists of cartilaginous plates (rings) which are hyaline cartilage surrounded by perichondrium. There is fibroelastic tissue between the rings called anular ligaments. The relevance for performing a tracheotomy in a ruminant is that the tracheal rings are relatively wider and the space between the rings is relatively smaller when compared to the horse where the procedure is more frequently performed.[24] Therefore, as we will describe in the technique, one will need to remove part of the rings to have an adequate opening to insert a tube into the trachea.

Indications

While not uncommon, upper respiratory obstruction is certainly a life-threatening condition in ruminants. Conditions such as traumatic or infectious pharyngitis appear to cause significant anxiety to cattle. Laryngeal edema will occasionally be seen in cattle presented with increased respiratory noise. A tracheotomy will establish a patent airway while the primary condition is determined and treated.

Anesthesia and Surgical Preparation

The skin over the trachea in the middle of the cervical region is clipped and surgically scrubbed. Appropriate restraint is determined by the size and temperament of the animal. Many calves can be safely restrained by one attendant while larger cattle need to be in a squeeze chute or head catch at least. The nose should be extended to allow access to the ventral neck. Local anesthesia of the skin and subcutaneous tissue in a line block on the midline is effective.

Instrumentation

1. General surgery pack
2. Tracheotomy tube

Surgical Technique

The skin of the neck is tensed over the trachea with the thumb and index finger of the surgeon's left hand on either side of the trachea. A ventral midline incision approximately 5 cm long is then made through the skin and subcutaneous tissue to expose the trachea. In *Bos Indicus* cattle, the excessive dewlap may be reflected to one side to allow the skin incision to be made over the trachea. A hemostat or finger is then used to palpate the tracheal rings and anular ligaments. A stab incision is made through the anular ligament in the center of the incision. This should create immediate airflow. In order to place a tracheotomy tube to maintain an airway, one needs to resect part of the tracheal rings on each side of the anular ligament incised. This is most easily done by grasping the middle of the ring with forceps and carefully cutting the ring on a curved line to take approximately one-third of the width of the ring. Do not excise more than half of the ring. Repeat the ring excision on the opposite side of the annular ligament incision. This should create an opening through which one can easily place a tube to maintain a patent airway. It also allows a large enough opening to facilitate changing the tube as needed. In the absence of a tracheotomy tube in life-threatening situations, one may use an endotracheal tube, syringe casing, or any available item that will maintain a patent airway for the immediate period of time. The tracheotomy tube may be secured with tape or tied to suture loops placed in the skin.

Postoperative Management

The primary cause of the respiratory distress must be treated and hopefully resolved. The ruminant produces more respiratory secretions than other animals. Therefore, the tracheotomy tube must be changed more frequently (at least twice a day) than in other species in order to keep it clean and patent. When the primary problem has resolved and the alternative airway is no longer needed, the tracheotomy tube can simply be removed and the wound cleaned daily while it heals by secondary intention.

Complications and Prognosis

The prognosis in these cases depends more on the primary lesion than the tracheotomy.

Umbilical Surgery

Relevant Anatomy

The external umbilical cord of a new born calf consists of the umbilical vein and urachus. The umbilical vein trans-ports oxygen-rich blood to the fetal calf from the placenta, and the urachus is an extension of the bladder that carries fetal waste to the placenta. Other components of the fetal circulation are the paired umbilical arteries, which carry oxygen-poor blood from the fetal calf to the placenta. The thick-walled arteries normally contract within the abdominal cavity at the time of birth. The umbilical vein runs from the umbilicus to the liver and becomes the falciform ligament. The urachus normally regresses totally. The paired umbilical arteries travel from the umbilicus on either side of the urachus then the bladder. They normally become the lateral ligaments of the bladder. The umbilicus itself is located closer to the preputial orifice in male calves than in males of other species. This is relevant when making the skin incision for umbilical surgery in male cattle.[25]

Indications

Cattle (usually calves) will have umbilical hernias that are either simple reducible hernias or partially reducible hernias, which are complicated by abscess of a remnant of the fetal circulation. Some calves will have swelling of the umbilical area that is not reducible and may even exhibit purulent discharge. Some will have abscessed remnants of fetal circulation without external abnormalities of the umbilicus. Occasionally calves with pollakiuria will have a persistent urachal remnant that mechanically prevents the bladder from totally emptying thus causing the clinical signs of frequent urination of small volumes.

Anesthesia and Surgical Preparation

Umbilical surgery is performed with the patient in dorsal recumbency with general anesthesia, sedation and local anesthesia or a high epidural anesthesia. It is wise to clip a broad area to allow an incision caudally to resect the urachus or umbilical arteries or cranially toward the xiphoid if marsupialization of the umbilical vein is necessary. The area is scrubbed for aseptic surgery.

Instrumentation

1. General surgery pack

Surgical Technique

The skin incision in heifers is a simple elliptical incision around the umbilical mass. Any draining tract should be oversewn to prevent contamination of the surgical site prior to making the incision. In the case of a very large umbilical mass, care should be taken to assure adequate skin is available for closure with minimal tension. The incision is continued through the subcutaneous tissue to the level of the external rectus sheath. Then a midline incision is made just immediately cranial (or caudal) to the mass (hernia or abscess) to allow the surgeon to place one finger into the peritoneal cavity to palpate for any structures associated with the umbilicus. This allows one to complete the elliptical body wall incision without unintentionally incising any abdominal structures. At this point any abscessed or persistent fetal remnants can be resected. The umbilical arteries are ligated as deep in the abdomen as possible. If the urachus is present, the tip of the bladder and the urachal remnant are resected. The bladder should be packed off from the abdomen with wet sterile towels. Stay sutures are placed in the bladder to hold it while the urachus is excised along with the tip of the bladder. There are many methods and materials for closing the bladder. We suggest using no. 2-0 absorbable suture in a simple continuous pattern to close the seromuscular layer including but not penetrating the mucosa. A second layer uses an inverting pattern such as a Cushing to close the seromuscular layer. The end result should be a closure that prevents any urine leakage. If the umbilical vein is abscessed and enlarged into the liver so that the surgeon does not feel safe simply ligating the vein, then it must be marsupialized through the body wall to facilitate drainage. The umbilical vein will exit the body wall at a site to the right of midline, just caudal to the last rib, such that the vein remnant is nearly vertical from the liver to the ventral body wall in the standing calf. A circular incision, approximately the size of the enlarged vein, is made at this exit site through the skin, subcutaneous tissue, and external rectus sheath to excise the circular piece of these structures. The rectus abdominus muscle and peritoneum are separated to facilitate passage of the umbilical vein. The distal aspect of the vein is dissected from the umbilicus and covered with a surgical sponge or part of a glove to prevent contamination of the peritoneum when the vein is pulled through the exit site with forceps. The vein is secured to the skin under minimal tension with absorbable suture in an interrupted pattern incorporating the wall of the vein but not obstructing the lumen in any way. The excess length of vein outside the body wall is excised. The vein usually drains and resolves. Owners should be warned that a second surgery to resect the vein may be needed; however, in most cases the vein regresses and does not need further intervention.

The elliptical skin incision that works well in heifers is not always practical in males due to the close proximity of the preputial orifice to the umbilicus. A crescent-shaped, or semilunar, skin incision is useful in male calves.[25] The middle of the two curvilinear incisions is rostral to the umbilicus and between the umbilicus and preputial orifice respectively. The concave part of the incision surrounds the preputial orifice, and the points of the connected curvilinear incisions are directed caudally. For simple hernias, retracting the sheath caudally may provide adequate exposure to make the elliptical body-wall incision to dissect the hernia. When more exposure is needed for any reason one may extend one end of the semilunar skin incision caudally and reflect the sheath to the con-tralateral side. This allows access to lengthen the elliptical body wall incision on the midline.

The body wall incision is closed in a routine fashion dependent on the size of the calf and the tension on the closure. One method would be to use no. 2 absorbable suture with one (or possibly more in a longer incision under tension) near-far-far-near suture to counteract tension, followed by separate lines of a simple continuous pattern between the tension sutures. The subcutaneous layer and skin in the elliptical heifer incision is likewise closed routinely according to surgeon preference. In the semilunar skin incision used in males, the body wall incision is still elliptical and therefore closed in the same manner. The subcutaneous layer is done in a transverse direction with some interrupted sutures to close the dead space created. The skin is closed with two separate simple continuous suture lines. Both will start at the center of the initial curvilinear incisions, immediately rostral to the preputial orifice, and continue caudally to the tips of the incision.

Postoperative Management

Antibiotic therapy may be appropriate dependent on the surgical findings. The calf should be housed in a clean dry area for 7–10 days to limit any environmental contamination of the incision. Exercise may be limited for a longer period if there is concern for body wall healing because of the size of the calf or length of the incision. Skin sutures should be removed in 14 days.

Complications and Prognosis

This umbilical surgery section has covered several different conditions. The potential complications and prognosis vary with the conditions. A simple hernia should have a good prognosis as well as a very low complication rate. Umbilical masses that consist of abscessed umbilical remnants understandably have a higher rate of incisional complications, even when there is no apparent contamination at surgery. Some of these calves will require additional surgeries to clear all infections and achieve a normally healed body wall.

References

1. Dyce, K.M., Sack, W.O., and Wensing, C.J.G. Textbook of Veterinary Anatomy, 2nd Ed. Philadelphia, W.B. Saunders, 1996.
2. Desrochers, A., and St. Jean, G. Surgical management of digit disorders in cattle. *Vet. Clin. Food Anim. Pract.*, 12:277–298, 1996.
3. Pejsa, T.G., St. Jean, G., Hoffsis, G.F., and Musser, J.M.B. Digit amputation in cattle: 85 cases (1971–1990). *J. Am. Vet. Med. Assoc.*, 202:981–984, 1993.
4. Desrochers, A., St-Jean, G., and Anderson, D.E. Use of facilitated ankylosis in the treatment of septic arthritis of the distal

interphalangeal joint in cattle: 12 cases (1987–1992). *J. Am. Vet. Med. Assoc.*, *206*(12):1923–1927, 1995.

5. Nuss, K., and Weaver, M.P. Resection of the distal interphalangeal joint in cattle: An alternative to amputation. *Vet. Rec.*, *128*:540–543, 1991.

6. Knight, A.P. Personal communication, 1980.

7. Greenough, P.R., MacCallum, F.J., and Weaver, A.D. Treatment and control of digital disease. *In* Lameness in Cattle, 2nd Ed. Edited by A.D. Weaver. Philadelphia, J.B. Lippincott, 1981, p. 228.

8. Guard, C. Personal communication, 2010.

9. Bicalho, R.C., Cheong, S.H., Warnick, L.D., Nydam, D.V., and Guard, C.L. The effect of digit amputation or arthrodesis surgery on culling and milk production in holstein dairy cows. *J. Dairy Sci.*, *89*:2596–2602, 2006.

10. Gelatt, K.N., and Titus, R.S. The special sense organs. *In* A Textbook of Large Animal Surgery. Edited by F.W. Oehme, J.E. Prier. Baltimore, MD, Williams & Wilkins, 1974.

11. Welker, B. Ocular surgery. *Vet. Clin. Food Anim. Pract.*, *11*:149–157, 1995.

12. Schulz, K.L., and Anderson, D.E. Bovine enucleation: A retrospective study of 53 cases (1998–2006). *Can. Vet. J.*, *51*(6):611–614, 2010.

13. Greenough, P.R. The integumentary system: Skin, hoof, claw and appendages. *In* Textbook of Large Animal Surgery. Edited by F.W. Oehme, J.E. Prier. Baltimore, MD, Williams & Wilkins, 1974.

14. Wallace, C.E. Cosmetic dehorning. *In* Bovine Medicine and Surgery. Vol. II, 2nd Ed. Edited by H.E. Amstutz. Santa Barbara, CA, American Veterinary Publications, 1980, p. 1240.

15. Hoffsis, G. Surgical (cosmetic) dehorning in cattle. *Vet. Clin. Food Anim. Pract.*, *11*:159–169, 1995.

16. Rings, D.M. Surgical treatment of pleuritis and pericarditis. *Vet. Clin. Food Anim. Pract.*, *11*:177–182, 1995.

17. Mason, T.A. Suppurative pericarditis treated by pericardiotomy in a cow. *Vet. Rec.*, *105*:350, 1979.

18. Noordsy, J.L. The cardiovascular system. *In* Textbook of Large Animal Surgery. Edited by F.W. Oehme, J.E. Prier. Baltimore, MD, Williams & Wilkins, 1974.

19. Horney, F.D. Surgical drainage of the pericardial sac. *Can. Vet. J.*, *1*:363, 1960.

20. Couture, Y., and Mulon, P.Y. Procedures and surgeries of the teat. *Vet. Clin. Food Anim.*, *21*:173–204, 2005.

21. Ghamsari, S.M., Acorda, J.A., Taguchi, K., Abe, N., and Yamada, H. Effect of different suture patterns of wound healing of the teat in dairy cattle. *J. Vet. Med. Sci.*, *57*:819–824, 1995.

22. Makady, F.M., Whitmore, H.L., Nelson, D.R., and Simon, J. Effect of tissue adhesives and suture patterns on experimentally induced teat lacerations in lactating dairy cattle. *J. Am. Vet. Med. Assoc.*, *11*:34–1991, 1932.

23. Diesem, C. The organ of vision: Ruminant sense organs and common integument. *In* Sisson and Grossman's the Anatomy of Domestic Animals, 5th Ed. Edited by R. Getty. Philadelphia, Saunders, 1975, p. 1180.

24. Hare, W.C.D. Ruminant respiratory system. *In* Sisson and Grossman's the Anatomy of Domestic Animals, 5th Ed. Edited by R. Getty. Philadelphia, Saunders, 1975, p. 916.

25. Baird, A.N. Umbilical surgery in calves. (Field surgery of cattle, Part II). *Vet. Clin. Food Anim. Pract.*, *24*(3):467–477, 2008.

Chapter 16

SMALL RUMINANT SURGERY

A. N. Baird, DVM, MS, DACVS

Objectives

1. Describe dehorning procedures for adult goats and disbudding young goats.
2. Describe surgical procedures for obstructive urolithiasis and vasectomy in males.
3. Describe cesarean section and mastectomy techniques in females.
4. Describe a technique for resection of a rectal prolapse.

Dehorning the Mature Goat

Relevant Anatomy

Unlike cattle, the horns of the goat are innervated by two separate cornual branches, one originating from the lacrimal nerve and the other from the infratrochlear nerve. The cornual branch of the lacrimal nerve runs superficially across the supraorbital process and may be blocked halfway between the lateral canthus of the eye and the lateral base of the horn.[1] The infratrochlear nerve may be blocked in between the medial canthus of the eye and the base of the horn on the medial side.[1] The cornual artery branches, located at the ventral edge of the horns, are of particular concern for hemorrhage during this procedure.

Indications

The mature goat is dehorned either to reduce the danger to man and other animals or if its horn(s) are broken. Some breed societies require dehorning to register the goat, although flock goats are generally left horned as protection from predators. Dehorning of male goats is sometimes combined with removal of the scent (horn) glands to reduce odor.[2,3]

Anesthesia and Surgical Preparation

As with other ruminants, food should be withheld from the goat for 12–24 hours before surgery to avoid ruminal tympany, regurgitation, and possible aspiration pneumonia if general anesthesia is administered.

Goats do not tolerate pain associated with even minor surgical procedures and can die of shock if sufficient analgesia is not provided. Although the exact cause of this shock is not known, it is believed to be a reaction to intense fear or fright from a combination of restraint and pain.[2] All goats should be anesthetized or deeply sedated before dehorning; refer to Chapter 2 for details of anesthetic techniques in goats.

Sedation needs to be supplemented with local analgesia of the horn. Once the goat is recumbent, the head region is clipped and prepared for a cornual nerve block and infratrochlear nerve block. The cornual branch of the lacrimal nerve is blocked by injecting 2 ml of local anesthetic as close as possible to the caudal ridge of the root of the supraorbital process to a depth of 1–1.5 cm. The cornual branch of the infratrochlear nerve is also blocked by injecting 2 ml of local anesthetic at the dorsomedial margin of the orbit. In larger goats, a ring block around the entire base of the horn may be necessary (Figure 16.1A). Lidocaine should be used judiciously in goats to avoid toxicity; the minimal dose should be used (see Chapter 2). While the anesthesia is taking effect, the area around the horn is prepared for aseptic surgery.

Instrumentation

1. General surgery pack
2. Obstetric wire saw, Gigli wire saw, or dehorning saw
3. Rongeur (for cosmetic dehorning)
4. Hemostats

Turner and McIlwraith's Techniques in Large Animal Surgery, 4th Edition. Dean A. Hendrickson and A. N. (Nickie) Baird.

Fig. 16.1. Dehorning the mature goat.

A

Horn (scent) gland

Clipped area

Cornual branch of lacrimal nerve

Cornual branch of infratrochlear nerve

Skin incision

Clipped area

B

Gigli wire

C

Antibacterial powder

Frontal sinus opening

D

Bandage

E

Surgical Technique

The skin is incised 1 cm from the base of the horn. Enough skin must be removed from the caudolateral and caudomedial areas, where scurs are likely to occur (Figure 16.1B). While an assistant supports the goat's head, the surgeon seats an obstetric wire saw or Gigli wire saw in the caudomedial aspect of the incision and removes the horn by directing the saw in a craniolateral direction (Figure 16.1C). Some surgeons prefer a dehorning saw, because it has less tendency to break and is less likely to leave a protuberance in the middle of the horn that may grow back.[2]

In male goats, the scent glands are located at the base of each horn (caudal and medial) and generally are removed during the dehorning procedure. Hemorrhage from the superficial temporal artery can be severe and should be stopped by ligating the artery or by pulling and twisting it with a hemostat.

When a goat is dehorned correctly, its frontal sinuses are exposed because of the extensive communication between the lumen of the cornual process and the frontal sinus. The head may be bandaged postoperatively to prevent both myiasis and the collection of foreign material in the sinus. Prior to bandaging, a topical antibacterial powder is dusted onto the dehorning site (Figure 16.1D,E). Bandaging is not accepted by everyone. Some surgeons believe that the wound should not be covered and should be allowed to remain dry. If the wound is neglected, myiasis can develop under the bandage, and the consequences may be more serious than if the wound was left open.

Cosmetic dehorning has been described as a method to avoid the need for extensive postoperative management of an open sinus with bandages and wound monitoring. The dehorning is performed as described above. After horn removal, a rongeur is used to remove frontal bone to thus allow skin closure over the surgical site. The skin at the incision edges is undermined; release incisions may also be needed in the skin between where the horns were located in order to relieve enough tension to allow primary closure of the surgical site. The skin incisions are then closed with near-far-far-near or simple interrupted sutures. In some cases it is difficult to completely close the surgical site. However, the open segment of the partially closed wound left to heal by secondary intention is greatly reduced in size and the healing is much quicker.[4] Skin sutures should be removed in 3 weeks.

Postoperative Management

Tetanus prophylaxis should be performed. If the animal's head is bandaged, the first bandage should be changed on the second postoperative day and replaced. The second bandage is left on for an additional 5–6 days. Many animals will require bandages for extended periods before the sinus closes.

In the summer, when flies are a problem, prevention of myiasis is important for several more weeks. The goat should be housed in an area free of dust and isolated from dirty surroundings. It is also advisable that the goat not mix with other members of the herd until the wound has healed. Any abnormal odor, purulent nasal discharge, head shaking, or rubbing is often an indication of frontal sinusitis, which necessitates removal of the bandage and treatment.

Complications and Prognosis

Dehorning can result in a reduction in milk production, impairment of spermatogenesis, sinusitis, myiasis, and loss of social status in the herd. The surgery should be planned to minimize these effects. For prevention of myiasis, the procedure should be reserved for the cooler months.[2] Life threatening complications are rare and the prognosis is good.

Disbudding the Young Goat

Anesthesia and Surgical Preparation

The hair around the horn buds should be clipped. The kid may be restrained in a dehorning box or held by an assistant. Sedation and local anesthesia are appropriate to limit pain and stress to the kid, although some producers will perform the disbudding with physical restraint only.

Instrumentation

1. Dehorning iron

Surgical Technique

Each iron is different as far as the temperature and how quickly it reaches that temperature. It is wise to test the iron on a board where it should leave a slightly depressed black ring. Some irons will turn cherry red when ready. The dehorning iron should be placed over the bud in a rocking motion. The ring of skin around the horn bud should be copper colored all around. One should also burn the cap of the horn to destroy the central core.

Postoperative Management

The kid should be given tetanus antitoxin when disbudded. The postoperative management simply involves observing the kid for complications.

Complications and Prognosis

The most common complication is scur formation when inadequate heat does not totally destroy the germinal tissue. More-serious, heat-induced complications result from overzealous burning of the horn. This thermal injury can lead to meningitis or cerebral malacia.

Obstructive Urolithiasis

Relevant Anatomy

The urinary tract of the male goat is like other ruminants in that the penis has a sigmoid flexure with the two bends. There is a urethral process (also called a vermiform appendage) that makes up the distalmost part of the urethra. The urethral process is approximately 3 cm long. The diameter of the urethral process is smaller than the proximal urethra.[5]

Indications

Urinary calculi will most frequently cause obstructions of the urethral appendage and at the distal bend of the sigmoid flexure.

Anesthesia and Surgical Preparation

Obstructed small ruminants may be treated while sedated with the addition of local anesthesia. When using lidocaine one must be conscious of the sensitivity of small ruminants and avoid toxic doses. Alternatively, one may choose to use general anesthesia to avoid lidocaine toxicity and have the benefit of working with a more relaxed patient.

Instrumentation

1. General surgery pack
2. Foley catheter

Surgical Technique

The first procedure done for any small ruminant with obstructive urolithiasis is to remove the urethral appendage. One may be able to extend the penis in a docile animal without sedation. However, most are more easily done with the aid of sedation or general anesthesia. The patient should be supported in a sitting position to flex the lumbosacral spine. This position makes extension of the penis much easier. The sigmoid flexure is straightened with one hand while the other (or an assistant) grasps the extended penis. Alternatively, one may use sponge forceps to retrieve the penis from within the preputial cavity. In animals castrated prior to puberty, the prepuce will be adhered to the penis. In this case the prepuce must be retracted from the penis to expose the complete urethral appendage for resection and to see the resulting urethral opening. The urethral appendage is frequently full of calculi and is often discolored. The urethral appendage is

simply removed at the free portion of the penis with scissors. This is the first step in treatment. The practitioner who is not comfortable with more-involved surgical procedures may consider this technique prior to referral in an effort to make the patient more comfortable.

There will frequently be some passage of urine when the appendage is removed. However, many obstructed animals will have other calculi, and the passage of urine is short term rather than curative. It is suggested to attempt passing a urinary catheter carefully, realizing that the sigmoid flexure is difficult to pass and the urethral diverticulum makes the passage of a catheter into the bladder unlikely.

A tube cystostomy provides a means of passing urine while temporarily bypassing the urethra, and urethral inflammation is treated.[6] Some consider the tube cystostomy combined with urine acidification to be the most successful treatment for obstructive urolithiasis.[7] The patient is positioned in dorsal recumbency. A caudal paramedian laparotomy incision is made approximately 6 cm long on either side of the sheath. When the abdomen is entered, the bladder should be very prominent in the obstructed animal. In addition to being distended, it may be dark in color and friable. There is often urine in the abdominal cavity, even in the absence of a rent in the bladder, via diapedesis through the wall of the distended bladder. The bladder is packed off from the peritoneal cavity with wet towels, and urine is suctioned from the bladder if needed. If the bladder is not too distended to work with, one may place stay sutures in the bladder, perform a cystotomy, and suction the urine as the bladder is opened. The bladder should be checked digitally for calculi. It may be repeatedly flushed and suctioned. It is often helpful to scoop calculi out of the bladder using a gallbladder spoon, a large dull curette, or even a sterile teaspoon. When the bladder is emptied of calculi, one should attempt to pass a polyurethane catheter normograde into the urethra. This is best done by putting tension on the bladder and filling the trigone region of the bladder with a finger or a syringe to help guide the catheter into the proximal urethra. If the catheter is passed into the urethra, one should gently flush the urethra to establish patency.

The Foley catheter is placed through a stab incision in the contralateral caudal paramedian site. A hemostat is placed from the peritoneum bluntly through the muscular body wall to tent the skin that is incised. The Foley is drawn into the abdominal cavity. The hemostat is then pleated through the omentum 3–5 times, and the tip of the Foley is pulled through the omentum. The cystotomy may be closed prior to or after placement of the Foley in the bladder, according to the surgeon's preference. The cystotomy is closed with no. 2-0 absorbable suture in a simple continuous line being careful not to penetrate the bladder lumen, then a second layer of an inverting pattern such as a Lembert. A purse-string suture that is large enough to accommodate the Foley is placed on the ventrolateral aspect of the bladder on the contralateral side to the original body wall incision. A stab incision is made inside the purse string, and the Foley is inserted followed by tightening and tying of the purse string. The Foley balloon is filled with sterile saline and then positioned at the bladder wall. The portion of the catheter outside the body wall is retracted so the portion inside the abdominal cavity is straight but not under tension. The catheter is secured to the body wall, and the abdominal incision is closed in a routine fashion. The catheter may need to be sutured to the skin cranial to the exit from the body wall in order to keep it off the pen floor. A finger of a surgical glove with a hole in the tip may be taped to the end of catheter to create a one-way valve.

Bladder marsupialization is another technique for management of obstructive urolithiasis.[8] It should be considered when there is a urethral rupture, in cases that require a less-expensive treatment than the tube cystostomy and prolonged postoperative management either as a first choice or after urethral patency cannot be established at surgery. The surgery is as described for the tube cystostomy to the point of placement of the Foley catheter. At that point, a 3-cm incision is made through the body wall at the contralateral paramedian site. A part of the bladder is pulled through this incision. It is sutured to the external rectus sheath with no. 2-0 or no. 3-0 absorbable suture in a simple interrupted pattern. The bladder is then incised and the mucosal layer is sutured to the skin with the same material and pattern.

These animals may be treated by urethrostomy as described in steers in Chapter 14. The urethral opening created by this technique is subject to stricture in a matter of months, so it is not a good long-term option for pet goats. It also does not allow for a cystostomy to remove calculi that are likely to be present in the bladder.

Postoperative Management

Management of the tube cystostomy is prolonged and intense. The patient should receive antibiotics and anti-inflammatories as well as IV fluids and treatment of any metabolic disorders. The catheter should be left open 24–48 hours. It can be closed for short periods after that while the patient is monitored closely. The Foley should be opened at any sign of discomfort. If urethral patency is established at surgery, the patient should be expected to start normal urination soon after surgery. If the urethra is still obstructed, the Foley may be required for weeks before the calculi are passed. When the patient is urinating normally with the Foley closed for 2–3 days, one can feel comfortable removing the catheter. The catheter should be left in place at least 7–10 days regardless of how quickly the animal is urinating in order for a fibrinous track to form around the catheter. This track helps prevent urine contamination of the abdominal cavity when the catheter is pulled since the balloon is

simply deflated, retention sutures are cut, and the catheter is pulled.

Postoperative management of the marsupialization is much less involved. The animal should be treated for any metabolic disorders, but the surgical site is simply monitored for urine flow and healing.

When the urethral appendage is removed and urine flow occurs, one must monitor closely for another obstruction. It may also be useful to treat the penis topically with an antiinflammatory ointment if adhesions of the prepuce were torn to facilitate the treatment.

Walpole's solution may be used in the bladder to dissolve calculi as part of the postoperative management with a tube cystostomy. This solution has been reported to be useful even when used via ultrasound guidance to percutaneously drain the bladder then instill Walpole's. This provided at least temporary relief in 80% of the cases, though 30% reobstructed.[9]

Complications and Prognosis

Very few animals will respond to removal of the urethral appendage alone, as most have other calculi that will cause another obstruction.

The tube cystostomy requires intensive management until normal urethral urine flow develops. Unfortunately this may take weeks for some to respond, and some may not respond quickly enough that decisions to euthanize the animal or pursue marsupialization are made.

The marsupialization may stricture over time causing the patient discomfort if the urethra is not patent. Some cases also suffer from prolapse of the bladder mucosa through the ostomy site or stricture of the site.[8,10]

In one review, 75% of the small ruminants treated for obstructive urolithiasis were discharged from the hospital. One year later, 75% of the discharged animals in which owners instituted a change of diet to minimize concentrate were alive, while only 25% of the animals that remained on high concentrate diets were alive.[11] In another review, reobstruction occurred in 20% of the cases treated by tube cystostomy.[12]

Mastectomy

Relevant Anatomy

The small ruminant udder is comprised of two mammary glands, as opposed to the cow which has four. The glands are relatively large. The arterial blood supply to the udder is by the external pudendal arteries and the perineal arteries. Venous return is by way of the external pudendal veins, perineal veins, and the subcutaneous abdominal veins that course cranially from each side of the udder. The pudendal vessels are found at the external inguinal ring. The perineal vessels are smaller and located near the midline caudal to the mammary gland.[5]

Indications

Goats tend to have more udder conditions requiring mastectomy than sheep. Mastectomy is a procedure largely for pet goats for obvious production reasons. Mastectomy is used to treat goats with gangrenous mastitis, precocious udder, or any mammary condition eliminated by removal.[13,14] Some udders become so large and pendulous that they become traumatized by dragging the ground.

Anesthesia and Surgical Preparation

The radical mastectomy is performed with the goat under general anesthesia in dorsal recumbency. The goat is milked to empty the udder to reduce the mass of the mammary gland as much as possible for ease of dissection. The skin of the udder and surrounding area is clipped and prepped for sterile surgery.

Instrumentation

1. General surgery pack
2. Penrose drain

Surgical Technique

The udder is very vascular; however, careful dissection with an understanding of the anatomy allows the radical mastectomy to be performed with minimal blood loss.

An elliptical skin incision around the udder has been described.[15] However, we prefer an inverted cloverleaf skin incision.[13] This is a series of four curvilinear incisions with the convex side toward the teats making cranial, caudal, and two lateral skin flaps respectively. These flaps are dissected off the mammary tissue to expose the vessels as described above. The vessels are ligated then transected before the mammary gland is dissected off the body wall. The mammary gland can be bluntly separated from the external rectus sheath. There is very little subcutaneous tissue to incorporate in the closure. There is considerable dead space under the skin flaps. The skin is closed in an "X" shape or as a double "Y" with the lateral flaps making a midline closure and the cranial and caudal flaps making the "Y" on each end. A Penrose drain is placed under the skin closure. Occasional interrupted sutures can be placed to tack the skin to the external rectus sheath in an effort to obliterate some of the dead space.

Alternatively, one may simply ligate and transect the pudendal vessels with the aid of local anesthesia and allow the udder to slough by avascular necrosis. This may be suggested in very toxic animals to avoid general anesthesia. However, the cosmetic appearance during the slough is not appreciated by many owners.

Postoperative Management

Perioperative antibiotics and antiinflammatory medications are appropriate. The Penrose is removed when drainage is minimal. This is usually in 2–3 days. Skin sutures are removed in 14 days if the surgical wound has healed adequately. One may leave the skin sutures in place a few more days if healing is questionable. One should have conversations with the owner about preventing the patient from becoming pregnant. Many are pet animals and are not exposed to a male. Others may need an ovariohysterectomy or ovariectomy if in a place that breeding is possible. That procedure would be done preferably during a second anesthetic episode rather than lengthening the surgery time and risking peritoneal contamination by combining procedures. While the correlation is not fully understood, there have been reports of dystocia in does that were allowed to carry a pregnancy after having a mastectomy performed.[14]

Complications and Prognosis

If vessels are not identified and securely ligated, intraoperative hemorrhage is a possible complication. Postoperative hematomas or seromas may form, and there may be delayed healing of the skin incision. However, the complication rate is very low when the procedure described is used, and the prognosis is generally good.

Vasectomy

Relevant Anatomy

The scrotal anatomy of the bull has been described in Chapter 14 does not vary significantly from that of the small ruminant. The vas deferens is easily palpated in the spermatic cord in the cranial aspect at the neck of the scrotum in small ruminants.

Indications

In some settings, the vasectomy is used to render male small ruminants infertile for the purpose of heat detection. More often, the teaser is placed with the females prior to the planned breeding season to stimulate them to start cycling. When the fertile males are placed in the flock of cycling females, the resultant birthing will be completed in a short time period.[16] Vasectomy may be done laparoscopically, but we will describe the conventional surgical approach.

Anesthesia and Surgical Preparation

The vasectomy may be done in tractable animals with local anesthesia as an assistant holds the animal sitting on the hindquarters or in lateral recumbency. Some less tractable animals will require sedation as well. In some situations the surgeon may choose to use general anesthesia but it is seldom required.

Small ruminants have more hair on the scrotum than bulls, so clipping the area of the neck of the scrotum where the vas deferens can be palpated is advised. The area is prepped prior to administering the local anesthesia followed by a final prep before the procedure is performed.

Instrumentation

1. General surgery pack

Surgical Technique

An incision approximately 4 cm long is made over the palpable vas deferens on the cranial part of the neck of the scrotum. The incision is continued through the skin and vaginal tunic to expose the vas deferens. A hemostat is used to elevate the vas out of the incision where two ligatures are placed as far apart as can be accomplished through the incision. The segment of vas deferens between the ligatures is then removed. The vaginal tunic is closed with no. 3-0 absorbable suture in a simple continuous pattern. The skin is closed with material and pattern of choice. The procedure is repeated on the other side. In some large operations, the teaser males have a vasectomy on one testicle and the other testicle is removed for ease of identification. This unilateral castration is done as described the bull in Chapter 13. The penile translocation technique for the bull, which is described in Chapter 13, may be used in small ruminants to create teaser animals, but it is more frequently performed in small ruminants as a surgical training procedure.

The penile translocation technique for the bull described in Chapter 13.

Postoperative Management

Minimal postoperative management is required beyond normal incision concerns of a relatively clean and dry pen to limit environmental contamination. Skin sutures are removed in 10–14 days. The male can be used in 1–2 weeks. If using earlier than 2 weeks, it is suggested that a semen exam is done to insure there are no sperm present in the ejaculate.

Complications and Prognosis

There are few short term complications associated with this procedure. In the long term, sperm granulomas are common but of little clinical significance.

Cesarean Section

Relevant Anatomy

Laparotomy principles and anatomy in cattle are described in Chapter 13, and cesarean section in the cow is described in Chapter 14. The elements previously described apply to the small ruminant with a few exceptions, which we will discuss here. The muscular body wall of small ruminants is much thinner than that of cattle, which may be problematic when administering local anesthetic or making too bold of an incision. Sheep will have more retroperitoneal fat than goats or cattle. Multiple fetuses are the rule rather than the exception in small ruminant pregnancy. Therefore, an incision in each uterine horn is often required.

Indications

Dystocia in small ruminants may be due to relative or absolute fetal oversize, pregnancy toxemia, malpositioning, or failure of cervical dilation. It is difficult to provide assistance to correct malpositioning and achieve vaginal delivery in smaller sheep and goats because of the size of the vagina.

Anesthesia and Surgical Preparation

Any of the techniques described for cows may be used but we prefer the recumbent left flank approach for small ruminants. Some practitioners perform standing flank laparotomy for selected cases when the female is of large stature. The left flank is clipped and prepped for administration of local anesthesia which is followed by a final surgical scrub. The anesthetic method of choice is usually a line block, though a paravertebral block is also acceptable. The lidocaine may be diluted to 1% and no more than 6 mg/kg body weight should be given to avoid toxicity. Some animals may require sedation in addition to the local anesthesia to facilitate the surgical procedure.

Instrumentation

1. General surgery pack

Surgical Technique

The left-flank incision should be large enough to allow the surgeon to place a hand into the abdominal cavity to manipulate and exteriorize the uterus. In some cases multiple fetuses can be delivered via one uterine incision near the uterine body. However, often it is easier and safer to make an incision in each uterine horn. The uterine incision may be made over the fetal hind limb as in cattle or directly over the head of the fetus which can then be delivered with the forelimbs back without detriment. The uterus is usually closed sufficiently by a single layer of an inverting pattern such as the Utrecht using no. 2-0 absorbable suture. The body wall is closed in routine fashion.

Postoperative Management

Perioperative antibiotics should be administered to these patients. Skin sutures may be removed in 14 days. Management is otherwise dependent on the metabolic state of the female, which usually correlates with the duration of the dystocia prior to surgical intervention. Animals suffering from pregnancy toxemia will require extensive postoperative care in the form of IV fluids, antiinflammatories and often tube feeding to provide needed energy. Skin sutures should be removed in 14 days.

Complications and Prognosis

Retained placenta is the most common postoperative complication following dystocia. Antibiotic treatment has been shown to decrease complications after cesarean section in small ruminants.[17] The prognosis is good for successful breeding following cesarean section for non-complicated dystocias.[17] The prognosis is fair to poor when the patient is toxemic from either the pregnancy itself or from a prolonged duration of dystocia.

Rectal Prolapse Resection in Small Ruminants

Relevant Anatomy

The rectum is caudal to the small colon. Much of it is retroperitoneal as it progresses to the anal canal which is only approximately 1 cm long in small ruminants. The rectococcygeus muscle bundles arise from the distal rectum and insert on the ventral aspect of the coccygeal vertebrae.[18] One may speculate that this anatomy contributes to the increased incidence of rectal prolapse when tail docking has been done very short.

The blood supply to the distal colon and rectum is located dorsally, which is important to remember as one dissects the rectal tissue for resection and anastomosis. There can be significant hemorrhage if one transects the vasculature without being prepared to clamp and ligate the vessels.

Indications

A persistent rectal prolapse that does not respond to nonsurgical treatment—including cleaning, topical anti-inflammatory ointments, repeated reduction, and/or reduction with purse-string retention suture—is one that may require surgical resection. There are a number of potential causes of rectal prolapse in small ruminants beyond tail docking. These include but are not limited to coughing, straining associated with diarrhea, parasites, or even urinary obstruction.

Anesthesia and Surgical Preparation

Epidural anesthesia is adequate in most cases. Some fractious animals may require sedation as well. The prolapsed tissue and area around the anus should be cleaned.

Instrumentation

1. General surgery pack
2. Spinal needles (4–6 inches long)
3. A section of endotracheal tube

Surgical Technique

A rectal prolapse ring may be used as a salvage procedure in most food animals; the reader is referred to Chapter 18 for a description of that technique in the pig. We will describe the surgical resection here; it may be applied to any food animal species. A tube small enough to be placed in the rectum without creating further trauma, yet large enough to provide as large a stoma as possible, is placed in the rectum extending proximal to the anal sphincter. The rectal tissue is secured to the retention tube with two spinal needles at right angles to each other. Each needle is inserted into the skin approximately 4 mm rostral to the visible prolapsed rectal mucosa, then insertion continues sequentially through the inner layer of prolapsed rectal tissue, both walls of the retention tube and the opposite inner layer of the prolapsed rectal tissue and finally exits the skin just rostral to the prolapsed mucosa 180 degrees from where it entered (Figure 16.2A). These needles prevent the rectal tissue from retracting into the abdomen when it is incised. In order to avoid the major blood supply, do not place a needle at the 12 o'clock position. The prolapsed tissue will be excised by a circular incision made as close as possible to the anus through both layers of the prolapse down to the retention tube. It is advised to make the incision for less than one-fourth the circumference of the prolapsed tissue secured to the retention tube. The incised segment is closed with absorbable suture in a simple continuous pattern opposing the rectal mucosa, while including deeper muscular tissue in the suture. The resection is completed by making the incision in 4–5 separate segments followed by closure with separate continuous suture lines using no. 2-0 absorbable suture material (Figure 16.2B). The dorsalmost aspect of the incision is made carefully so the blood supply may be ligated prior to transection. Upon completion of the resection, the needles and tube are removed and the prolapse should be resolved. Rarely, the tissue is edematous enough that reduction and purse-string suture retention is needed.

Postoperative Management

The animal may be returned to grazing. Dry feedstuffs such as hay should be limited for 48 hours in an effort to maintain relatively loose feces.

Fig. 16.2. A. Tube stent placement for rectal prolapse resection. **B.** Rectal prolapse resection partially complete with tube stent in place.

Complications and Prognosis

A failure of the suture line will lead to a catastrophic breakdown of the closure and peritonitis. However, this is a rare occurrence. The most common complication is stricture of the rectum leading to difficulty with defecation. Abscesses may also occur. The prognosis is good provided any predisposing condition that led to the prolapse has resolved.

References

1. Hull, B.L. Dehorning the adult goat. *Vet. Clin. Food Anim.*, *11*:183–185, 1995.
2. Bowen, J.S. Dehorning the mature goat. *J. Am. Vet. Med. Assoc.*, *171*:1249, 1977.
3. Guss, S.B. Management and Diseases of Dairy Goats. Scottsdale, AZ, Dairy Goat Journal Publishing, 1977.
4. Hague, B.A., and Hooper, R.N. Cosmetic dehorning in goats. *Vet. Surg.*, *26*(4):332–334, 1997.
5. Sisson, S. Ruminant urogenital system. *In* Sisson and Grossman's The Anatomy of Domestic Animals, 5th Ed. Edited by R. Getty. Philadelphia, Saunders, 1975, p. 937.
6. Rakestraw, P.C., Fubini, S.L., Gilbert, R.O., and Ward, J.O. Tube cystostomy for treatment of obstructive urolithiasis in small ruminants. *Vet. Surg.*, *24*(6):498–505, 1995.
7. Tarunbir Singh Amarpal Kinjavdekar, P., Aithal, H.P., and Pawde, A.M. Comparison of four surgical techniques for the management of obstructive urolithiasis in male goats. *Ind. J. Vet. Surg.*, *31*(1):15–20, 2010.
8. May, K.A., Moll, H.D., Duncan, R.B., Moon, M.M., Pleasant, R.S., and Howard, R.D. Experimental evaluation of urinary bladder marsupialization in male goats. *Vet. Surg.*, *31*(3):251–258, 2002.
9. Janke, J.J., Osterstock, J.B., Washburn, K.E., Bissett, W.T., Roussel, A.J., and Hooper, R.N. Use of Walpole's solution for treatment of goats with urolithiasis: 25 cases (2001–2006). *J. Am. Vet. Med. Assoc.*, *234*(2):249–252, 2009.
10. May, K.A., Moll, H.D., Wallace, L.M., Pleasant, R.S., and Howard, R.D. Urinary bladder marsupialization for treatment of obstructive urolithiasis in male goats. *Vet. Surg.*, *27*(6):583–588, 1998.
11. Baird, A.N. Unpublished data, 2012.
12. Ewoldt, J.M., Anderson, D.E., Miesner, M.D., and Saville, W.J.: Short- and long-term outcome and factors predicting survival after surgical tube cystostomy for treatment of obstructive urolithiasis in small ruminants. *Vet. Surg.*, *36*(5):417–422, 2006.
13. Plummer, J.P., and Plummer, C. Diseases of the mammary gland. *In* Sheep and Goat Medicine, 2nd Ed. Edited by D.G. Pugh, A.N. Baird. Maryland Heights, MO, Saunders, 2012, p. 442.
14. Whitlock, B.K., Coffman, E.A., and Pugh, D.G. Diseases of the endocrine system. *In* Sheep and Goat Medicine, 2nd Ed. Edited by D.G. Pugh, A.N. Baird. Maryland Heights, MO, Saunders, 2012, p. 231.
15. Cable, C.S., Peery, K., and Fubini, S.L. Radical mastectomy in 20 ruminants. *Vet. Surg.*, *33*(3):263–266, 2004.
16. Edmondson, M.A., Roberts, J.F., Baird, A.N., and Pugh, D.G. Theriogenology of sheep and goats. *In* Sheep and Goat Medicine, 2nd Ed. Edited by D.G. Pugh, A.N. Baird. Maryland Heights, MO, Saunders, 2012, p. 150.
17. Brounts, S.H., Hawkins, J.F., Baird, A.N., and Glickman, L.T. Outcome and subsequent fertility of sheep and goats undergoing cesarean section because of dystocia: 110 cases (1981–2001). *J. Am. Vet. Med. Asssoc.*, *224*(2):275–279, 2004.
18. Schummer, A., Nickel, R., and Sack, W.O. Alimentary canal of ruminants. *In* The Viscera of the Domestic Mammals, 2nd Ed. Edited by A. Schummer, R. Nickel, W.O. Sack. New York, Springer-Verlag, 1979, p. 171.

Chapter 17

CAMELID SURGERY

A. N. Baird, DVM, MS, DACVS

Objectives

1. Discuss different techniques for castration of camelids.
2. Describe a method of cesarean section in camelids.
3. Describe common management of fighting teeth, as well as more involved cheek tooth removal in camelids.

Castration of the Llama

Relevant Anatomy

The scrotum of camelids is nonpendulous and relatively small. The scrotal skin is very thick. The testes of llamas are reported to be approximately 4–7 cm long. The tail of the epididymis is tightly adhered to the testes and is more difficult to palpate than in ruminants with pendulous testicles.[1]

Indications

Hand-raised male camelids that may imprint on humans should be castrated at about 2 months of age in an effort to decrease the occurrence of berserk male syndrome. Other indications for castration of camelids are for prevention of the spread of poor genetics and for management reasons to allow males and females to be housed together without the possibility of unwanted pregnancy. Not all agree on the best age to castrate camelids, but at least one recommendation is after 12 months of age but before sexual maturity in order to avoid intact male behavior.[2]

Anesthesia and Surgical Preparation

Standing castration is performed with the animal sedated and local anesthetic injected into the testicle, spermatic cord, and scrotal skin. Approximately 3 ml of diluted 1% lidocaine is adequate for each testicle. The animal is restrained in a camelid chute or is tied to a sturdy object and pushed against a wall or door way. The tail is wrapped to prevent tail hairs from contaminating the incisions.

General anesthesia is used for recumbent castrations either as will be described in the standing patient or for closure of the skin incision in order for it to heal by first-intention healing.[3,4] Clipping is not usually necessary; the scrotum is prepped for sterile surgery.

Instrumentation

1. General surgery pack
2. Emasculators

Surgical Technique

Standing Castration

The testicles are pushed dorsally in the scrotum and an incision the length of the testicle is made through the skin and fascia to expose the common vaginal tunic. Blunt dissection to free the testicle from surrounding fascia is less difficult if the common vaginal tunic remains intact. After blunt dissection of the testicle, the spermatic cord may be crushed with hemostats and ligated. A single ligature is adequate in most cases, although one may choose to double ligate with one transfixing and one circumferential suture. One may alternatively use an emasculator on the cord for hemostasis. If an emasculator is used, be sure it is of the appropriate size to adequately crush the small spermatic cord of the camelid. Those used on larger species may not crush the small cord well enough to achieve hemostasis. The procedure is repeated on the

Turner and McIlwraith's Techniques in Large Animal Surgery, 4th Edition. Dean A. Hendrickson and A. N. (Nickie) Baird.
© 2013 John Wiley & Sons, Inc. Published 2013 by John Wiley & Sons, Inc.

opposite side and the skin incisions are left open to heal by secondary intention.

Recumbent Castration

The camelid may be castrated under general anesthesia using the same technique as described for the standing castration. However, we will describe a recumbent procedure that closes the skin for primary healing. The animal is placed in dorsal recumbency in a frog-leg position with a rope or hobbles over the dorsosacral region securing the hind limbs in a flexed position. One testicle is pushed forward of the scrotum approximately 12–15 cm. A 5–cm incision is made through the skin and subcutaneous tissue over that testicle to expose the common vaginal tunic. Care must be taken to avoid incising the penis, which is easily palpated. After blunt dissection of the testicle, the spermatic cord is double ligated and the testicle is removed. The contralateral testicle is then pushed into position, and hemostats are used to bluntly dissect deep to the penis to exteriorize the testicle through the previous skin incision. That spermatic cord is then ligated, and the testicle is removed. The subcutaneous tissue is then closed in a caudal–to-cranial direction with no. 3-0 absorbable material in a simple continuous pattern. The tail of the suture at the starting knot is left long. The loop of suture is cut from the cranial subcutaneous knot and a subcuticular closure is started from the tag of suture of the cranial knot progressing caudally. At the caudal extent of the closure the suture is tied to the long tag of the first knot and thus buried.

Postoperative Management

Antibiotics should be given if the primary healing technique is used. The incision should be kept free of flies in hot weather. The new gelding should be exercised. The surgical site should be observed closely for up to 10 days.

Complications and Prognosis

Postoperative hemorrhage may occur if proper hemostasis is not achieved. The incisions should be monitored for signs of infection. The primary closure surgical sites tend to heal well with less swelling than those left open to heal by secondary intention. However, should the primary closure site become infected, it is a more significant problem since drainage should be established, which will likely require a second anesthesia.

Cesarean Section in the Camelid

Relevant Anatomy

The camelid uterus is bicornate and grossly resembles that of a mare more than that of small ruminants. The body is short but looks longer because of the horns being fused for a distance with a septum dividing them. We will describe a ventral midline approach for cesarean section. The linea is narrow and the surgeon will incise the rectus abdominus muscle when straying the slightest off the midline. Many surgeons are happy with a flank laparotomy for this procedure. However, there are unique variations of the abdominal wall musculature that should be reviewed before one chooses to use a flank approach to the camelid abdomen.

Indications

Fortunately the frequency of dystocia in camelids is low. However, cesarean section is indicated to relieve dystocia for any reason. The most common fetal cause of dystocia is a cranial presentation with the head retained. Dystocia may also be due to other fetal malpositions, fetal monsters, or uterine torsion to name a few.[5,6] The animals are small enough that extensive vaginal manipulation to relieve a dystocia is not feasible nor in the best interest of the animal. Therefore, one should quickly choose to perform surgery when initial attempts at manipulation are not successful.

Anesthesia and Surgical Preparation

Cesarean section may be performed successfully in camelids via a number of approaches and anesthetic protocols. General anesthesia is our method of choice with the animal in dorsal recumbency for the midline incision. Sedation, local anesthesia and physical restraint may be used for the midline or flank approaches. Animals that are easily managed may be operated via a standing flank while restrained in a llama chute. The surgical site should be clipped and prepped for sterile surgery.

Instrumentation

1. General surgery pack

Surgical Technique

The midline incision is made from the just cranial to the mammary gland continuing cranially for approximately 40 cm. The uterus is located and exteriorized through the body wall incision. The uterus is positioned to allow an incision in the greater curvature of the gravid horn (usually the left) and packed off from the peritoneum with wet sterile towels if possible to limit contamination. The cria is delivered and handed to an assistant for resuscitation as needed. The placenta is frequently removed with minimal traction. The uterus is closed with absorbable suture in an inverting pattern. The condition of the tissue will allow the surgeon to determine if one- or two-layer closure is required. The uterus is rinsed with sterile saline and returned to the abdominal cavity. The body

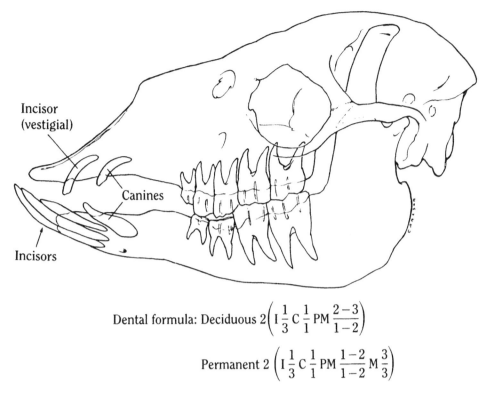

Dental formula: Deciduous $2\left(I\,\dfrac{1}{3}\,C\,\dfrac{1}{1}\,PM\,\dfrac{2-3}{1-2}\right)$

Permanent $2\left(I\,\dfrac{1}{3}\,C\,\dfrac{1}{1}\,PM\,\dfrac{1-2}{1-2}\,M\,\dfrac{3}{3}\right)$

Fig. 17.1. Dentition of the llama (Lama glama).

wall incision is closed in a routine fashion. We prefer to use three equally placed near-far-far-near sutures for tension with simple continuous suture lines between the tension sutures in the linea. This is followed by a simple continuous pattern in the subcutaneous layer and the same in the skin.

Postoperative Management

Perioperative antibiotics and antiinflammatory drugs are given. The animal is confined to a clean, dry area for at least 10 days. Skin sutures are removed in 14 days.

Complications and Prognosis

There are few complications, and the prognosis is good if the dystocia is resolved quickly. A prolonged dystocia and resultant patient compromise lead to toxemia and metabolic disorders which understandably are associated with postoperative complications and a poorer prognosis.

Tooth Removal in the Llama

Relevant Anatomy

The dental formula of the adult llama is I(1/3) − C(1/1) − PM (1-2/1-2) − M(3/3).[7] The shape and direction of the root of the canine teeth in llamas are important considerations to facilitate atraumatic removal of these teeth.

The dentition of the llama is shown in Figure 17.1. The root of the canine follows a caudal direction, a factor important at the time of tooth removal.

Indications

As a management tool to prevent injury when fighting, removal of canine teeth of the llama may be necessary. The other indication for removal of canine teeth is a tooth root abscess. A root abscess may occur secondary to partial removal in which the crown has been amputated and the pulp cavity is exposed. Partial amputation is done to minimize injuries inflicted to other herd members. Infection subsequently migrates down the pulp cavity. Removal of molar teeth is usually to resolve a root abscess. The common causes of root abscesses of the molars are broken teeth. Some abscesses are caused by actinomycosis (resembling "lumpy jaw" in cattle), whereas others are spontaneous, with no apparent cause. Signs of a tooth problem include swelling of the mandible, pain, head shyness, a draining fistula, or impaired mastication. Radiographs of the affected tooth show varying degrees of bone lysis at the tooth root. Animals with chronic cases have radiographic evidence of increased bone density (sclerosis) surrounding the tooth root.

As with horses, endodontic therapy is an alternative to tooth removal that may be used in camelids as well. This technique is considered advanced, however, and is not described here.

Anesthesia and Surgical Preparation

Tooth removal in the llama is performed with the animal under general anesthesia. Xylazine, in combination with local anesthesia, has been used by some surgeons, but inhalation anesthesia (halothane) is preferred. The llama is given a guaifenesin-ketamine or guaifenesin-thiamylal combination intravenously to effect, an endotracheal tube is placed, and halothane-oxygen is administered. The llama is positioned in lateral recumbency with the affected tooth uppermost. A mouth speculum, similar to that used in dogs, is positioned to allow the surgeon free access to the incisor teeth or the ability to palpate the affected molar tooth. If a canine tooth is to be removed, the mucosa around the tooth is surgically prepared. If a molar tooth is to be removed, the hair over the surgical site is clipped, and routine surgical preparation is performed. The exact location of the surgical site is determined by the position of the affected molar on radiographs. Markers on the skin such as skin staples or placement of a malleable probe into the draining tract associated with an abscessed tooth when taking intraoperative radiographs will help with proper location of the buccotomy incision for removal of cheek teeth.

Instrumentation

1. General surgery pack
2. Mouth speculum (canine mouth gag)
3. Small mallet
4. Chisel (approximately ¼-inch width)
5. Curette
6. Dental punch
7. Small periosteal elevator
8. Forceps
9. Air drill

Surgical Technique

Removal of Canine Teeth

For removal of a canine tooth, a fusiform incision is made through the mucous membrane around the tooth and is extended down to the mandibular bone (Figure 17-2A and B). A second incision is made directly over the tooth root, curving caudad, in the direction of the long axis of the tooth (Figure 17-2B). Using a periosteal elevator, the surgeon reflects the gingiva and periosteum away from the lateral surface of the mandible, in the direction of the tooth root. Similar elevation is performed on the medial side of the tooth extending about one-eighth of an inch from the gum–tooth margin. A segment of bone on the lateral side of the tooth is then removed (Figure 17-2C). Periosteum may first be reflected from this region; this is not critical. This lateral bone is removed because this is the direction in which the tooth will be extracted. The use of a chisel on the lingual side of the tooth facilitates removal of the tooth. Knowledge of the direction of the canine tooth root is important for atraumatic removal of this tooth. As bone is removed, the tooth should be grasped periodically and moved in a side-to-side motion to ascertain when it is ready for extraction. Eventually, the tooth can be extracted without risking fracture of the mandible. The alveolus is then curetted, to remove all diseased bone associated with the root abscess (Figure 17-2D). Debris is flushed from the site with sterile saline solution. The gingiva is then apposed over the empty socket using no. 2-0 synthetic, absorbable, monofilament suture (Figure 17-2E).

If the equipment is available, a Hall air drill with the appropriate bur can be used to remove the bone from the lateral surface of the canine tooth. Most important is the position of the canine tooth root within the bone. The tooth root is extensive and follows a marked caudal direction.

Removal of the Crown of Canine Teeth

It is a common management tool to partially remove the canine (fighting teeth) in males to prevent injury to other animals or humans. Trimming the canines too closely may lead to exposure of the pulp cavity and subsequent abscessation. However, this is a rare complication. The llama is restrained in a chute with the head secured or sedated and restrained in hand by an assistant. A Gigli wire is used to saw the teeth as close to the gum line as possible without damaging the oral mucosa. This will leave blunted teeth just a few mm long. A Dremel or small equine float is used to smooth any sharp edges on the teeth.

Removal of Molar Teeth

The exact location of the affected tooth is confirmed on the radiographs and by palpation of the crown of the tooth with the fingertips. A straight incision is made directly over the longitudinal axis of the tooth (Figure 17-2F). The periosteum is reflected (optional). The bone lateral to the tooth is removed, but the bone immediately ventral to the tooth is preserved (Figure 17-2G). The tooth should be freed of bone at its rostral and caudal surfaces using a chisel. A dental punch is placed on the tooth root; and with gentle tapping, it seats itself into the root of the tooth. The surgeon should place his fingertips over the crown of the tooth and guide the punch with the other hand. An assistant then delivers the blows to the punch. The surgeon feels the vibrations of the blows transmitted through the tooth to his fingertips. Occasionally, the punch has to be redirected. The tooth gradually loosens, and the blows of the mallet should then become less forceful. Conversely, a hole can be made over the affected roots with a trephine or Hall air drill.

When a single root of a cheek tooth is abscessed, the tooth may be split and only the crown associated with the

A

Outline of
canine tooth

Incision in
mucosa

B

Lateral
surface
of mandible

C

Empty
socket

Curette

D

Closure
of mucosa

E

Fig. 17.2.   **A–H.** Tooth removal in the llama.

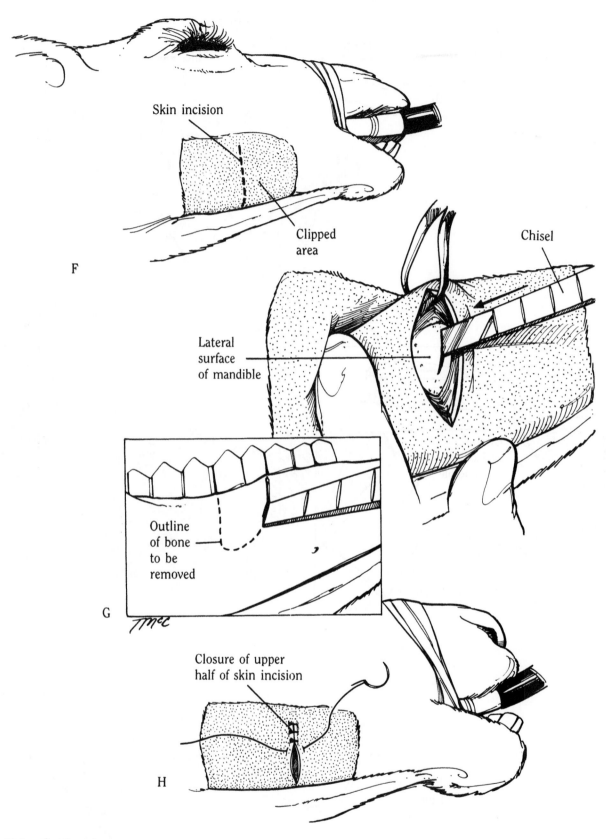

F

Skin incision

Clipped
area

Chisel

Lateral
surface
of mandible

Outline
of bone
to be
removed

G

Closure of upper
half of skin incision

H

Fig. 17.2.   Continued.

infected root is removed. This allows the surgeon to save much of the occlusal surface of the cheek teeth.

Following repulsion of the tooth, any small fragments of bone or teeth are removed. The alveolus is curetted and is flushed. The ventral half of the incision is left open, to provide ventral drainage of the alveolus. The upper half is closed with simple interrupted sutures with nonabsorbable suture material (Figure 17-2H).

Postoperative Management

The llama should be placed on antibiotics preoperatively and for approximately 1–2 weeks following surgery. The wound where the canine tooth has been removed usually requires little postoperative care. Following molar extraction, the alveolus can be flushed daily with a mild antiseptic solution or until granulation tissue has begun to fill the defect. Long-term care will involve monitoring and the occasional floating of the opposing teeth which will not wear normally in the absence of the removed tooth (or teeth).

Complications and Prognosis

We have seen uncomplicated healing after removal of canine and molar teeth. Daily flushing of the alveolus seems to keep food and debris from lodging in the wound in the case of molar teeth. This sort of aftercare can be performed by the owner. Reports of success and complication rates of tooth extraction in llamas are rare, but one study showed a unanimous success of surgical extraction for treatment of tooth abscesses with very few complications.[8] Another study showed that animals in poor body condition at the time of surgery had a higher complication rate than those in good body condition. Complications included chronic draining tracts, reinfection, or osteomyelitis.[9] Medical treatment of tooth abscessation resulted in recurrence of symptoms in some animals.

References

1. Carson, R.L., Powe, T.A., and Pugh, D.G. Examination and special diagnostic procedures of the scrotum and testes. *In* Large Animal Urogenital Surgery, 2nd Ed. Edited by D.F. Wolfe, H.D. Moll. Baltimore, MD, Williams & Wilkins, 1999, p. 273.
2. Nickolmann, S., Hoy, S., and Gauly, M. Effects of castration on the behavior of male llamas (Lama glama). *Tieraerztl. Prax. G. N.*, 36(5):319–323, 2008.
3. Baird, A.N., Pugh, D.G., Wenzel, J.G.W., and Lin, H.C. Comparison of two techniques for castration of llamas. *J. Am. Vet. Med. Assoc.*, 208(2):261–262, 1996.
4. Pugh, D.G., Baird, A.N., Wolfe, D.F., Wenzel, J.G.W., and Lin, H.C. A prescrotal castration technique for llamas. *Eq. Pract.*, 16(4):26–28, 1994.
5. Anderson, D.E. Uterine torsion and cesarean section in llamas and alpacas. (Special Issue: Alpaca and llama health management). *Vet. Clin. Food Anim. Pract.*, 25(2):523–538, 2009.
6. Pearson, L.K., Rodriguez, J.S., and Tibary, A. Uterine torsion in late gestation alpacas and llamas: 60 cases (2000–2009). *Small Rum. Res.*, 105, 1–3:268–272, 2012.
7. Turner, A.S. Surgical conditions in the llama. *Vet. Clin. Food Anim.*, 5:81–99, 1989.
8. Cebra, M.L., Cebra, M.K., and Garry, F.B. Tooth root abscesses in New World camelids: 23 cases (1972–1994). *J. Am. Vet. Med. Assoc.*, 209:819–822, 1996.
9. Niehaus, A.J., and Anderson, D.E. Tooth root abscesses in llamas and alpacas: 123 cases (1994–2005). *J. Am. Vet. Med. Assoc.*, 231(2):284–289, 2007.

Chapter 18

SWINE SURGERY

A. N. Baird, DVM, MS, DACVS

Objectives

1. Describe basic techniques for castration and inguinal herniorrhaphy in the piglet.
2. Describe procedures for ablation of the preputial diverticulum.
3. Describe a technique for cesarean section in the sow and ovariohysterectomy in pot-bellied pigs.
4. Describe the prolapsed ring technique of treating rectal prolapse.

Castration of the Piglet

Relevant Anatomy

The testes of the boar are large in comparison to the bull, which is a direct reflection of sperm production. Located caudal to the thighs and ventral to the anus, the testes normally range from 10–15 cm in length and 5–9 cm in diameter.[1] The spermatic cord, usually 20–25 cm long, is comprised of the ductus deferens, testicular artery, testicular vein, lymphatics, the testicular plexus of autonomic nerves, cremaster muscle, and the visceral layer of the vaginal tunic. The epididymis is closely associated with the ventral aspect of the testis and terminates in the cauda epididymis at the dorsum of the testis where it becomes the ductus deferens.[1]

Indications

Generally, castration of the piglet is performed to improve the manageability of the herd; it also improves carcass quality because it removes taint. It is preferable to castrate piglets within the first 3 weeks of life. Research indicates that pain-associated behavioral responses do not differ between pigs castrated at 1, 5, 10, and 20 days. However, recorded data on pig weaning weights and weight gain appears to favor castration at 14 days rather than 1 day.[2,3] Although generally regarded as poor management, castration of larger pigs is occasionally indicated. The litter of piglets scheduled to be castrated should be clean and in good physical condition. If piglets in a litter are scouring, castration should be postponed. The area in which the castration is to be performed should be relatively clean and free of dust. If castration is to be performed in hot weather, it should be done early in the morning.

Anesthesia and Surgical Preparation

Surgical castration of piglets is a painful procedure at any age. The cutting of the spermatic cord has been identified as the most painful event. Appropriate anesthetic protocols are limited, however, due to cost effectiveness, ease and quickness of administration, and the quality of recovery. Recovery must be rapid and complete so the piglet does not develop postoperative hypothermia or so that it is not crushed by the sow.[4] For economical reasons, surgical castration of piglets less than 3 weeks old is often performed without anesthesia. The herdsman restrains the piglet in a vertical position by the hind legs by the hocks and securing the animal either against the herdsman's body or in a clean V-trough. Local analgesia is certainly indicated at this point and will help to reduce stress on the animal. Intratesticular and intrafunicular administration of 2% lidocaine (4 mg/kg) were shown to be equally effective in reducing nociceptive pain responses in castrated piglets less than 28 days old.[4] One study judged lidocaine reduced the pain response of piglets during castration and also failed to determine any positive effect of meloxicam.[5] Another study showed evidence that piglets given meloxicam showed signs of decreased pain after castration when compared to piglets given local anesthesia for the procedure or those castrated without

Turner and McIlwraith's Techniques in Large Animal Surgery, 4th Edition. Dean A. Hendrickson and A. N. (Nickie) Baird.
© 2013 John Wiley & Sons, Inc. Published 2013 by John Wiley & Sons, Inc.

lidocaine.[6] Researchers will rightfully continue to investigate the use of analgesics to relieve stress and pain during castration. We are not comfortable with the benefit of any specific analgesic protocol at this time. A technique for inhalational anesthesia in piglets has also been described with isoflurane, isoflurane/N_2O, and carbon dioxide as well.[7] It is important to note that, to date, the Food and Drug Administration has not approved an analgesic for use in meat-producing pigs in the United States. Furthermore, withdrawal times and food residues are not documented for these drugs. The practitioner is ultimately responsible for using these drugs judiciously in pigs destined for market.

Before beginning castration, the inguinal area should be carefully inspected for any evidence of inguinal hernia. Then, the inguinal and scrotal areas are scrubbed with a suitable disinfectant (Figure 18.1A).

Instrumentation

1. General surgery pack
2. No. 12 scalpel blades

Surgical Technique

By pressing the fingers of the left hand into the animal's scrotum, the testes are pushed craniad into the inguinal area. A longitudinal incision through the skin, subcutaneous tissue, and fascia is made directly over each testis with a no. 12 scalpel blade (Figure 18.1B). (Figure 18.1C shows the method of holding the no. 12 scalpel blade and handle.) Using blunt dissection with fingers, the surgeon grasps the testis in one hand while applying sufficient traction to break the scrotal ligament; this delivers the tunic-covered testis through the wound (Figure 18.1D). If the incision results in an open vaginal tunic, the tunic should be retrieved immediately to reduce the incidence of scirrhous cord. Traction on the testis is maintained by the left hand while a sterile scalpel blade is used to scrape and sever the tunic and cord structures. The scraping should be performed as proximal as possible on the cord, so the severed end of the cord retracts into the inguinal region. This reduces the chances of infection and scirrhous cord formation. To minimize the chances of accidentally lacerating the piglet in some other area, the scraping should be performed in a direction *away* from the animal (Figure 18.1E). This procedure is repeated on the opposite testis. The resulting incisions are located cranial to the normal position of the testes to provide adequate ventral drainage. The left-handed operator uses the right hand to press the testis forward and holds the scalpel in his left hand.

Postoperative Management

Some surgeons prefer to dust the surgical site with an antibacterial powder; this is generally unnecessary if piglets can be turned into a clean, dry pen. The piglets should not be allowed into dirty quarters until healing is complete, usually within 5–7 days. If there is evidence of inguinal-scrotal hernia, then the entire spermatic cord should be transfixed and ligated before it is severed. (See the discussion in this chapter of inguinal herniorrhaphy in the piglet.)

If intratesticular anesthesia is used to castrate boars, the testes must be disposed of carefully.

Complications and Prognosis

The prognosis for this procedure is very good. Occasionally, death may result due to intestinal prolapse from an undetected inguinal hernia. Complications most commonly associated with this procedure are abscess and behavioral side effects including reductions in suckling time and increased lying time.[3]

Inguinal Herniorrhaphy in the Piglet

Relevant Anatomy

The inguinal canal is described as a potential space communicating between the internal and external abdominal oblique muscles.[8] The internal inguinal ring, formed by the internal oblique muscle and the inguinal ligament, leads from the canal into the abdominal cavity. An invagination of peritoneum into the scrotum, the vaginal ring, extends into the internal ring. A larger–than–normal vaginal ring is believed to predispose some male piglets to inguinal hernias. The superficial inguinal ring is formed by an opening in the external oblique muscle near the pecten pubis. Anatomical differences specific to swine include a larger deep (internal) ring and a relatively short inguinal canal.[8]

Indications

Frequently, inguinal hernias are discovered in piglets at the time of castration. These hernias generally do not reduce spontaneously; and when the ordinary castration procedure is used, evisceration is a frequent postcastration complication. The economics of hernia repair in the pig should be discussed with the client before surgery is undertaken.

Anesthesia and Surgical Preparation

For practical and economic reasons, no anesthetic is used routinely for small piglets; however, larger pigs require anesthesia similar to that used for castration of large pigs. The pig is restrained in a vertical position by the herdsman or by ropes in a clean V-trough if the pig is too large.

Gauze

Skin
incision

Location
of testes

A

B

C

TMCC

D

E

Testis

Scrotal
ligament

Fig. 18.1. **A–E.** Castration of the piglet.

The skin of the inguinal and scrotal areas is scrubbed with a suitable antiseptic.

Instrumentation

1. General surgery pack

Surgical Technique

An incision approximately 7 cm long is made through the skin, subcutaneous tissues, and fascia over the external inguinal ring (Figure 18.2A). Extensive hernias may require a larger incision. The testis, spermatic cord, and surrounding fascia are isolated using blunt dissection. Steady traction is exerted on the testis, tunics, and cord, pulling them loose from their attachment in the scrotum (scrotal ligament) (Figure 18.2B). The freed vaginal tunic should not be incised. By grasping the testis, the surgeon twists the vaginal sac, to return the intestines to the abdomen. Fingers may be used to "milk" the intestines into the abdomen. A pair of Kelly forceps is used to grasp the sac while a transfixation ligature is applied on the proximal end of the cord just distal to the inguinal ring (Figure 18.2C). Generally, the ligature is of strong, absorbable suture material, such as no. 0 or no. 1 synthetic absorbable suture (Figure 18.2D). At this point, some operators prefer to anchor the hernia sac to the inguinal ring with the ends of the transfixation ligature. The testis and excess spermatic cord are removed (Figure 18.2E).

The skin incision may be partially closed with absorbable suture material, or it may be left completely open to allow ventral drainage. Because hernias may be hereditary, the bilateral castration of hernia-affected pigs is recommended. Hernias may be bilateral, so one should also transfix the cord of the opposite side to prevent postoperative herniation.

Postoperative Management

The surgical site may be dusted with a suitable antibacterial powder. This is generally unnecessary if piglets can be turned into a clean, dry pen. The piglets should not be allowed in dirty quarters until healing is complete. A heat lamp is also recommended.

Complications and Prognosis

The prognosis of this procedure depends on the extent of the hernia. Eviscerated inguinal hernias where the intestine has become edematous have a high rate of complications. Chronic inguinal hernias can result in intestinal incarceration and strangulation, which would necessitate resection and anastomosis. Other complications included wound infection and peritonitis.

Cryptorchid Castration of Piglets

Relevant Anatomy

The anatomy of the normal testes and inguinal ring has been described above. We suggest a parainguinal approach to remove retained testicles in the pig. The anatomy of the ventral abdomen and parainguinal area is not appreciably different from other large animal species with the exception of an abundance of retroperitoneal fat in older pigs.

Indications

Pigs occasionally present for castration with one scrotal testicle and the other not palpable externally. Economically, the margins may preclude treatment of such a pig in commercial operations. However, pigs intended for show may warrant surgery to prevent the development of smell and developmental changes associated with intact boars.

Anesthesia and Surgical Preparation

The pig is placed in dorsal recumbency in a V-trough as described. We use general anesthesia to perform this procedure but sedation and local anesthesia is just as acceptable. The skin of the inguinal and scrotal areas is scrubbed with a suitable antiseptic.

Instrumentation

1. General surgery pack

Surgical Technique

The skin incision is made obliquely between the inguinal canal and the midline approximately 2–4 cm in length dependent on the size of the patient and anticipated size of the retained teste. The surgeon should insert one finger into the abdominal cavity and sweep near the internal inguinal ring. The retained testicle is usually located near the internal inguinal ring. If the sweep of the inguinal ring fails to discover the testicle, a more extensive digital exploration of the abdomen should follow. The testicle can generally be removed from the abdominal cavity with little tension and is ligated with absorbable suture material. The muscular body wall is closed with a simple continuous pattern. The external rectus sheath, which is the holding layer of the abdominal closure, may be closed with a simple continuous pattern unless tension on the incision dictates a different pattern. This is not often the case. The subcutaneous tissue and skin are closed in a routine fashion. The contralateral scrotal testicle is removed as described for standard castration earlier.

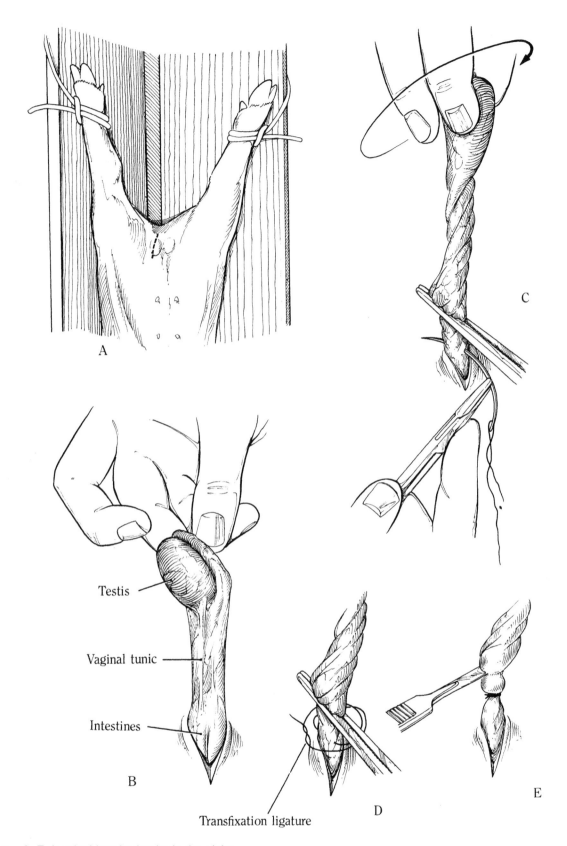

Testis

Vaginal tunic

Intestines

Transfixation ligature

A

B

C

D

E

Fig. 18.2. **A–E.** Inguinal herniorrhaphy in the piglet.

Postoperative Management

One may give perioperative antibiotics for this abdominal surgery. However, it is probably not necessary if attention is paid to aseptic technique and the procedure is done in a clean environment. The animal should be housed in a clean area for 5 days following surgery to minimize incisional complications.

Complications and Prognosis

Complications are not likely as long as technique is not compromised and postoperative care is appropriate. The prognosis is good.

Preputial Diverticulum Ablation

Relevant Anatomy

The preputial diverticulum is a bilobed structure that communicates with the preputial cavity dorsally just caudal to the preputial orifice. There is no known function of this diverticulum. It can hold up to 2 L of material including semen, urine, and smegma.[9]

Indications

Some boars develop a habit referred to as "balling," which is masturbating into the diverticulum. Some will actually prefer this to natural cover of a female. Occasionally the diverticulum becomes ulcerated which causes pain, making the boar hesitant to breed. Some believe the contaminated environment of the diverticulum may be a source of infection contributing to ascending cystitis infections.[10] Some boars present because of breeding failure, which may or may not be related to the diverticulum. The anesthesia allows a thorough examination of the penis and prepuce in an attempt to identify any abnormalities. Some owners will opt for a diverticulum ablation regardless of findings as a relatively inexpensive and minimally invasive way to eliminate a potential reason for breeding failure. More recently ablation of the preputial diverticulum has become popular for animals used in boar studs to eliminate contamination of the ejaculate by bacterial organisms found in the fluid stored in the diverticulum.[11,12]

Anesthesia and Surgical Preparation

The boar is placed under general anesthesia in dorsal recumbency. The fluid accumulated in the diverticulum is squeezed out through the preputial cavity and orifice. After the diverticulum is emptied, it is flushed with antimicrobial solution. If the diverticulum cannot be everted for ablation as described below, one will then clip and surgically prepare the area for a paramedian incision over the diverticulum on one side as the surgeon chooses.

Instrumentation

1. General surgery pack (including 2 oschner forceps and sponge forceps)

Surgical Technique

The sponge forceps are placed into the preputial cavity to gently grasp the penis and extend it for examination. The penis is returned into the preputial cavity, and the oschner forceps are the placed into the preputial cavity. The opening to the preputial diverticulum is found in the dorsal aspect of the preputial cavity just caudal to the preputial orifice. The forceps can be used to outline the diverticulum. One can frequently place two forceps into the diverticulum, one in each lobe (Figure 18.3A). The forceps are then used to grasp the deepest part of the diverticulum on each side and roll the forceps to evert the sac like diverticulum. Care must be taken not to tear the tissue. When both sides of the bilobed structure are everted, the stalk connecting the diverticulum to the preputial cavity is ligated with a transfixation ligature using no. 1 absorbable suture being careful not to compromise the lumen of the preputial cavity (Figure 18.3B).

Another, more involved procedure for ablation of the preputial diverticulum has been described via a paramedian incision. The author uses this technique when eversion is not successful for reasons such as tearing of tissue or scarring. The diverticulum is packed with roll gauze soaked in an antimicrobial solution to help outline the structure. A paramedian incision approximately 4 cm long approximately 2 cm off midline is made over one side of the packed diverticulum. The skin and subcutaneous tissue is incised to expose the very thin preputial diverticulum that has been packed with gauze. The diverticulum is then dissected free and the stalk connecting with the preputial cavity is ligated. The dead space created is closed as well as the subcutaneous layer and skin. Care must be taken not to damage the prepuce.

Postoperative Management

The boar should be given 3 weeks of sexual rest before be used for breeding.

Complications and Prognosis

Complications with either procedure described are not common. The prognosis for return to breeding is good if the real problem was the preferential ejaculation into the diverticulum. This procedure will obviously not improve other conditions that may cause breeding failure.

Fig. 18.3. **A.** Forceps placed into the preputial diverticulum. **B.** The everted preputial diverticulum.

Cesarean Section in the Sow

Relevant Anatomy

Sows can farrow up to 25 fetuses with 12–13 in each horn. At the end of pregnancy, the uterine horns may occupy most of the ventral half of the abdomen. In this species, the uterine body is short but may appear longer in vivo because the uterine horns continue cranially a few centimeters before bifurcating. During a cesarean section, the surgeon should be aware of the thick layer of adipose tissue encountered before peritoneum. The neophyte surgeon may confuse the extensive subperitoneal fat for omentum with adhesions.

Indications

Cesarean section in the sow is indicated for the relief of dystocia. The following are common causes of dystocia: uterine inertia; excessive adipose tissue around the birth canal; relative fetal oversize in small, immature sows; transverse presentation of a piglet; fetal monsters; and malformation of the birth canal due to previous pelvic fractures or injuries during previous parturitions. Cesarean section is also indicated for the production of specific-pathogen-free (SPF) piglets.

The operation is successful if done early in the parturition process; however, the large animal surgeon frequently is presented with an exhausted animal subjected to numerous attempts to remove the piglets manually. Generally, tissue damage to the birth canal is considerable, and emphysematous fetuses may be present in such cases. These sows are frequently in a state of endotoxic shock and are poor risks for surgery.

Instrumentation

1. General surgery pack

Anesthesia and Surgical Preparation

The sow is positioned in lateral recumbency, and ropes are tied to its feet if necessary. Adequate restraint is essential, so aseptic technique is not compromised. Once the

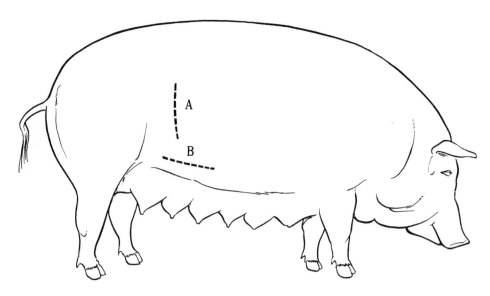

Fig. 18.4. Cesarean section in the sow.

sow has been placed in either left- or right-lateral recumbency, the surgical site is prepared. Local or regional anesthesia in the form of a line block, an inverted L block, or an epidural block may be administered at this time. (Alternate sedative and general anesthetic techniques are presented in Chapter 2.) Azaperone may be used for chemical restraint of the sow as well. This drug does cross the placental barrier, resulting in minor sedation of the piglet. However, respiratory depression in the piglet is usually low, and the prognosis for survival is good. To avoid serious complications, the dose should be kept minimal (maximum dose 8 mg/kg IM). If additional sedation is needed, thiopental or metomidate may be administered intravenously.

Three basic types of incisions are used for cesarean section in sows. The first is a vertical incision, either in the left or right paralumbar fossa and flank region; and the second is a horizontal incision in the ventral paralumbar area about 6–8 cm above the well-developed mammary tissue (Figure 18.4). The third, ventral midline incision, which we do not describe in this chapter, allows access to both uterine horns; but it is awkward to position the sow for this incision. Some surgeons are also concerned about potential disruption of the midline incision site by nursing piglets.

The surgical site is clipped, but shaving is generally unnecessary. Local anesthetic is administered, depending on which approach is to be used (we prefer the vertical incision). The surgical site is given an additional scrub and is prepared for aseptic surgery in a routine manner.

Surgical Technique

The following technique is for the vertical incision. The surgeon makes a 20-cm vertical skin incision that commences 6–8 cm ventral to the transverse processes of the lumbar vertebrae, midway between the last rib and the thigh muscles. The incision is continued through the skin, subcutaneous adipose tissue, muscles of the flank, subperitoneal adipose tissue, and peritoneum. The abdominal cavity is explored for the bifurcation of the uterus. The surgeon makes a 15- to 20-cm incision through the uterine wall, as close to the body of the uterus as possible, being careful not to cut one of the piglets. If the bifurcation can be located, the entire litter can be brought out through one incision. This leaves only one uterine incision to close and decreases surgery time. If this is not possible, an incision is made in each uterine horn close to the bifurcation; and the piglets are removed from each horn separately. If an assistant is present, the piglets can be massaged down the uterine lumen toward the incision as the others are removed; but it is generally necessary for the surgeon to reach up into each uterine horn in search of more piglets while pulling the uterine walls up the surgeon's arms as one would pull on the arms of a thick woolen sweater. Great care should be exercised in exposing the ovarian end of each uterine horn. Its attachment is friable in the sow; and if one is not careful, the ovarian artery may be easily torn, possibly resulting in fatal hemorrhage. One should be sure to explore the vaginal canal for remaining piglets and to remove any loose placentae.

Dead and emphysematous piglets usually have their corresponding placentae detached and are easily removed. Prior to closure of the uterine incisions, any intrauterine medication is administered. The uterus is closed with any of the inverting patterns described in the discussion of bovine cesarean section in Chapter 14. If infection is present, a two-layer closure is recommended.[13] The uterine horns are placed in the abdominal cavity individually, making sure they are not twisted.

The combined muscle and subcutaneous layers are closed as one, using no. 0 or no. 1 synthetic absorbable suture material in a simple continuous pattern. The skin is closed with an interlocking pattern using polymerized caprolactam in a manner similar to closure of the bovine flank.

Postoperative Management

During closure of the uterus and body wall, an assistant should dry the piglets vigorously and should place them in warm surroundings. Once surgery is completed, the sow is moved to a clean, dry pen, and the piglets are placed beside the sow.

Toxic patients should receive pre- and postoperative antibiotics, as well as other forms of supportive therapy for shock, such as intravenous fluids. Oxytocin can aid in contraction of the uterus and in milk letdown.

Complications and Prognosis

As mentioned previously, incorrect surgical technique or manipulation of the uterine horns may result in rupture of the ovarian artery and hemorrhage. Other potential complications include wound infection and peritonitis. To the author's knowledge, there are no reports of survival rates for this procedure. However, assuming aseptic technique is used and little contamination occurs, the prognosis for the sow is good and most of the piglets should be successfully recovered.

Ovariohysterectomy in the Pot-Bellied Pig

Relevant Anatomy

The anatomy of the gravid uterus has been described for cesarean section. The nongravid uterus is obviously much smaller and the horns are curled upon themselves much like that of many ruminants. The pot-bellied pig will generally have a lot of subcutaneous fat which may complicate the procedure. The uterus and mesometrium of the pot-bellied pig is more friable than tissues with which most large animal surgeons are familiar, so one should take special care in dissection and ligation during this surgery.

Indications

Owners of pet pigs often wish to have them rendered infertile because they simply have no desire to ever raise a litter of piglets. Therefore, they also wish to avoid any behavioral issues of a pig exhibiting signs of estrus.

Anesthesia and Surgical Preparation

The surgery is performed with the pig in dorsal recumbency under general anesthesia. The ventral abdomen is clipped and prepped for a surgical incision on the ventral midline between the umbilicus and pelvic brim.

Instrumentation

1. General surgery pack

Surgical Technique

A ventral midline incision is made from just caudal to the umbilicus toward the pelvic brim for a distance determined by the size of the patient. The subcutaneous fat can be dissected bluntly with surgical sponges to expose the linea alba while causing less hemorrhage than sharp dissection would yield. A horn of the uterus is located with a finger within the abdominal cavity. The uterine horn is followed to the ovary. The ovarian pedicle is ligated with absorbable suture. The uterus is then followed to the contralateral ovary which is also ligated and transected. The body of the uterus is then ligated with transfixation and circumferential sutures caudal to the cervix. The uterus and ovaries are removed, and the all ligatures are examined closely for any hemorrhage. The incision is then closed in a routine fashion using suture material and pattern of choice.

Alternatively, one may perform an ovariectomy without hysterectomy. This procedure accomplishes the same goals while being quicker and technically easier. The author has used ovariectomy on many young pigs without complications. However, some believe that uterine tumors are common enough that the uterus should be removed at surgery.[14]

Postoperative Management

Routine incision observation and care are practiced. The pig may be confined for a few days to limit activities that might stress the abdominal incision such as jumping on and off of furniture. Pain medications may be given if needed.

Complications and Prognosis

Complications are rare if attention is paid to technique. The prognosis is generally good with the possible exception of animals that undergo an ovariectomy only and develop uterine disease years later.

Rectal Prolapse Ring Placement

Relevant Anatomy

The pig rectum is surrounded by fat and enlarges just before becoming the anal canal which is very short. The anal muscles include the internal anal sphincter muscles, which are made of smooth muscle, and the external anal sphincter muscle, which is made of striated muscle.[15]

Indications

A piglet (or adult swine) with a rectal prolapse is a candidate for placement of a rectal prolapse ring to facilitate resection of the prolapsed tissue. In piglets, respiratory disease causing a cough, as well as the behavior of piling on, may cause rectal prolapse. Adult swine are occasionally affected by rectal prolapse as well. The condition is complicated in group-housed animals as some will show cannibalistic behavior in the presence of prolapsed tissue.

Anesthesia and Surgical Preparation

An epidural is useful especially in adult swine. Piglets would benefit from an epidural anesthetic as well, but many smaller piglets have rings placed by lay people on the farm, with physical restraint only. The prolapsed tissue should be cleaned to remove as much organic debris as possible.

Instrumentation

1. Prolapse ring
2. Elastrator bands and/or umbilical tape
3. Grasping forceps

Surgical Technique

The surgical technique of resection of the rectal prolapse with primary closure is described in the small ruminant in Chapter 16. That technique may be used in swine for selected cases, but for economic reasons the prolapse ring technique described here will be used more commonly. This is especially true for young commercial piglets. A commercially available prolapse ring of the largest size that fits into the prolapsed rectum without causing more trauma is selected. In the absence of a commercially available ring, some lay people will use PVC couplings or reducers used with pipe for plumbing as a prolapse ring. The ring is lubricated and one may wish to attach a suture tag on the ring in case during positioning the ring advances proximally beyond reach of the practitioner. The ring is advanced so that the smaller external diameter center of the ring is at the anus. It may be advanced with a finger or grasping forceps. Then the ring is secured in place with umbilical tape and/or elastrator bands. The umbilical tape has good knot security and can be placed when the prolapsed tissue is too large for elastrator bands to be used. The tissue distal to the suture will slough in 3–5 days, and the ring will also be passed. If there is excessive tissue, one may excise it after 24 hours. The piglet will pass a reduced volume of feces through the ring. The ring will often become plugged but the piglet can survive the plugged

ring for up to 7 days.[16] The tissue layers at the suture will adhere together forming an anastomosis.

Postoperative Management

Swine treated in this manner may be given reduced feedings until the ring sloughs just to create less fecal matter. They should be isolated to avoid cannibalistic behavior of other pigs.

Complications and Prognosis

There is potential for the site to dehisce if the ring dislodges for any reason. The more common complication is healing with some stricture formation. This is seldom clinically significant as most of these pigs are destined for slaughter and will reach top weight before having problems from any stricture.

References

1. Powe, T.A. Anatomy of the scrotum, testes, epididymis, and spermatic cord in swine. In Large Animal Urogenital Surgery. Edited by D.F. Wolfe, H.D. Moll. Baltimore, MD, Williams & Wilkins, 1999, p. 217.
2. McGlone, J.J., and Hellman, J.M. Local and general anesthetic effects on behavior and performance of two- and seven-week-old castrated and uncastrated piglets. J. Anim. Sci., 66:3049–3058, 1988.
3. McGlone, J.J., Nicholson, R.I., Hellman, J.M., and Herzog, D.N. The development of pain in young pigs associated with castration and attempts to prevent castration-induced behavioral changes. J. Anim. Sci., 71:1441–1446, 1993.
4. Haga, H.A., and Ranheim, B. Castration of piglets: the analgesic effects of intratesticular and intrafunicular lidocaine injection. Vet. Anaes. Analg., 32:1–9, 2005.
5. Kluivers-Poodt, M., Houx, B.B., Robben, S.R.M., Koop, G., Lambooij, E., and Hellebrekers, L.J. Effects of a local anaesthetic and NSAID in castration of piglets, on the acute pain responses, growth and mortality. Animal, 6(9):1469–1475, 2012.
6. Hansson, M., Lundeheim, N., Nyman, G., and Johansson, G.: Effect of local anaesthesia and/or analgesia on pain responses induced by piglet castration. Acta Vet. Acand., 53:34, 2011.
7. Walker, B., Jaggin, N., Doherr, M., and Schatzmann, U. Inhalational anaesthesia for castration of newborn piglets: experiences with isoflurane and isoflurane/N₂O. J. Vet. Med., 51:150–154, 2004.
8. Sack, W.O. Essentials of Pig Anatomy. Ithaca, Veterinary textbooks, 1982.
9. Wolfe, D.F., Beckett, S.D., and Carson, R.L. Acquired conditions of the penis and prepuce. In Large Animal Urogenital Surgery, 2nd Ed. Edited by D.F. Wolfe, H.D. Moll. Baltimore, MD, Williams & Wilkins, 1999, p. 237.
10. Lawhorn, B., Jarret, P.D., Lackey, G.F., Crabill, M., Peloso, J.G., and Steiner, A. Removal of the preputial diverticulum in swine. J. Am. Vet. Med. Assoc., 205(1):92–96, 1994.
11. Cuesta Guillen, A.F., Reyes Avila, I.R., Dominguez Fernandez de Tejerina, J.C., and da Silva Gonzalez, S. Ablation of the

preputial diverticulum in the pig like prevention of the seminal contamination. *REDVET*, *12*(2):021105, 2011.

12. Vieira Pinto, M.M., Ramalho, S., Rodriques, J., and Perestrelo-Vieira, R. The importance of the prepuce diverticulum as a source of contamination of the semen collected for artificial insemination. *Vet. Tech.*, *9*(4):44–48, 1999.

13. Hokanson, J.F. Surgery; female genital tract; experimental and miscellaneous. *In* Diseases of Swine, 4th Ed. Edited by H.W. Dunn, A.D. Leman. Ames, IA, Iowa State University Press, 1975.

14. Baumwart, C.A., Prado, T.M., Anderson, M.P., Coffman, E.A., Simpson, K.M., and Campbell, G.A. Successful treatment of a Vietnamese potbellied pig with an ovarian leiomyoma. *J. Am. Vet. Med. Assoc.*, *236*(5):558–561, 2010.

15. Schummer, A., Nickel, R., and Sack, W.O. The alimentary canal of the pig. *In* The Viscera of the Domestic Mammals, 2nd Ed. Edited by A. Schummer, R. Nickel, W.O. Sack. New York, Springer-Verlag, 1979, p. p147.

16. Douglas, R.G.A. A Simple method for correcting rectal prolapse in pigs. *Vet. Rec.*, *117*(6):129, 1985.

INDEX

Page references followed by f denote figures. Page references followed by t denote tables.

Aanes' method of repair of third-degree
    perineal laceration, 169–174,
    171f–173f
Abdominal exploration
    in cattle, 212–215, 213f–214f
    in horses, 196–202, 197f–200f
Abomasopexy
    left-flank, 222, 225, 226f–227f
    paramedian, 221–222, 228,
        229f–230f
    right-flank, 222, 225, 228
Abomasum
    left-side displacement (LDA),
        221–222, 224, 226f, 228, 230
    right-side displacement (RDA),
        221–222, 224–225, 230–231
    right torsion (RTA), 221–222, 224,
        228, 230
Acepromazine (acetylpromazine)
        maleate, for tranquilization and
        sedation
    in horses, 16, 17t
    in small ruminants, 16, 18t
Acid-base imbalance, diagnosis of,
        24–26
Adhesions, equine castration
        complication, 146, 152
Adhesives, tissue, 67
Alexander chisel, 49f
Alexander gouge, 49f
Allis tissue forceps, 37, 42f
Amputation
    of digit in cattle, 273–276, 275f
    of the penis in the horse, 166–169,
        167f–169f
    preputial in cattle, 245–248, 247f
    of splint bones in the horse, 131–134,
        132f–133f
    via disarticulation, 274, 276

Analgesia
    infiltration, 7–8
    intravenous local, 14–16, 15f
    regional, 7–16
        epidural analgesia, 10–11, 11f–12f,
            13t–14t
        eye, 14
        horn, 14
        inverted L block, 8, 8f
        limb, 14–16, 15f
        paravertebral block, 9–10, 9f
Anastomosis, 231–232
Anesthesia. See also Regional analgesia;
        specific surgical techniques
    general, 16–23
        induction, 19–21, 19t–21t
        maintaining, 21–23, 22t
        overview, 16, 18
        preanesthetic evaluation, 18
        premedication, 18–19
    local and regional, 7–16, 8f–9f,
        11f–12f, 13t–14t, 15f
    monitoring, 23
    tranquilization and sedation, 16,
        16t–18t
    for wound exploration, 95
Anion gap, 26
Annular ligament of the fetlock,
        transection of, 127–129, 128f
Antibiotics
    antimicrobial impregnated suture
        materials, 65
    role in surgery, 5
    topical, 5
Anticholinergic drugs, 19
Antiinflammatory drug use in wound
        exploration, 95–96
Antimicrobial therapy, in traumatic
        wounds, 95

Antiseptic agents, 94
Arthrotomy, fetlock joint, 134–136,
        135f
Asepsis, principles of, 4
Aseptic surgery, 6
Atropine, 19
Autoclaving, 38
Azaperone
    for cesarean section in swine, 292
    for tranquilization and sedation in
        swine, 16, 18t

Babcock intestinal forceps, 43f
Backhaus towel clamps, 42f
Balfour retractor, 38, 48f
Balling behavior of boars, 316
Balling gun, 58f
Bandages, stent, 88, 88f
Bandage scissors, 36, 40f
Bandaging skin grafts, 109
Barnes dehorner, 280
Base deficit/excess, 25–26, 28
Bennett's speculum, 55f
Benzotropine mesylate, for priapism, 146
Bicarbonate
    administration of, 28
    concentration in acid-base
        diagnosis, 25–26
Bistoury (tenotomy) knife, 114,
        115f–116f
Bladder marsupialization, 297
Bloat, 11, 18, 23, 219
Blood gases, 25, 25t, 26
Bone-holding forceps, Kern, 48f
Bone rasp, 48f, 50f
Bone rongeurs, 50f
Bovine. See Cattle
Bowed tendon, 127
Braided absorbable sutures, 62, 65

Turner and McIlwraith's Techniques in Large Animal Surgery, 4th Edition. Dean A. Hendrickson and A. N. (Nickie) Baird.
© 2013 John Wiley & Sons, Inc. Published 2013 by John Wiley & Sons, Inc.

Breeder's stitch, 159
Brown-Adson forceps, 42f
Buhner method of repair for vaginal
　　prolapse, 265–266, 267f–268f
Buhner tape needle, modified, 57f
Bulb syringe, 51f
Bulls
　castration
　　of calf, 235–236, 237f
　　unilateral, 257–258
　corpus cavernosum penis (CCP)
　　thrombosis, 251–252
　epididymectomy, 252, 253f
　hematoma evacuation of penis,
　　241–245, 243f–244f
　inguinal herniorrhaphy, 252, 254–257,
　　255f–256f
　penile fixation, 250f, 251
　penile translocation, 248, 249f, 251
　preputial resection and
　　anastomosis, 245–248, 247f
　teaser bull preparation, 248–252,
　　249f–250f
　urethrostomy, 236, 238, 239f–240f,
　　241
Bupivacaine, 7–8
Butorphanol, for tranquilization and
　　sedation
　in cattle, 16t
　in horses, 17t

Calculi, urinary
　in cattle, 238
　in small ruminants, 296–297
Calf castration, 235–236, 237f
Camelid surgery, 303–309
　castration of the llama, 303–304
　cesarean section, 304–305
　tooth removal in the llama, 305–309,
　　307f–308f
Cannula, teat, 58f
Capillary refill time, 24
Caprolactam, polymerized, 64t, 66–67
Carbon dioxide, measurement of, 25–26
Caslick's operation for pneumovagina in
　　the mare, 156–159, 157f–158f
Castration
　cattle
　　calf, 235–236, 237f
　　unilateral in bull, 257–258
　horse, 139–152, 141f–144f
　　complications, 145–146, 152
　　cryptorchidectomy, 147f–152f,
　　　152–156
　llama, 303–304
　swine, 311–312, 313f
　　cryptorchid castration of
　　　piglets, 314, 316
Catgut, 62
Catheter
　cow, 55f
　epidural, 11

mare, 56f
stud, 56f
Cattle
　abdominal exploration, 212–215,
　　213f–214f
　dehorning, 277, 279–280, 281f–282f
　digit amputation, 273–276, 275f
　epidural anesthesia, 10–11, 11f
　eye enucleation, 276–277, 278f–279f
　fluid balance evaluation, normal values
　　for, 25t
　gastrointestinal surgery, 211–232
　　for abomasal displacement/
　　　torsion, 221–231, 223f, 226f–227f,
　　　229f–230f
　　abomasopexy, left-flank, 222, 225,
　　　226f–227f
　　abomasopexy, paramedian,
　　　221–222, 228, 229f–230f
　　abomasopexy, right-flank, 222, 225,
　　　228
　　cecal dilatation/volvulus, 231
　　laparotomy, flank, 212–215,
　　　213f–214f
　　laparotomy, principles of, 211
　　omentopexy, right-flank, 221–224,
　　　223f
　　pyloro-omentopexy, 224–225
　　rumenostomy (rumen
　　　fistulation), 219–221, 220f
　　rumenotomy, 215–219, 217f–218f
　　small intestinal resection and
　　　anastomosis, 231–232
　general anesthesia in, 16–24, 20t, 22t
　intubation in, 20
　regional analgesia, 8–11, 8f–9f, 11f,
　　13t, 14, 15f
　rib resection and pericardiotomy, 280,
　　282–283, 284f–285f
　surgical site preparation, 6
　teat laceration repair, 283, 285–288,
　　287f
　third eyelid resection, 288
　tracheotomy, 288–289
　tranquilization and sedation, 16, 16t
　umbilical surgery, 289–290
　urogenital surgery, 235–270
　　castration of calf, 235–236, 237f
　　cervicoplexy for vaginal
　　　prolapse, 266, 268–270, 269f
　　cesarean section, 258–265,
　　　260f–264f
　　corpus cavernosum penis (CCP)
　　　thrombosis, 251–252
　　epididymectomy, 252, 253f
　　hematoma evacuation of
　　　penis, 241–245, 243f–244f
　　inguinal herniorrhaphy, 252,
　　　254–257, 255f–256f
　　penile fixation, 250f, 251
　　penile translocation, 248, 249f,
　　　251

preputial resection and anastomosis
　　in bull, 245–248, 247f
retention suturing of vulva, 265–
　　266, 267f–268f
teaser bull preparation, 248–252,
　　249f–250f
urethrostomy, 236, 238, 239f–240f,
　　241
Cattle leader, 52f
CCP (corpus cavernosum penis)
　　thrombosis, 251–252
Cecal dilatation/volvulus, in cattle,
　　231
Cervical prolapse, 265
Cervicopexy for vaginal prolapse, in
　　cattle, 266, 268–270, 269f
Cervix, laceration of, 170
Cesarean section
　in camelids, 304–305
　in cow, 258–265, 260f–264f
　in mare, 160, 162–164, 163f
　in small ruminants, 299–300
　in swine, 317–319, 318f
Chains, obstetric, 56f
Cheek tooth repulsion, in horses,
　　191–196, 193f–194f
Chemical sterilization, 38
Chip fractures, fetlock joint, 134–136,
　　135f
Chisel
　Alexander, 49f
　U.S. Army, 49f
Chlorhexidine, 6, 94
Chloride, serum, 27
Chromic catgut, 62
Circumcision
　in bull, 245–248, 247f
　in horses, 164–166, 165f–166f
Clamp, towel, 37, 42f
Cleaning wounds, 94
Clipping, preoperative, 5–6
Closure
　delayed primary, 96
　primary closure, 96
　secondary-intention healing, 96–97
　using tension-relieving incisions,
　　103–104, 104f
Clubfoot, treatment of, 120, 122
Coffin (distal interphangeal) joint,
　　flexure deformities of, 120, 122,
　　126–127
Cold (chemical) sterilization, 38
Collagen, 62
Connell suture, 85–86, 85f
Continuous horizontal mattress
　　suture, 79, 79f
Continuous Lembert suture, 84–85, 84f
Continuous lock stitch (Ford interlocking
　　suture), 83, 83f
Contrast agents, 95
Corneal reflex, 23
Cornual block, 14

Corpus cavernosum penis (CCP)
    thrombosis, 251–252
Cotton, 64t, 66
Counterirritants, 113
Crile forceps, 43f
Cruciate (cross mattress) suture, 81,
    82f
Cryptorchidectomy
    in horses, 147f–152f, 152–156
        inguinal approach, 147f–149f,
            153–154
        laparoscopic, 152f, 155–156
        parainguinal approach, 150f–151f,
            154
        standing flank approach, 151f, 154
    in swine, 314, 316
Curette, 49f
Cushing suture, 85, 85f
Cyanoacrylate, 67
Cystostomy, tube, 296–297

Dacron, 67
DDSP (dorsal displacement of the soft
    palate), in horse, 184
Dead space, 96–98
Debridement, 95, 97
Deep digital flexor accessory ligament,
    desmotomy of, 119–122, 121f
Deep digital flexor tenotomy, 126–127
Dehorner
    Barnes-type, 52f
    gouge, 53f
    keystone, 53f
Dehorning
    cosmetic in cattle, 277, 279–280,
        281f–282f
    of mature goat, 293–295, 294f
    regional analgesia for, 14
Dehydration, 23–24, 24t
Delayed primary closure, 96
Dental elevator, 50f
Dental float, 53f
Dental formula
    horse, 191
    llama, 305, 305f
Dental punch, 53f, 192, 193f–194f,
    195–196
Dental surgery
    repulsion of cheek teeth in
        horses, 191–196, 193f–194f
    tooth removal in the llama, 305–309,
        307f–308f
Desflurane, 21
Desmitis
    deep digital flexor accessory
        ligament, 119
    suspensory, 124, 131
Desmotomy, in horses
    annular ligament, 127–129, 128f
    inferior (distal) check ligament,
        119–122, 121f
    medial patellar, 113–114, 115f–116f

superior check ligament, 122–124,
    123f
Detomidine
    for anesthetic maintenance, 22t
    epidural use of, 10–11, 13t–14t
    for tranquilization and sedation
        in cattle, 16t
        in horses, 16, 17t
Dexon, 63t, 65
Diazepam (Valium)
    for anesthetic induction, in cattle and
        small ruminants, 20t
    for convulsion control, 8
    for tranquilization and sedation
        in small ruminants, 16
        in swine, 18t
Digit amputation in cattle, 273–276,
    275f
    via disarticulation, 274, 276
Disarticulation, digit amputation
    via, 274, 276
Disbudding young goat, 295–296
Distal (inferior) check ligament
    desmotomy, 119–122, 121f
Dobutamine, for hypotension, 22
Dopamine, for hypotension, 22
Dorsal displacement of the soft palate
    (DDSP), in horse, 184
Dose syringe, 59f
Double-layer inverting suture
    patterns, 87–88
Doyen (Gillmann) compression
    forceps, 43f
Drains, 97–101
    active, 99, 100f–101f
    fenestrated tube, 99, 100f
    for hygromas, 98, 98f
    indications, 97
    passive, 97–98
    Penrose, 98, 98f
    for peritoneal drainage, 99, 101f
    sump-Penrose, 99, 101f
Draping, 4, 6
Dressing, tie over, 88, 88f
Droperidol, for tranquilization and
    sedation in swine, 16, 18t
Dystocia
    in camelids, 304–305
    in cow, 258
    in mare, 160, 162–164, 163f
    in small ruminants, 299–300
    in sow, 317–319

Écraseur, 59f
Ectropion, Z-plasty for relief of
    acquired, 105, 106f
Edema, in equine castration, 145
Electrolyte abnormalities, diagnosis
    of, 26–27
Elevator, dental, 50f
Elliptical excision undermining for repair
    of an elongated defect, 103, 104f

Emasculator, 52f
Empyema, guttural pouch, 186, 189
Endotracheal intubation, 18
    in cattle, 20
    in swine, 20–21
Endotracheal tube, 59f
Enucleation of the eye, in cattle,
    276–277, 278f–279f
Ephedrine, for hypotension, 22
Epididymectomy, 252, 253f
Epidural analgesia, 10–11, 11f–12f,
    13t–14t
Epineural capping, in palmar digital
    neurectomy, 129
Epithelialization, 93
Equine. See Horses
Equine molar forceps, 54f
Ethylene oxide, for sterilization, 38
Eventration, post-castration in
    horse, 145–146
Excision, sharp of wounds, 95
Eye
    enucleation in cattle, 276–277,
        278f–279f
    regional analgesia of, 14
    third eyelid resection, 288
Eyeball rotation, for anesthetic
    monitoring in cattle, 23

Feed, withholding prior to surgery, 18
Femoral nerve paresis, 22
Fenestrated tube drain, 99, 100f
Fetlock (metacarpophalangeal) joint
    annular ligament transection,
        127–129, 128f
    arthrotomy, 134–136, 135f
    flexure deformities of, 120, 122,
        124–126
Fetotomy, 162
Finochietto rib spreader, 38, 48f
Fistulation, rumenal, 219–221, 220f
Flank laparotomy, in cattle, 212–215,
    213f–214f
Flexure deformity, treatment of
    deep digital flexor tenotomy,
        126–127
    inferior check ligament
        desmotomy, 119–122, 121f
    superficial digital flexor
        tenotomy, 124–126, 125f
    superior check ligament
        desmotomy, 122–124, 123f
Float, dental, 53f
Fluid balance, normal values used in the
    evaluation of, 25t
Fluid therapy, 23–29
    in anesthetized patient in elective
        surgery, 27
    composition of fluids for, 28t
    in compromised patient
        according to requirements, 27–29
        without preliminary data, 29

Fluid volume deficits
    diagnosis of, 23–24, 24t
    treatment of, 27–29
Foals
    inducing anesthesia in, 19
    preanesthetic agents, contraindication
        for, 18
    umbilical herniorrhaphy, 207–210,
        208f–209f
Foerster sponge forceps, 45f
Foley catheter, 296–297
Forceps
    Allis tissue, 37, 42f
    Babcock intestinal, 43f
    Brown-Adson, 42f
    Crile, 43f
    Doyen (Gillmann) compression, 43f
    equine molar, 54f
    Foerster sponge, 45f
    grasping, 37
    Halsted mosquito, 37, 45f
    hemostatic, 37, 37f, 43f, 45f
    Kelly, 37, 44f
    Kern bone-holding, 48f
    Michel clip, 43f
    Mixter, 45f
    Ochsner, 46f
    Rochester-Carmalt, 45f
    sponge, 37
    thumb, 37, 37f
    tissue, 37, 42f
    use of, 37, 37f
    uterine biopsy, 56f
    Vulsellum, 37, 45f
Ford interlocking suture, 83, 83f
Foreign body, in traumatic
        wound, 94–95
Foreign-body reaction, 62
4-S modified Roeder knot, 73, 73f

Galt trephine, 53f
Gambee suture, 87, 88f
Gas sterilization, 38
Gastrointestinal surgery
    in cattle, 211–232
    in horse, 196–210
Gelpi retractor, 38, 47f
General anesthesia, 16–23
    induction, 19–21, 19t–21t
    maintaining, 21–23, 22t
    overview, 16, 18
    preanesthetic evaluation, 18
    premedication, 18–19
Gigli wire and handles, 51f
Gillmann (Doyen) compression
        forceps, 43f
GKX. See Guaifenesin, ketamine, and
        xylazine
Gloves, surgical, 4, 5
Glycomer 631 (Biosyn), 63t, 65
Glycopyrrolate, 19

Goats
    cesarean section, 299–300
    dehorning of mature, 293–295, 294f
    disbudding young, 295–296
    general anesthesia in, 18–23, 20t,
        22t
    mastectomy, 297–298
    obstructive urolithiasis, 296–297
    regional analgesia in, 8–11, 13t, 14
    tranquilization and sedation, 16, 18t
    urethral appendage removal, 296–297
    vasectomy, 298–299
Gouge, 49f
Grafting. See Skin grafting
Gram stain, 6
Granny knot, 71, 72f
Granulation tissue, 94, 96–97
Grasping forceps, 37
Guaifenesin
    for anesthetic induction
        in cattle and small
            ruminants, 19–20, 20t
        in horses, 19, 19t
    for anesthetic maintenance, 22t
Guaifenesin, ketamine, and xylazine
        (GKX), 19–20
    for anesthetic induction in cattle and
        small ruminants, 20t
    for anesthetic induction in swine, 21t
Gut, surgical, 62, 63t
Guttural pouches, surgical entry and
        drainage of, 186–189, 187f–188f

Hair, presurgical removal, 5–6
Halothane, 23
Halsted mosquito forceps, 37, 45f
Harleco CO$_2$ apparatus, 25, 26
HCG (human chorionic
        gonadotropin), 146
Healing, 96–97
    delayed primary, 96
    moist wound, 96–97
    primary, 96
    secondary-intention, 96–97
Heel pain
    inferior (distal) check ligament
        desmotomy, 119–122, 121f
    palmar digital neurectomy for, 129
Hematoma evacuation of the bovine
        penis, 241–245, 243f–244f
Hemorrhage, in equine castration, 145
Hemostatic forceps, 37, 37f, 43f, 45f
Herniation, in equine castration
        complication, 145–146
Herniorrhaphy
    inguinal in bull, 252, 254–257,
        255f–256f
    inguinal in piglet, 312, 314, 315f
    umbilical in foal, 207–210, 208f–209f
H-flap, sliding, 105, 105f
Hibbs gouge, 49f

Hobday's roaring bur, 56f
Hollow organs, suturing patterns for
        closure of, 83–88
Hoof groover, Hughes, 55f
Hoof knife, German, 55f
Hoof nippers, 54f
Horn
    dehorning in cattle, 277, 279–280,
        281f–282f
    dehorning in goats, 293–295,
        294f
    regional anesthesia, 14
Horses
    abdominal exploration, 196–202,
        197f–200f
    check teeth, repulsion of, 191–196,
        193f–194f
    epidural anesthesia, 10–11, 12f
    fluid balance evaluation, normal values
        for, 25t
    gastrointestinal surgery, 196–210
        laparotomy, standing flank,
            202–206, 203f–206f
        laparotomy, ventral midline,
            196–202, 197f–200f
        umbilical herniorrhaphy in
            foals, 207–210, 208f–209f
    general anesthesia, 16–23, 22t
    orthopedic surgery, 113–136
        amputation of splint bones,
            131–134, 132f–133f
        arthrotomy of fetlock joint,
            134–136, 135f
        deep digital flexor
            tenotomy, 126–127
        inferior (distal) check ligament
            desmotomy, 119–122, 121f
        lateral digital extensor
            tenotomy, 114, 116–119,
            117f–118f
        medial patellar desmotomy,
            113–114, 115f–116f
        palmar digital neurectomy,
            129–131, 130f
        sectioning of palmar (plantar)
            annular ligament of the
            fetlock, 127–129, 128f
        superficial digital flexor
            tenotomy, 124–126, 125f
        superior check ligament
            desmotomy, 122–124, 123f
    preoperative evaluation, 3
    regional analgesia, 7–11, 12f, 13t
    skin staple use in, 67
    surgical site preparation, 5
    tetanus prophylaxis, 5
    tranquilization and sedation, 16, 17t
    upper respiratory tract surgery,
        177–189
        guttural pouch surgery/
            drainage, 186–189, 187f–188f

laryngotomy, laryngeal
ventriculectomy, and
ventriculocordectomy, 179–183,
181f–183f
soft palate, partial resection,
183–184, 185f
tracheostomy, 177–179, 178f
urogenital surgery, 139–174
Aanes' method of repair of third-
degree perineal laceration,
169–174, 171f–173f
amputation of penis, 166–169,
167f–169f
Caslick's operation for
pneumovagina, 156–159,
157f–158f
castration, 139–152, 141f–144f
cesarean section, 160, 162–164,
163f
circumcision, 164–166, 165f–166f
cryptorchidectomy, 147f–152f,
152–156
urethroplasty, 159–160, 161f–162f
wound exploration in, 95
wound healing in, 94
Human chorionic gonadotropin
(HCG), 146
Hydrogen peroxide, 38, 94
Hygromas, use of Penrose drains to
treat, 98, 98f
Hyovertebrotomy approach, to guttural
pouch, 186–189, 187f–188f
Hypercapnia, 23
Hypercarbia, 23
Hyperkalemia, 27
Hypernatremia, 26, 28
Hyperthermia, malignant, 21
Hypokalemia, 27, 28
Hypotension, during anesthesia, 22
Hypovolemia, 24
Hypoxema, 23

Incisions, tension-relieving, 103–104,
104f
Infection
antibiotic use, 5
antimicrobial impregnated suture
materials, 65
in castration, 146
postoperative, managing, 6
prevention, 4
skin staple use and, 67
Inferior (distal) check ligament
desmotomy, 119–122, 121f
Infiltration analgesia, 7–8
Inguinal herniorrhaphy
in bull, 252, 254–257, 255f–256f
in piglet, 312, 314, 315f
Inhalation anesthesia
for anesthetic induction in foals, 19
for anesthetic maintenance, 21–23, 22t

Instruments, 33–59. See also specific
instruments
forceps, 37, 37f, 42f–46f
general surgery pack, 38
miscellaneous, 48f–59f
needle holders, 36–37, 36f, 39f–40f
photo gallery of, 39f–59f
preparation of, 38
retractors, 37–38, 47f–48f
scalpel, 33, 34f–35f, 35, 39f
scissors, 35–36, 35f, 40f–41f
towel clamp, 37, 42f
use of, 33–38
Insurance, 4
Interrupted horizontal mattress
suture, 79, 79f
Interrupted Lembert suture, 84, 84f
Intravenous limb anesthesia of
ruminants, 14–16, 15f
Intubation, endotracheal, 18
in cattle, 20
in swine, 20–21
Intussusception, 232
Inverted L block, 8, 8f
Iowa pig snare, 52f
Isoflurane, 21, 22t

Jaw tone, 23

Kelly forceps, 37, 44f
Kern bone-holding forceps, 48f
Ketamine
for anesthetic induction
in cattle and small ruminants, 20,
20t
in horses, 19, 19t
in swine, 20, 21t
for anesthetic maintenance, 21,
22t
Ketamine/midazolam, for tranquilization
and sedation
in small ruminants, 18t
in swine, 17t
Knots
granny, 71, 72f
Miller's, 72f, 73, 76
principles of tying, 71–73
slipknot (two half-hitches), 71, 72f
4-S modified Roeder, 73, 73f
square, 71, 72f
surgeon's, 72f, 73
tying with needle holder, 73, 74f

Laceration
perineal, 169–174, 171f–173f
teat, 283, 285–288, 287f
Lactate, as bicarbonate source, 28
Lactic acidosis, 26
Lactomer 9-1 (Polysorb-Tyco), 63t, 65
Laminitis, deep digital flexor tenotomy
for, 126–127

Laparoscopy, for cryptorchidectomy in
horses, 152f, 155–156
Laparotomy
in cattle
flank, 212–215, 213f–214f
principles, 211
in horse
standing flank, 202–206, 203f–206f
ventral midline, 196–202, 197f–200f
Laryngeal spasm, 20
Laryngeal ventriculectomy, in
horse, 179–183, 181f–183f
Laryngotomy, in horse, 179–183,
181f–183f
Laser ventriculectomy/
ventriculocordectomy, 183, 183f
Lateral digital extensor tenotomy, 114,
116–119, 117f–118f
Lavage, for wound cleaning, 94
Leader, cattle, 52f
Lembert suture
continuous, 84–85, 84f
interrupted, 84, 84f
Lichty teat knife, 57f
Lidocaine hydrochloride
convulsions in sheep from, 8
for epidural analgesia, 10–11, 13t–14t
with epinephrine, 14
for local and regional analgesia, 7–8,
10, 14
Ligatures, 73, 75f, 76
Limb anesthesia, intravenous, 14–16, 15f
Line block, 8, 14
Lister scissors, 40f
Littauer stitch scissors, 40f
Llama, 303–309
castration of, 303–304
cesarean section, 304–305
dental formula, 305, 305f
tooth removal, 305–309, 307f–308f
Locking-loop tendon suture, 89, 89f, 91
Lock stitch, continuous, 83, 83f

Malignant hyperthermia, 21
Mallet, 49f
Mare
Aanes' method of repair of third-
degree perineal laceration,
169–174, 171f–173f
Caslick's operation for
pneumovagina, 156–159,
157f–158f
cesarean section, 160, 162–164, 163f
urethroplasty, 159–160, 161f–162f
Masculine behavior, persistent after
castration, 146
Mastectomy, in small
ruminants, 297–298
Mattress suture
continuous horizontal, 79, 79f
cross, 81, 82f

Mattress suture (*cont'd*)
    interrupted horizontal, 79, 79f
    vertical, 79, 80f, 81, 105
Maxillary flap sinusotomy for tooth
        repulsion, 194f, 195
Mayo-Hegar needle holder, 39f
Mayo scissors, 35, 40f
McPherson speculum, 53f
Medetomidine
    for anesthetic maintenance, 22t
    epidural use of, 10, 13t
    for tranquilization and sedation
        in cattle, 16t
        in horses, 16, 17t
Medial patellar desmotomy, in the
        horse, 113–114, 115f–116f
Memory, suture, 66
Mepivacaine hydrochloride
    for epidural analgesia, 13t
    for local and regional analgesia, 7,
        14
Mesh expansion technique, 103–104,
        104f
Metabolic acidosis, 25–28
Metabolic alkalosis, 25–29
Metacarpal bones, amputation of, 131–
        134, 132f–133f
Metatarsal bones, amputation of, 131–
        134, 132f–133f
Metzenbaum scissors, 35, 41f
Michel clip, 43f
Michel trephine, 51f
Miller's knot, 72f, 73, 76
Minchev technique, 265
Mixter forceps, 45f
Moist wound healing, 96–97
Molar cutter, 54f
Molar forceps, equine, 54f
Molars, repulsion in horses, 191–196,
        193f–194f
Monofilament sutures, absorbable, 65
Morphine
    epidural use of, 11, 13t
    for tranquilization and sedation in
        horses, 17t
Mouth gag, canine, 54f
Mouth wedge, Bayer, 53f
Myopathy, postanesthesia, 22

Navicular disease, palmar digital
        neurectomy for, 129
Near-far-far-near suture, 81, 81f, 105
Needle holder
    knot tying with, 73, 74f
    Mayo-Hegar, 39f
    Olsen-Hegar, 40f
    use of, 36, 36f
Needle(s), 67–69
    for hollow-organ surgery, 83
    swaged, 68, 68f
    taper cut, 68, 69f
    types, 67–69, 68f, 69f

Nerve blocks, 7, 14, 16. *See also specific*
        techniques
Neurectomy, palmar digital, 129–131,
        130f
Neuroma, formation with palmar digital
        neurectomy, 131
Newberry knife, 236
Nippers, 54f
Nylon (Dermalon, Ethilon,
        Supramid), 64t, 66

Obstetric chains, 56f
Obstructive urolithiasis, in small
        ruminants, 296–297
Ochsner forceps, 46f
Ocular reflexes, 23
Olsen-Hegar needle holder, 40f
Omentopexy, right-flank, 221–224, 223f
Opioids, 16, 17t
Orthopedic surgery, equine, 113–136
Osteotome set, U.S. Army, 48f
Ovariohysterectomy in the pot-bellied
        pig, 319
Oxygen supplementation, 20, 23

Packed cell volume (PCV), 24, 25t, 27
Palate, partial resection of soft in
        horses, 183–184, 185f
Palmar digital neurectomy, 129–131,
        130f
Palmar/plantar annular ligament
        transection, 127–129, 128f
Palpebral reflexes, 23
Paralumbar block, 10
Paramedian abomasopexy, 221–222, 228,
        229f–230f
Paraphimosis, 146, 252
Paravertebral block, 9–10, 9f
Parker-Kerr oversew, 86, 86f
Patella, medial desmotomy of, 113–114,
        115f–116f
PDS (polydioxanone), 63t, 65
Penile paralysis, 146
Penis
    cattle
        corpus cavernosum penis (CCP)
            thrombosis, 251–252
        hematoma evacuation, 241–245,
            243f–244f
        penile fixation, 250f, 251
        penile translocation, 248, 249f, 251
        preputial resection and anastomosis
            in bull, 245–248, 247f
        urethrostomy, 236, 238, 239f–240f,
            241
    horse
        amputation, 166–169, 167f–169f
        circumcision, 164–166, 165f–166f
Pennyback rongeurs, 50f
Penrose drain, 98, 98f
Pericardectomy in cattle, 280, 282–283,
        284f–285f

Perineal laceration, Aanes' method of
        repair, 169–174, 171f–173f
Periodontal probe, 50f
Peritoneal drainage, 99, 101f
Peritonitis, 83, 218–219, 270
Peroneal nerve paresis, 22
Peterson block, 14
PH, blood, 25
Physical examination, preoperative, 3
Pigs. *See* Swine
Pig snare, 52f
Pneumovagina, Caslick's operation
        for, 156–159, 157f–158f
Poliglecaprone 25 (Monocryl), 64t, 65
Polydioxanone (PDS), 63t, 65
Polyesters, 64t, 67
Polyethylene, 64t, 66
Polyglactin 910 (Vicryl-Ethicon), 63t, 65
Polyglycolic acid (Dexon-Tyco), 63t, 65
Polyglyconate (Maxon), 63t, 65
Polyglytone 6211 (Caprosyn), 64t, 65
Polymerized caprolactam (Supramid,
        Vetafil), 64t, 66–67
Polypropylene (Prolene and
        Surgilene), 64t, 66
Polysorb, 63t, 65
Potassium
    abnormalities, 27
    administration of, 28–29
Pot-bellied pig, ovariohysterectomy
        in, 319
Povidone-iodine, solution/scrub, 6, 94
Premedication, 18–19
Preoperative evaluation, 3–4
Preputial diverticulum ablation, in
        swine, 316, 317f
Preputial resection and anastomosis in
        bull, 245–248, 247f
Presurgical considerations, 3–6
    antibiotic use, 5
    infection, postoperative, 6
    infection prevention, 4
    preoperative evaluation, 3–4
    preoperative planning, 5
    surgical classification, 4–5, 4t
    surgical judgment, 4
    surgical site preparation, 5–6
Priapism, 146
Primary closure, 96
Probe, periodontal, 50f
Propofol, 20–21, 20t
Proud flesh, 97
Proximal sesamoid bones, chip
        fracture, 134–136, 135f
Pupillary dilation, 23
Purse-string suture, 86, 87f
Putti double-ended bone rasp, 48f
Pyloro-omentopexy, 224–225

Reconstructive surgery. *See* Wounds,
        reconstructive surgery of
Record keeping, 3–4

Rectal prolapse
    resection in small ruminants, 300–301,
       301f
    ring placement in swine, 319–320
Reefing, 164–166, 165f–166f, 245–246
Referral, 4
Regional analgesia, 7–16
    epidural analgesia, 10–11, 11f–12f,
       13t–14t
    eye, 14
    horn, 14
    inverted L block, 8, 8f
    limb, 14–16, 15f
    paravertebral block, 9–10, 9f
Regurgitation, 18, 20
Reimer emasculator, 52f
Respiratory acidosis, 25
Respiratory alkalosis, 25
Respiratory tract surgery in the
      horse, 177–189
Retention suturing of the bovine
      vulva, 265–266, 267f–268f
Reticulum, exploration of, 215–219,
      217f–218f
Retractor
    Balfour, 38, 48f
    Finochietto rib spreader, 38, 48f
    Gelpi, 38, 47f
    malleable, 37, 47f
    Senn, 37, 47f
    United States Army, 37, 47f
    use of, 37–38
    Volkmann, 37, 47f
    Weitlaner, 38, 47f
Retrobulbar (four-point) block, 14
Rib resection, in cattle, 280, 282–283,
      284f–285f
Rib spreader, Finochietto, 38, 48f
Richter's hernia, 207
Roaring, 179
Roaring bur
    French-model, 57f
    Hobday's, 56f
    strawberry, 57f
Rochester-Carmalt forceps, 45f
Roeder knot, 4-S modified, 73, 73f
Roeder towel clamps, 42f
Romifidine
    for anesthetic maintenance, 22t
    for tranquilization and sedation in
      horses, 16, 17t
Rongeurs, 50f
Rumenostomy (rumen fistulation), 219–
      221, 220f
Rumenotomy, 215–219, 217f–218f
Rumenotomy board, 56f

Savage technique, 91, 91f
Scalpel, 33, 34f, 39f
Scalpel blade, 33, 34f, 35, 35f, 39f
Scar tissue, removal of excessive, 105,
      107f

Scissors
    bandage, 36, 40f
    Lister, 40f
    Littauer stitch, 40f
    Mayo, 35, 40f
    Metzenbaum, 35, 41f
    operating, 41f
    use of, 35, 35f
    wire-cutting, 41f
Scrubbing, surgical site preparation, 6
Secondary-intention healing, 96–97
Sedation
    in cattle, 16, 16t
    in horses, 16, 17t
    purposes for, 16
    in small ruminants, 16, 18t
    in swine, 16, 18t
Senn retractor, 37, 47f
Serra emasculator, 52f
Sesamoid chip fracture, 134–136, 135f
Sevoflurane, 21
Sheep. *See also* Small ruminant surgery
    convulsion with lidocaine, 8
    fluid balance evaluation, normal values
      for, 25t
    general anesthesia in, 18–23, 20t, 22t
    regional analgesia in, 8–11, 13t
    surgical site preparation, 6
    tranquilization and sedation, 16, 18t
Shirley wound drain, 99
Silastic drains, 97–98
Silk, 64t, 65–66
Simple continuous suture, 77–78, 78f, 87
Simple interrupted suture, 77, 78f, 87,
      87f
Sinusotomy, maxillary flap
      sinusotomy, 194f, 195
Skin elasticity, estimating, 23
Skin grafting, 105–111
    bandaging, 109
    overview, 105, 107
    pinch-skin, 107, 108f, 109
    postgrafting, 109
    punch-skin, 109, 110f
    random pattern flaps, 109, 111
    recipient bed preparation, 107
    tunnel grafting, 109, 111f
Skin punch, Keyes, 50f
Skin staples, 67
Sliding H-flap, 105, 105f
Slipknot (two half-hitches), 71, 72f
Small intestinal resection and
      anastomosis, 231–232
Small ruminants. *See also* Goats; Sheep
    epidural anesthesia, 13t
    surgery, 293–301
      cesarean section, 299–300
      dehorning of mature goat, 293–295,
        294f
      disbudding young goat, 295–296
      mastectomy, 297–298
      obstructive urolithiasis, 296–297

      rectal prolapse resection, 300–301,
        301f
      vasectomy, 298–299
    tranquilization and sedation, 16, 18t
Sodium, serum, 24
Sodium ion abnormalities, 26–27
Soft palate, partial resection in
      horses, 183–184, 185f
Sow, cesarean section in the, 317–319,
      318f
Speculum
    Bennett's, 55f
    heavy-swine mouth, 53f
    McPherson, 53f
    thoroughbred vaginal, 54f
Splint bones, amputation of, 131–134,
      132f–133f
Sponge forceps, 37
Square knot, 71, 72f
Stainless steel, 64t, 67
Standing flank laparotomy, in
      horse, 202–206, 203f–206f
Stent bandages, 88, 88f
Sterilization of instruments, 38
Still-Luer bone rongeurs, 50f
Stitch scissors, Littauer, 40f
Stomach pump, 59f
Strawberry roaring bur, 57f
Stringhalt, 114, 116, 119
Strong ion gap, 26
Subcuticular suture, 81, 82f
Suction tip, Yankauer suction, 51f
Sump-Penrose drain combination, 99,
      101f
Superficial digital flexor tendinitis,
      treatment of, 122, 124
Superficial digital flexor tenotomy,
      124–126, 125f
Superior check ligament
      desmotomy, 122–124, 123f
Surgeon's knot, 72f, 73
Surgery pack, general, 38
Surgical classifications, 4–5, 4t
Surgical conscience, 5
Surgical gut, 62, 63t
Surgical instruments. *See* Instruments
Surgical judgment, 4
Surgical preparation. *See specific surgical
      techniques*
Surgical site, preparation of, 5–6
Suspensory desmitis, 124, 131
Suspensory ligament, 134–136, 135f
Suture materials, 61–67
    absorbable, 62, 65
      braided, 62, 65
      collagen, 62
      monofilament, 65
      surgical gut (catgut), 62, 63t
    antimicrobial impregnated, 65
    Buhner perivaginal tape, 265–266,
      267f–268f
    clinical application, 61–62

Suture materials, (cont'd)
  common, table of, 63t–64t
  ideal, properties of, 61
  nonabsorbable, 65–67
    cotton, 64t, 66
    nylon, 64t, 66
    polyesters, 64t, 67
    polymerized caprolactam, 64t,
      66–67
    polypropylene and
      polyethylene, 64t, 66
    silk, 64t, 65–66
    skin staples, 67
    stainless steel, 64t, 67
  in traumatic wounds, 96
Suture patterns, 77–91. See also specific
      techniques
  basic patterns, 77–83
    continuous horizontal mattress, 79,
      79f
    continuous lock stitch (Ford
      interlocking), 83, 83f
    cruciate (cross mattress), 81, 82f
    interrupted horizontal mattress, 79,
      79f
    near-far-far-near, 81, 81f, 105
    simple continuous, 77–78, 78f
    simple interrupted, 77, 78f
    subcuticular, 81, 82f
    vertical mattress, 79, 80f, 81, 105
  Buhner's method, 265–266, 267f–268f
  buried purse-string, 265–266,
      267f–268f
  for closure of hollow organs, 83–88
    Connell, 85–86, 85f
    continuous Lembert, 84–85, 84f
    Cushing, 84, 85f
    double-layer inverting, 87–88
    Gambee, 87, 88f
    interrupted Lembert, 84, 84f
    Parker-Kerr oversew, 86, 86f
    purse-string, 86, 87f
    simple continuous, 87
    simple interrupted, 87, 87f
  for severed tendons, 88–91
    locking-loop tendon suture, 89, 89f,
      91
    Savage technique, 91, 91f
    three-loop pulley pattern, 90f, 91
  stent bandage (tie-over dressing), 88,
      88f
  Utrecht method of uterine
      closure, 259, 262f–264f
Suturing traumatic wounds, 96
Swine
  castration of the piglet, 311–312, 313f
  cesarean section, 317–319, 318f
  cryptorchid castration of piglets, 314,
      316
  epidural anesthesia, 10–11, 14t
  fluid balance evaluation, normal values
      for, 25t

general anesthesia in, 18–23, 21t, 22t
  inguinal herniorrhaphy the piglet, 312,
      314, 315f
  intubation, 20–21
  ovariohysterectomy in the pot-bellied
      pig, 319
  premedication in, 19
  preputial diverticulum ablation, 316,
      317f
  rectal prolapse ring
      placement, 319–320
  surgical site preparation, 6
  tranquilization and sedation, 16, 17t
Synovitis, digital sheath, 127
Syringe
  bulb, 51f
  dose, 59f

Tail docking, rectal prolapse and, 300
Tape needle, modified Buhner, 57f
Teaser bull preparation, 248–252,
      249f–250f
  anesthesia and surgical
      preparation, 248
  complications and prognosis, 252
  corpus cavernosum penis (CCP)
      thrombosis, 251–252
  epididymectomy, 252, 253f
  indications, 248
  penile fixation, 250f, 251
  penile translocation, 248, 249f, 251
  postoperative management, 252
Teat bistoury, Udall, 57f
Teat cannula, 58f
Teat curette, Cornell, 57f
Teat knife, 57f
Teat lacerations, repair of, 283, 285–288,
      287f
Teat slitter, 58f
Teat tube, 286
Teat-tumor extractor, Hugs, 57f
Telazol. See Tiletamine/zolazepam
      (Telazol), for anesthetic induction
Tendinitis
  in digital sheath, 127
  superficial digital flexor, 122, 124
Tendons, suture patterns for
      severed, 88–91, 89f–91f
Tenotomy
  deep digital flexor, 126–127
  lateral digital extensor, 114, 116–119,
      117f–118f
  superficial digital flexor, 124–126,
      125f
Tenotomy knife, 50f
Tension-relieving skin incisions, 103–
      104, 104f
Tension suture
  interrupted horizontal mattress, 79,
      79f
  near-far-far-near, 81, 81f, 105
  vertical mattress, 79, 80f, 81, 105

Testicle
  cattle
    calf castration, 235–236, 237f
    unilateral castration in
      bull, 257–258
  horse
    castration, 139–152, 141f–144f
    cryptorchidectomy, 147f–152f,
      152–156
  llama castration, 303–304
  swine
    castration, 311–312, 313f
    cryptorchid castration of
      piglets, 314, 316
Testosterone, measuring levels of, 146
Tetanus prophylaxis, 5, 95
Third eyelid resection, 288
Three-forceps method of tissue
      ligation, 73, 75f, 76
3-loop pulley suture, 90f, 91
Thumb forceps, 37, 37f
Tie-over dressings, 88, 88f
Tiletamine/zolazepam (Telazol), for
      anesthetic induction
  in cattle and small ruminants, 20t
  in horses, 19t
  in swine, 21t
Tissue adhesives, 67
Tissue forceps, 37, 42f
Tooth
  anatomy, 191
  removal in llama, 305–309, 307f–308f
  repulsion of cheek teeth in
      horses, 191–196, 193f–194f
Total plasma protein (TPP), 24, 25t, 27
Towel clamps, 37
  Backhaus, 42f
  Roeder, 42f
Tracheostomy, in horse, 177–179, 178f
Tracheotomy, 288–289
Tracheotomy tube, 59f
Tranquilization
  in cattle, 16, 16t
  in horses, 16, 17t
  purposes for, 16
  in small ruminants, 16, 18t
  in swine, 16, 18t
Transfixation ligature, 73, 75f
Traumatic wounds, assessment of, 93–94
Trephination, in horses, 192, 193f–194f,
      195
Trephine
  Galt, 53f
  Michel, 51f
Triclosan, 63t, 65
Triple drip solution, 19–21, 21t–22t
Trocar, 99, 100f
  corkscrew, 58f
  wood-handle cattle, 58f
Tuohy spinal needle, 11
Twitch, 52f
Typhlotomy, 231

Udder infusion tube, 58f
Umbilical herniorrhaphy in the
        foal, 207–210, 208f–209f
Umbilical surgery, 289–290
Umbilical tape, 66
United States Army chisel, 49f
United States Army retractor, 37, 47f
Upper respiratory tract surgery in the
        horse, 177–189
Urethral appendage, removal of
        goat, 296–297
Urethroplasty by caudal relocation of the
        transverse fold, 159–160,
        161f–162f
Urethrostomy, in cattle, 236, 238,
        239f–240f, 241
Urine pooling, 159
Urogenital surgery
    in cattle, 235–270
    in horses, 139–174
Urolithiasis
    in cattle, 238
    obstructive in small
        ruminants, 296–297
Uterine biopsy forceps, Jackson, 56f
Utrecht method of uterine closure, 259,
        262f–264f

Vaginal prolapse, in cattle
    cervicoplexy for, 266, 268–270, 269f
    retention suturing (Buhner's
        method), 265–266, 267f–268f
Vaginal speculum, 54f
Vasectomy, in small ruminants, 298–299
Ventilatory compromise, in anesthetized
        horses, 23
Ventral midline laparotomy, in
        horse, 196–202, 197f–200f
Ventriculectomy/ventriculocordectomy,
        in horse, 179–183, 181f–183f
Vertical mattress suture, 79, 80f, 81,
        105

Vesicovaginal reflux, 159
Viborg's triangle approach, to guttural
        pouches, 186, 187f
Vicryl, 63t, 65
Visceral prolapse, in equine castration
        complication, 145–146
Volkmann double-ended curette, 49f
Volkmann retractor, 37, 47f
Volvulus
    abomasal, 221
    cecal, 231
Vulsellum forceps, 37, 45f
Vulva, retention suturing of, 265–266,
        267f–268f

Water, withholding prior to surgery, 18
Weingarth's ring, 216
Weitlaner retractor, 38, 47f
Whitehouse approach, to guttural
        pouches, 186
Wire-cutting scissors, 41f
Wound contraction, 93
Wound management, 93–101
    antibiotic therapy, 95
    antiinflammatory drug therapy,
        95–96
    assessment of traumatic
        wounds, 93–94
    closure and healing, 96–97
        delayed primary, 96
        primary, 96
        secondary-intention, 96–97
        wound care prior to closing, 97
    drains, 97–101
        active, 99, 100f–101f
        fenestrated tube, 99, 100f
        for hygromas, 98, 98f
        indications, 97
        passive, 97–98
        Penrose, 98, 98f
        for peritoneal drainage, 99, 101f
        sump-Penrose, 99, 101f

excision and debridement, 95
exploration of wound, 94–95
preparation of wound, 94
Wounds, reconstructive surgery
        of, 103–111
    closure using tension-relieving
        incisions, 103–104, 104f
    elliptical excision undermining for
        repair of elongated defect, 103,
        104f
    scar tissue removal, 105, 107f
    skin grafting, 105–111
        bandaging, 109
        meshed grafts, 107
        pinch-skin, 107, 108f, 109
        postgrafting, 109
        punch-skin, 109, 110f
        random pattern flaps, 109, 111
        recipient bed preparation, 107
        tunnel grafting, 109, 111f
    sliding H-flap, 105, 105f
    Z-plasty, 105, 106f

Xylazine
    for anesthetic induction
        in cattle and small ruminants, 20t
        in horses, 19t
        in swine, 21t
    for anesthetic maintenance, 22t
    epidural use of, 10, 13t–14t
    for tranquilization and sedation
        in cattle, 16t
        in horses, 16, 17t
        in small ruminants, 16, 18t
        in swine, 17t

Yankauer suction tip, 51f

Zolazepam. *See* Tiletamine/zolazepam
        (Telazol), for anesthetic
        induction
Z-plasty, 105, 106f

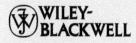